# Gynaecology by Ten Teachers

## 18th Edition

### Edited by

**Ash Monga** BMed(Sci) BM BS MRCOG
Consultant Gynaecologist, Princess Anne Hospital,
Southampton University Hospitals NHS Trust,
Southampton, UK

This book owes a great debt to Professor Stuart Campbell who, along with the present editor Ash Monga, was responsible for introducing the concepts and features to the seventeenth edition that are continued here.

## Hodder Arnold

A MEMBER OF THE HODDER HEADLINE GROUP

First published in Great Britain in 1919 as *Diseases of Women*
Eleventh edition published in 1966 as *Gynaecology*
Seventeenth edition published in 2000
This eighteenth edition published in 2006 by
Hodder Education, a member of the Hodder Headline Group,
338 Euston Road, London NW1 3BH
**http://www.hoddereducation.com**

Distributed in the United States of America by Oxford University Press Inc.,
198 Madison Avenue, New York, NY10016
Oxford is a registered trademark of Oxford University Press

*British Library Cataloguing in Publication Data*
A catalogue record for this book is available from the British Library

*Library of Congress Cataloging-in-Publication Data*
A catalog record for this book is available from the Library of Congress

ISBN-10 [normal]: 0 340 81662 7
ISBN-13 [normal]: 978 0 340 81662 2
ISBN-10 [ISE]: 0 340 81663 5 (International Students' Edition, restricted territorial availability)
ISBN-13 [ISE]: 978 0 340 81663 9

2 3 4 5 6 7 8 9 10

Commissioning Editors: Georgina Bentliff and Clare Christian
Development Editor: Heather Smith
Project Editor: Wendy Rooke
Production Controller: Jane Lawrence
Cover Design: Amina Dudhia

Typeset in 9.5/12 Minion by Charon Tec Pvt. Ltd, Chennai, India
www.charontec.com
Printed and bound in India

What do you think about this book? Or any other Hodder Arnold title?
Please visit our website at www.hoddereducation.com

**Gy**
**by**

# Contents

# The Ten Teachers

Keith Edmonds FRCOG FRANZCOG
Consultant in Obstetrics and Gynaecology,
Queen Charlotte's Hospital, London, UK

Ailsa E. Gebbie MFFP FRCOG
Consultant in Community Gynaecology, Dean,
Family Planning Centre, Edinburgh, UK

Phillip Hay MBBS MRCP
Reader in Genitourinary Medicine, St George's
Hospital Medical School, London, UK

Susan Ingamells BSc(Hons) PhD BM MRCOG
Consultant Gynaecologist and Subspecialist in
Reproductive Medicine, Princess Anne Hospital,
Southampton University Hospitals NHS Trust,
Wessex Fertility Clinic, Southampton, UK

Ash Monga BMed(Sci) BM BS MRCOG
Consultant Gynaecologist, Princess Anne Hospital,
Southampton University Hospitals NHS Trust,
Southampton, UK

Jane Norman MB ChB MD FRCOG
Reader in Obstetrics and Gynaecology, University of
Glasgow, Glasgow, UK

David W. Purdie MD FRCOG FRCP Ed
Consultant, Edinburgh Osteoporosis Centre,
Edinburgh, UK

Fran Reader MFFP FRCOG BASRT Accred
Consultant in Family Planning and Reproductive
Health Care, Ipswich Hospital NHS Trust,
Ipswich, UK

W. Patrick Soutter MD MSc FRCOG
Reader in Gynaecological Oncology,
Imperial College
Faculty of Medicine, Hammersmith Hospital,
London, UK

R. W. Stones MD FRCOG
Senior Lecturer in Obstetrics and Gynaecology,
University of Southampton, Southampton, UK

# Acknowledgements

The editor and the publishers would also like to thank the contributors to the previous edition who have not been directly involved in the preparation of this 18th edition:

Stuart Campbell

James Drife

William Dunlop

Jason Gardosi

Donald Gibb

JG Grudzinskas

Kevin Harrington

Des Holden

Richard Jonanson

Christoph Lees

Kypros Nicolaides

Margaret Oates

Michael Robson

Neil Sebire

Malcolm Symonds

Basky Thilaganathan

Guy Thorpe-Beeston

# Commonly used abbreviations

| | | | |
|---|---|---|---|
| ACTH | adrenocorticotrophic hormone | HSV | herpes simplex virus |
| AFP | alpha-fetoprotein | 5HT | 5-hydroxytryptamine |
| AIDS | acquired immunodeficiency syndrome | HWY | hundred woman-years |
| AUC | area under the curve | HyCoSy | hysterocontrast sonography |
| BEP | bleomycin and etoposide | ICSI | intracytoplasmic sperm injection |
| BNF | *British National Formulary* | Ig | immunoglobulin |
| BV | bacterial vaginosis | IGF | insulin-like growth factor |
| CI | confidence interval | IGFBP | insulin-like growth factor binding proteins |
| CIN | cervical intraepithelial neoplasia | | |
| CMV | cytomegalovirus | IL | interleukin |
| COCP | combined oral contraceptive pill | IUD | intrauterine contraceptive device |
| CT | computerized tomography | IUI | intrauterine insemination |
| CVS | chorionic villus sampling | IUS | intrauterine system |
| D&E | dilatation of the cervix and evacuation of the uterus | IVC | in-vitro culture |
| | | IVF | in-vitro fertilization |
| DFA | direct fluorescent antibody (test) | IVM | in-vitro maturation |
| DHEA | dihydroepiandrosterone | IVP | intravenous pyelogram |
| DI | donor insemination | LAM | lactational amenorrhoea method |
| DSM IV | *Diagnostic and Statistical Manual of Mental Disorders IV* of the American Psychiatric Association | LCR | ligase chain reaction |
| | | LDL | low-density lipoprotein |
| | | LGV | lymphogranuloma venereum |
| | | LH | luteinizing hormone |
| DUB | dysfunctional uterine bleeding | LLETZ | large loop excision of the transformation zone |
| DV | dysaesthetic vulvodynia | | |
| DVT | deep vein thrombosis | LNG-IUS | levonorgestrel intrauterine system |
| E2 | oestradiol | LSIL | low-grade squamous intraepithelial lesion |
| EC | emergency contraception | LUF | luteinized unruptured follicle syndrome |
| ED | every-day (preparations) | MAC | *Mycobacterium avium intracellulare* complex |
| EGF | epidermal growth factor | | |
| ELISA | enzyme-linked immunosorbent assay | MBL | menstrual blood loss |
| ESR | erythrocyte sedimentation rate | MCP-1 | macrophage chemotactic protein-1 |
| ET | embryo transfer | MESA | micro-epididymal sperm aspiration |
| FBC | full blood count | MMP | matrix metalloproteinase |
| FGF | fibroblast growth factor | MRI | magnetic resonance imaging |
| FSH | follicle-stimulating hormone | NETZ | LLETZ using a diathermy wire |
| FTA | fluorescent treponemal antibody (test) | NGU | non-gonococcal urethritis |
| GIFT | gamete intrafallopian transfer | NHS | National Health Service |
| GnRH | gonadotrophin-releasing hormone | NSAID | non-steroidal anti-inflammatory drug |
| GTD | gestational trophoblastic disorder | OHSS | ovarian hyperstimulation syndrome |
| GUM | genitourinary medicine | PCOS | polycystic ovarian syndrome |
| hCG | human chorionic gonadotrophin | PCP | *Pneumocystis carinii* pneumonia |
| HDL | high-density lipoprotein | PCR | polymerase chain reaction |
| HFEA | Human Fertilization and Embryology Authority | PESA | percutaneous sperm aspiration |
| | | PGF2$\alpha$ | vasoconstrictor prostaglandin |
| HIV | human immunodeficiency virus | PGE2 | vasodilator prostaglandin |
| HLA | human leukocyte antigen | PID | pelvic inflammatory disease |
| hMG | human menopausal gonadotrophin | PMB | postmenopausal bleeding |
| HOL | hairy oral leukoplakia | PMS | premenstrual syndrome |
| HPO | hypothalamo–pituitary–ovarian (axis) | POF | premature ovarian failure |
| HPV | human papillomavirus | POP | progestogen-only pill |
| HRT | hormone replacement therapy | PPNG | penicillinase-producing *Neisseria gonorrhoea* |
| HSG | hysterosalpingogram | | |
| HSIL | high-grade squamous intraepithelial lesion | | |

| | | | |
|---|---|---|---|
| RCOG | Royal College of Obstetricians and Gynaecologists | TOP | termination of pregnancy |
| REM | rapid eye movement (sleep) | TPHA | *Treponema pallidum* haemagglutination assay |
| RPR | rapid plasma reagin (test) | TPPA | *Treponema pallidum* particle agglutination |
| SARA | sexually acquired reactive arthritis | TVT | tension-free vaginal tape |
| SCJ | squamocolumnar junction | USI | urodynamic stress incontinence |
| SERM | selective oestrogen receptor modulator | UTI | urinary tract infection |
| SHBG | sex hormone binding globulin | VAIN | vaginal intraepithelial neoplasia |
| SSRI | selective serotonin reuptake inhibitor | VCU | videocystourethrography |
| STD | sexually transmitted disease | VDRL | Venereal Diseases Research Laboratory (test) |
| STI | sexually transmitted infection | VEGF | vascular endothelial growth factor |
| SUZI | subzonal insemination | VIN | vulval intraepithelial neoplasia |
| TA | transactional analysis | VTE | venous thromboembolism |
| TDF | testicular determining factor | VV | vulval vestibulitis |
| TESA | testicular sperm aspiration | WHO | World Health Organization |
| TGF | transforming growth factor | ZIFT | zygote intrafallopian transfer |

# The gynaecological history and examination

## OVERVIEW

A careful detailed history is essential before the examination of any patient. In addition to a good general history, focusing on the history of the presenting complaint will allow you to customize the examination to elicit the appropriate signs and make an accurate diagnosis.

## History

When interviewing a patient to obtain her history, the consultation should ideally be held in a closed room with no one else present. Enough time should be allowed for the patient to express herself, and the doctor's manner should be one of interest and understanding. It is important that a template is used for history taking, as this prevents the omission of important points. A sample template is given on page 2.

## Examination

It is important that the examiner smiles, introduces her/himself by name and, if appropriate, asks the patient's name. A handshake often helps to put the patient at ease.

Important information about patients can be obtained by watching them walk into the examination room; poor mobility may affect decisions regarding surgery. While obtaining a history, it is possible to assess the patient's affect. A history that is taken with sensitivity will often encourage the patient to reveal more details that are relevant to future management.

Before proceeding to abdominal examination, a general examination should be performed. This includes examining the hands and mucous membranes for evidence of anaemia. The supraclavicular node should always be examined, particularly on the left side, where, in cases of abdominal malignancy, one might palpate the enlarged Virchow's node (this is also known as Troissier's sign). The thyroid gland should be palpated.

The chest and breasts should always be examined; this is particularly relevant if there is a suspected ovarian mass, as there may be a breast tumour with secondaries

## S Symptoms

### History-taking template
The following outline is suggested.
- Name, age, occupation.
- A brief statement of the general nature and duration of the main complaints.

### History of presenting complaint
This section should focus on the presenting complaint, but certain important points should always be enquired about.
- Abnormal menstrual loss.
- Pattern of bleeding – regular or irregular.
- Intermenstrual bleeding.
- Amount of blood loss – greater or less than usual.
- Number of sanitary towels or tampons used.
- Passage of clots or flooding.
- Pelvic pain – site of pain, nature and relation to periods.
- Anything that aggravates or relieves the pain.
- Vaginal discharge – amount, colour, odour, presence of blood.

Obviously if the presenting complaint is one of subfertility or is urogynaecological, the history must be appropriately tailored (see Chapters 7 and 16).

### Usual menstrual cycle
- Age of menarche.
- Usual duration of each period and length of cycle.
- First day of the last period.

### Previous gynaecological history
This section should include any previous gynaecological treatments or surgery. The date of the last cervical smear should also be recorded.

### Previous obstetric history
- Number of children with ages and birth weights.
- Any abnormalities with pregnancy, labour or the puerperium.
- Number of miscarriages and gestation at which they occurred.
- Any termination of pregnancy with record of gestation age and any complications.

### Sexual and contraceptive history
- History of discomfort, pain or bleeding during intercourse.
- The use of contraception and type of contraception used.

### Previous medical history
- Any serious illnesses or operations with dates.
- Family history.

### Enquiry about other systems
- Appetite, weight loss, weight gain.
- Bowels.
- Micturition.
- Other systems.

### Social history
The history regarding smoking and alcohol intake should be obtained. It is important to ascertain whether the woman is married or has a sexual partner. Any family problems should be discussed, and it is especially important in the case of a frail patient to enquire about home arrangements if surgery is being considered.

### Summary
It is important to summarize the history in one or two sentences before proceeding to examination to alert the examiner to the salient features.

---

in the ovaries known as Krukenburg tumours. In addition, a pleural effusion may be elicited as a consequence of abdominal ascites. The next step should be to proceed to abdominal and pelvic examination.

## Abdominal examination

The patient should empty her bladder before the abdominal examination. She should be comfortable and lying semi-recumbent, with a sheet covering her from the waist down, but the area from the xiphisternum to the symphysis pubis should be left exposed. It is usual to examine the woman from her right-hand side. Abdominal examination comprises inspection, palpation, percussion and, if appropriate, auscultation.

### Inspection
The contour of the abdomen should be inspected and noted. There may be an obvious distension or mass (Fig. 1.1).

The presence of surgical scars, dilated veins or striae gravidarum (stretch marks) should be noted. It is important specifically to examine the umbilicus for laparoscopy scars and just above the symphysis pubis

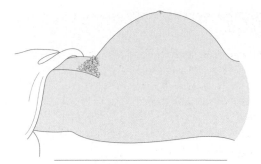

**Figure 1.1** Abdominal distension.

for Pfannenstiel scars (used for Caesarean section, hysterectomy, etc.). The patient should be asked to raise her head or cough and any herniae or divarication of the rectus muscles will be evident.

### Palpation

First, if the patient has any abdominal pain, she should be asked to point to the site. This area should not be examined until the end of palpation. It is usual to get the patient to cough, as she may show signs of peritonism. Palpation using the right hand is performed, examining the left lower quadrant and proceeding in a total of four steps to the right lower quadrant of the abdomen. Palpation should include examination for masses, liver, spleen and kidneys. If a mass is present but it is possible to palpate below it, it is more likely to be an abdominal mass rather than a pelvic mass. It is important to remember that one of the characteristics of a pelvic mass is that one cannot palpate below it.

If the patient has pain, her abdomen should be palpated gently and the examiner should look for signs of peritonism, i.e. guarding and rebound tenderness. The patient should also be examined for inguinal herniae and lymph nodes.

### Percussion

Percussion is particularly useful if free fluid is suspected. In the recumbent position, ascitic fluid will settle down into a horseshoe shape and dullness in the flanks can be demonstrated.

As the patient moves over to her side, the dullness will move to her lowermost side; this is known as 'shifting dullness'. A fluid thrill can also be elicited.

An enlarged bladder due to urinary retention will also be dull to percussion and this should be demonstrated

to the examiner (many pelvic masses have disappeared after catheterization).

### Auscultation

This method is not specifically useful for the gynaecological examination. However, a patient will sometimes present with an acute abdomen with bowel obstruction or a postoperative patient with ileus, and therefore listening for bowel sounds may be appropriate.

## Pelvic examination

Before proceeding to a vaginal examination, the patient's verbal consent should be obtained and a female chaperone should be present for any intimate examination.

The external genitalia are first inspected under a good light with the patient in the dorsal position, the hips flexed and abducted and the knees flexed. The left lateral position is used for examination of prolapse or to inspect the vaginal wall with a Sims' speculum (Fig. 1.2). The patient is asked to strain down to enable the detection of any prolapse and also to cough, as this will show the sign of stress incontinence. After this, a bivalve (Cusco's) speculum is inserted to visualize the cervix (Fig. 1.3). It is usual to warm the speculum to make the examination more comfortable for the patient. If taking a smear test, this is performed at the same time.

Bimanual digital examination is then performed (Fig. 1.4). This technique requires practice. It is customary to use the fingers of the right hand in the vagina and to place the left hand on the abdomen. In a virgin or a child, only a rectal examination should be performed. The left hand is used to separate the labia minora to expose the vestibule and the examining fingers of the right hand are inserted. The cervix is palpated and any hardness or irregularity noted. The hand on the abdomen is placed just below the umbilicus and the fingers of both hands are then used to palpate the uterus. The size, shape, position, mobility and tenderness of the uterus are noted. The tips of the vaginal fingers are then placed into each lateral fornix and the adnexae are examined on each side. Except in a very thin woman, the ovaries and Fallopian tubes are not palpable. The uterosacral ligaments can be palpated in the posterior fornix and may be scarred or shortened in women with endometriosis.

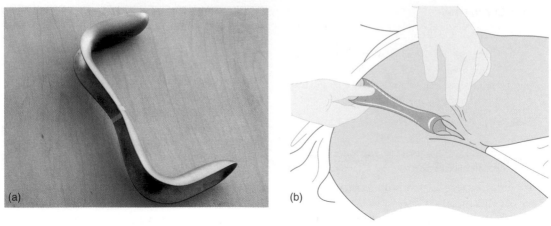

**Figure 1.2** (a) Sims' speculum. (b) Sims' speculum exposing anterior vaginal wall.

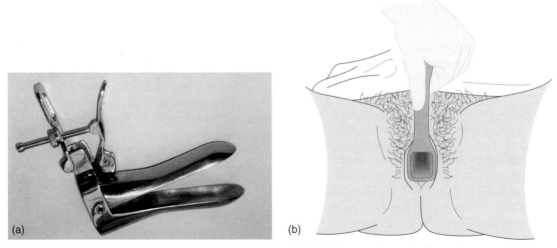

**Figure 1.3** (a) Cusco's speculum. (b) Cusco's speculum in position with the blades opened exposing the cervix.

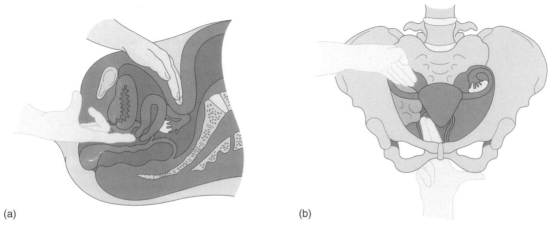

**Figure 1.4** (a) Bimanual examination of the pelvis, assessing uterine size. (b) Examining the lateral fornix.

## Rectal examination

A rectal examination may be used as an alternative to vaginal examination in a virgin or a child. In addition, it may be useful to differentiate between enterocele and rectocele and can be used to assess the size of a rectocele.

## Investigations

The appropriate investigation should be performed, e.g. swabs for discharge or cervical smear.

Other investigations are discussed in Appendix 1.

## Key Points

- The consultation should be performed in a private environment in a sensitive fashion.
- The student should introduce him/herself to the patient and be courteous.
- The student should be familiar with a template and use it regularly to avoid omissions.
- A chaperone should always be present for an intimate examination.
- The examination should begin with inspection of the patient's hands.
- The patient should be comfortable and at the end of the examination the student should cover the exposed section and help the patient to sit up.
- When presenting the history to the examiner, it should be succinct and should be summarized before presenting the examination.
- Remember the examiners will usually ask for a differential diagnosis.

# Embryology and anatomy

## OVERVIEW

An understanding of the development and anatomy of the female genital tract is important in the practice of gynaecology. Both the urinary and genital systems develop from a common mesodermal ridge running along the posterior abdominal wall. Although the development of the kidneys and bladder is outside of the realm of this chapter, it is important to remember that congenital anomalies of the genital tract may also be associated with congenital anomalies of the urinary tract. This chapter serves as a reminder and is not a comprehensive guide to the embryology and anatomy.

## EMBRYOLOGY

### Development of the genital organs

During the fifth week of embryonic life the nephrogenic cord develops from the mesoderm and forms the urogenital ridge and mesonephric duct (later to form the Wolffian duct) (Fig. 2.1). The mesonephros consists of a comparatively large ovoid organ on each side of the midline, with the developing gonad on the medial side of its lower portion. The paramesonephric duct later forms the Müllerian system. The fate of the mesonephric and paramesonephric ducts is dependent on gonadal secretion. Assuming female development, the two paramesonephric ducts extend caudally to project into the posterior wall of the urogenital sinus as the Müllerian tubercle. The Wolffian system degenerates.

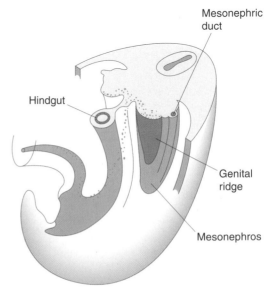

**Figure 2.1** Cross-sectional diagram of the posterior abdominal wall showing the genital ridge.

## Development of the uterus and Fallopian tubes

The lower end of the Müllerian ducts come together in the midline, fuse and develop into the uterus and cervix (Fig. 2.2). At first there is a septum separating the lumina of the two ducts, but later this disappears and a single cavity is formed, i.e. the uterus.

The upper parts of both ducts retain their identity and form the Fallopian tubes. The lower end of the fused Müllerian ducts beyond the uterine lumen remains solid, proliferates and forms a cord.

## Development of the vagina

During the ninth week of embryonic life, the cord does not open out into the sinus but makes contact with the sinovaginal bulbs, which are solid outgrowths from the sinus. As the pelvic region of the fetus elongates, the sinus and Müllerian tubercle become increasingly distanced from the tubular portions, the ducts. The solid epithelial cord provides the length of the future vagina. The current view is that most of the upper vagina is of Müllerian origin. The solid sinovaginal bulbs also have to canalize to form a lower vagina and this occurs above the level of the eventual hymen, so that the epithelia of both surfaces of the hymen are of urogenital sinus origin. Complete canalization of the vagina is a comparatively late event, occurring in the sixth and seventh months.

## Development of the external genitalia

There is overlap in the timing of the formation of the external genitalia and the internal duct system.

There is a common indifferent stage consisting of two genital folds, two genital swellings and a midline anterior genital tubercle. The female development is a simple progression from these structures:

- genital tubercle → clitoris
- genital folds → labia minora
- genital swellings → labia majora.

A male phenotype is dependent on the production of fetal testosterone. Agents or inborn errors that prevent the synthesis or action of androgens inhibit the formation of male external genitalia and the female phenotype will develop.

## Development of the ovary

The primitive gonad is first evident in embryos at 5 weeks. It forms as a bulb on the medial aspect of the mesonephric ridge and is of triple origin, from the coelomic epithelium of the genital ridge, the underlying mesoderm and the primitive germ cells. There is proliferation of cells in and beneath the coelomic epithelium of the genital ridge. By 5–6 weeks these cells are seen spreading as ill-defined cords (sex cords) into the ridge, breaking up the mesenchyme into loose strands. The primitive germ cells are seen at first lying between the cords and then within them (Fig. 2.3).

Morphological development of the ovary occurs about 2 weeks later than the testes and proceeds more slowly. The sex cords develop extensively and epithelial cells in this area are known as pregranulosa cells. The germ cells decrease in size by 14–16 weeks. The active growth phase causes enlargement of the gonad. The next stage involves the primitive germ cells (now known as oocytes) becoming surrounded by a ring of pregranulosa cells; stromal cells develop from the ovarian mesenchyme. Mitotic division, by which the

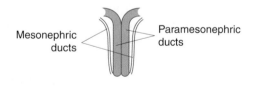

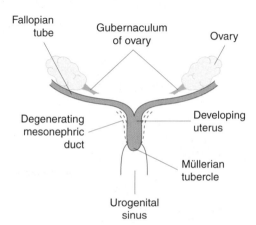

**Figure 2.2** Caudal growth of paramesonephric ducts (top). Fusion to form the uterus and Fallopian tubes (below).

germ cells have been increasing in numbers, then ceases and they enter the first stage of meiosis and prophase arrest. The number of oocytes is greatest before birth and thereafter declines. Approximately 7 million germ cells are present at 5 months, but at birth this has fallen to 2 million, half of which are atretic.

At the same time as the ovary descends extraperitoneally into the abdominal cavity, two ligaments develop and these appear to help control its descent, guiding it to its final position and preventing its complete descent through the inguinal ring, in contrast to the testes.

## ANATOMY

Anatomy is covered in some depth in the pre-clinical years. This is intended as a brief review.

## External genitalia

### The vulva

The female external genitalia, commonly referred to as the vulva, include the mons pubis, the labia majora and minora, the vestibule, the clitoris and the greater vestibular glands (Fig. 2.4). The mons pubis is composed of fibrofatty tissue, which covers the body of the pubic bones. Inferiorly it divides to become continuous with the labium majus on each side of the vulva. In the adult, the skin that covers the mons pubis bears pubic hair, the upper limit of which is usually horizontal.

The labia majora are two folds of skin with underlying adipose tissue bounding either side of the vaginal opening. They contain sebaceous and sweat glands and a few specialized apocrine glands. In the deepest part of each labium is a core of fatty tissue continuous with that of the inguinal canal and the fibres of the round ligament terminate here.

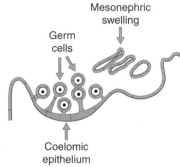

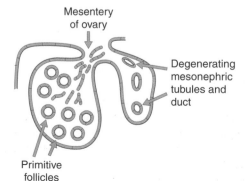

**Figure 2.3** Development of the ovary.

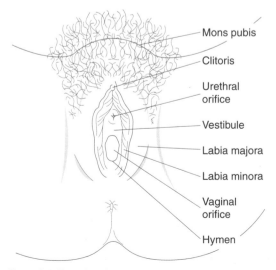

**Figure 2.4** The vulva of a virgin.

The labia minora are two thin folds of skin that lie between the labia majora. Anteriorly they divide into two to form the prepuce and frenulum of the clitoris. Posteriorly they fuse to form a fold of skin called the fourchette. They contain sebaceous glands but have no adipose tissue. They are not well developed before puberty, and atrophy after the menopause. Their vascularity allows them to become turgid during sexual excitement.

The clitoris is a small erectile structure. The body of the clitoris contains two crura, the corpora cavernosa, which are attached to the inferior border of the pubic rami. The clitoris is covered by the ischiocavernosus muscle; bulbospongiosus muscle inserts into its root. The clitoris is about 1 cm long but has a highly developed nerve supply and is very sensitive during sexual arousal.

The vestibule is the cleft between the labia minora. The urethra, the ducts of the Bartholin's glands and the vagina open in the vestibule. The vestibular bulbs are two oblong masses of erectile tissue that lie on either side of the vaginal entrance. They contain a rich plexus of veins within the bulbospongiosus muscle. Bartholin's glands, each about the size of a small pea, lie at the base of each bulb and open via a 2 cm duct into the vestibule between the hymen and the labia minora. These are mucus-secreting, producing copious amounts during intercourse to act as a lubricant.

The hymen is a thin fold of mucous membrane across the entrance to the vagina. There are usually openings in it to allow menses to escape. The hymen is partially ruptured during first coitus and is further disrupted during childbirth. Any tags remaining after rupture are known as carunculae myrtiformes.

### Age changes

In infancy the vulva is devoid of hair and there is considerable adipose tissue in the labia majora and pubis that is lost during childhood but reappears during puberty, at which time hair grows. After menopause the skin atrophies and becomes thinner. The labia minora shrink, subcutaneous fat is lost and the vaginal orifice becomes smaller.

## The internal reproductive organs

Figure 2.5 shows a sagittal section of the human female pelvis.

## The vagina

The vagina is a fibromuscular canal lined with stratified squamous epithelium that leads from the uterus to the vulva. It is longer in the posterior wall (around 9 cm) than anteriorly (approximately 7 cm). The vaginal walls are normally in apposition, except at the vault, where they are separated by the cervix. The vault of the vagina is divided into four fornices: posterior, anterior and two lateral (Fig. 2.6).

The midvagina is a transverse slit and the lower portion is an H shape in transverse section. The vaginal walls are rugose, with transverse folds. The vagina is kept moist by secretions from the uterine and cervical glands and by some transudation from its epithelial lining. It has no glands. The epithelium is thick and rich in glycogen, which increases in the postovulatory phase of the cycle. However, before puberty and after the menopause, the vagina is devoid of glycogen because of oestrogen deficiency.

Döderlein's bacillus is a normal commensal of the vagina that breaks down the glycogen to form lactic acid, producing a pH of around 4.5. This has a protective role for the vagina in decreasing the growth of pathogenic organisms.

The upper posterior vaginal wall forms the anterior peritoneal reflection of the pouch of Douglas. The middle third is separated from the rectum by pelvic fascia and the lower third abuts the perineal body. Anteriorly, the lip of the vagina is in direct contact with the base of the bladder; the urethra runs down the lower half in the midline to open to the vestibule. Its muscles fuse with the anterior vaginal wall. Laterally, at the fornices, the vagina is related to the attachment at the cardinal ligaments. Below this are the levator ani muscles and the ischiorectal fossae. The cardinal ligaments and the uterosacral ligaments, which form posteriorly from the parametrium, support the upper part of the vagina.

### Age changes

At birth, the vagina is under the influence of maternal oestrogens, so the epithelium is well developed. After a couple of weeks, the effects of the oestrogens disappear and the pH rises to 7 and the epithelium atrophies. At puberty the reverse occurs, and finally, at the menopause, the vagina tends to shrink and the epithelium atrophies.

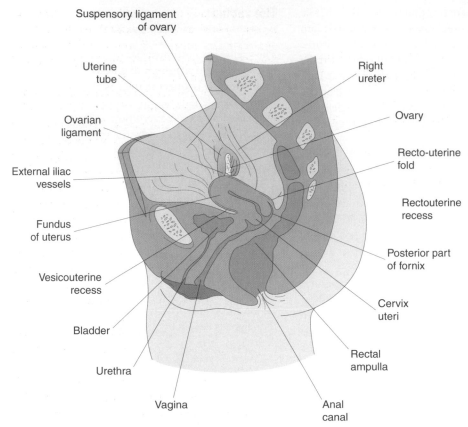

**Figure 2.5** Sagittal section of the human female pelvis.

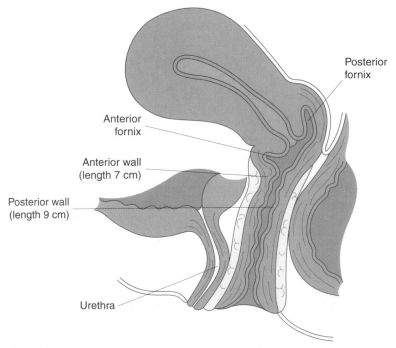

**Figure 2.6** Sagittal section of the vagina.

## The uterus

The uterus is shaped like an inverted pear, tapering inferiorly to the cervix, and in the non-pregnant state is situated entirely within the pelvis. It is hollow and has thick muscular walls. Its maximum external dimensions are approximately 7.5 cm long, 5 cm wide and 3 cm thick (Fig. 2.7).

An adult uterus weighs about 70 g. The upper part is termed the body or corpus. The area of insertion of each Fallopian tube is termed the cornu and the part of the body above the cornu, the fundus. The uterus tapers to a small central constricted area, the isthmus, and below this is the cervix, which projects obliquely into the vagina and can be divided into vaginal and supravaginal portions (Fig. 2.8).

The cavity of the uterus is the shape of an inverted triangle and, when sectioned coronally, the Fallopian tubes open at the lateral angles. The constriction at the isthmus where the corpus joins the cervix is the anatomical internal os. Seen microscopically, the site of the histological internal os is where the mucous membrane of the isthmus becomes that of the cervix.

The uterus consists of three layers: the outer serous layer (peritoneum), the middle muscular layer (myometrium) and the inner mucous layer (endometrium).

The peritoneum covers the body of the uterus and, posteriorly, the supravaginal portion of the cervix. The serous coat is intimately attached to a subserous fibrous layer except laterally, where it spreads out to form the leaves of the broad ligament.

The muscular myometrium forms the main bulk of the uterus and comprises interlacing smooth muscle fibres intermingling with areolar tissue, blood vessels, nerves and lymphatics. Externally these are mostly longitudinal, but the larger intermediate layer has interlacing longitudinal, oblique and transverse fibres. Internally they are mainly longitudinal and circular.

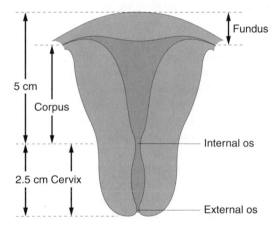

**Figure 2.7** Uterine dimensions.

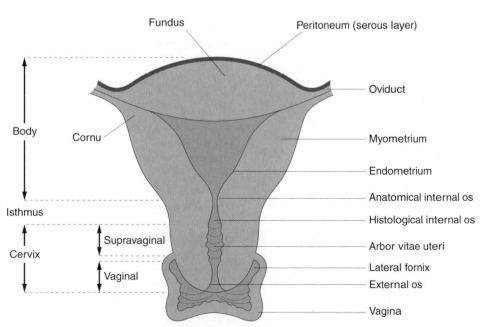

**Figure 2.8** Coronal section of the uterine cavity.

The inner endometrial layer has tubular glands that dip into the myometrium. The endometrial layer is covered by a single layer of columnar epithelium. Ciliated prior to puberty, this epithelium is mostly lost due to the effects of pregnancy and menstruation. The endometrium undergoes cyclical changes during menstruation and varies in thickness between 1 and 5 mm.

### The cervix

The cervix is narrower than the body of the uterus and is approximately 2.5 cm in length. Due to antiflexion or retroflexion, the long axis of the cervix is rarely the same as the long axis of the body of the uterus. Anterior and lateral to the supravaginal portion is cellular connective tissue, the parametrium. The posterior aspect is covered by peritoneum of the pouch of Douglas. The ureter runs about 1 cm laterally to the supravaginal cervix. The vaginal portion projects into the vagina to form the fornices.

The upper part of the cervix mostly consists of involuntary muscle, whereas the lower part is mainly fibrous connective tissue. The mucous membrane of the endocervix has anterior and posterior columns from which folds radiate out, known as the arbor vitae. It has numerous deep glandular follicles that secrete a clear alkaline mucus, the main component of physiological vaginal discharge. The epithelium of the endocervix is cylindrical and is also ciliated in its upper two-thirds and changes to stratified squamous epithelium around the region of the external os. This squamocolumnar junction is also known as the transformation zone and is an area of rapid cell division; approximately 90 per cent of cervical carcinoma arises in this area.

### Position of the uterus

The longitudinal axis of the uterus is, approximately, at right-angles to the vagina and normally tilts forwards. This is termed anteversion. The uterus is usually also flexed forwards on itself at the isthmus – anteflexion. In around 20 per cent of women, this tilt is not forwards but backwards – retroversion and retroflexion. This does not have a pathological significance.

### Age changes

The disappearance of maternal oestrogens after birth causes the uterus to decrease in length by around one-third and in weight by about one-half. The cervix is then twice the length of the uterus.

At puberty, however, the corpus grows much faster and the size ratio reverses. After the menopause, the uterus atrophies, the mucosa becomes very thin, the glands almost disappear and the wall becomes relatively less muscular. These changes affect the cervix more than the corpus; cervical loops disappear and the external os becomes more or less flush with the vault.

## The Fallopian tubes

Each Fallopian tube extends outwards from the uterine cornu to end near the ovary. At the abdominal ostium, the tube opens into the peritoneal cavity, which is therefore in communication with the exterior of the body via the uterus and the vagina. The tubes (oviducts) convey the ovum from the ovary towards the uterus, which provides oxygenation and nutrition for sperm, ovum and zygote should fertilization occur.

The Fallopian tube (Fig. 2.9) runs in the upper margin of the broad ligament, part of which, known as the mesosalpinx, encloses it so that the tube is completely covered with peritoneum except for a narrow strip along this inferior aspect. Each tube is about 10 cm long and is described in four parts:
1. the interstitial portion
2. the isthmus
3. the ampulla
4. the infundibulum, or fimbrial portion.

The interstitial portion lies within the wall of the uterus; the isthmus is the narrow portion adjoining the uterus. This passes into the widest and longest portion, the ampulla. This in turn terminates in the extremity known as the infundibulum, where the funnel-shaped opening of the tube into the peritoneal cavity is surrounded by finger-like processes, called fimbriae, into which the muscle coat does not extend. The inner surfaces of the fimbriae are covered by ciliated epithelium, which is similar to the lining of the Fallopian tube itself. One of these fimbriae is longer than the others and extends to, and partly embraces, the ovary. The muscle fibres of the wall of the tube are arranged in an inner circular and an outer longitudinal layer.

The tubal epithelium forms a number of branched folds, or plicae, which run longitudinally; the lumen of the ampulla is almost filled with these folds. The folds have a cellular stroma, but at their bases the epithelium is only separated from the muscle by a very scanty amount of stroma. There is no submucosa and there

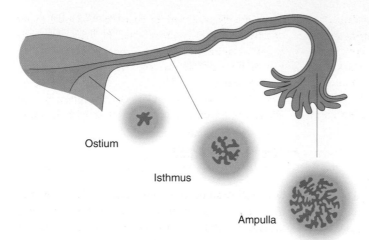

**Figure 2.9** The Fallopian tube.

Ostium

Isthmus

Ampulla

are no glands. The epithelium of the Fallopian tubes contains two functioning cell types: the ciliated cells, which act to produce a constant current fluid in the direction of the uterus; and the secretory cells, which contribute to the volume of tubal fluid. Changes occur under the influence of the menstrual cycle, but there is no cell shedding during menstruation.

## The ovaries

The size and appearance of the ovaries depend on both age and the stage of the menstrual cycle. In the young adult they are almond shaped, solid, a greyish-pink and approximately 3 cm long, 1.5 cm wide and 1 cm thick.

In the child, the ovaries are small structures, approximately 1.5 cm long. They have a smooth surface and at birth contain between 1 and 2 million primordial follicles, some of which will ripen into mature follicles in the reproductive years. The ovaries increase to adult size in the months preceding puberty. This considerable increase is brought about by proliferation of the stromal cells and by the commencing maturation of the ovarian follicles. After the menopause, no active follicles are present and the ovary becomes a small, shrunken structure with a wrinkled surface.

The ovary is the only intra-abdominal structure not to be covered by peritoneum. Each ovary is attached to the cornu of the uterus by the ovarian ligament, and at the hilum to the broad ligament by the mesovarium, which contains its supply of vessels and nerves. Laterally, each ovary is attached to the

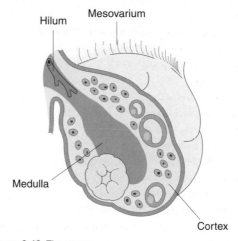

**Figure 2.10** The ovary.

suspensory ligament of the ovary with folds of peritoneum, which become continuous with that overlying the psoas major.

Anterior to the ovary lie the Fallopian tubes, the superior portion of the bladder and the uterovesical pouch. The ovary is bound behind by the ureter where it runs downwards and forwards in front of the internal iliac artery.

### Structure

The ovary (Fig. 2.10) has a central vascular medulla consisting of loose connective tissue containing many elastin fibres and non-striated muscle cells. It has an outer thicker cortex, denser than the medulla, consisting of networks of reticular fibres and fusiform cells, although there is no clear-cut demarcation between

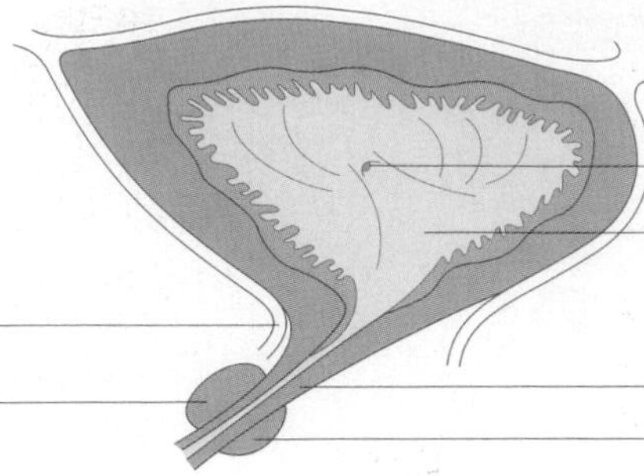

**Figure 2.11** The bladder and urethra.

Uteric opening

Trigone

Pubourethral

External sphincter

Urethral smooth muscle

External sphincter

the two. The surface of the ovaries is covered by a single layer of cuboidal cells, the germinal epithelium. Beneath this is an ill-defined layer of condensed connective tissue, the tunica albuginea, which increases in density with age. At birth, numerous primordial follicles are found, mostly in the cortex, but some are found in the medulla. With puberty, some form each month into Graafian follicles, which, at later stages of their development, form corpora lutea and ultimately atretic follicles, the corpora albicans.

### Vestigial structures

Vestigial remains of the mesonephric duct and tubules are always present in young children, but are variable structures in adults. The epoophoron, a series of parallel blind tubules, lies in the broad ligament between the mesovarium and the Fallopian tube. The tubules run to the rudimentary duct of the epoophoron, which runs parallel to the lateral Fallopian tube. Situated in the broad ligament, between the epoophoron and the uterus, are occasionally seen a few rudimentary tubules, the paroophoron. In a few individuals, the caudal part of the mesonephric duct is well developed, running alongside the uterus to the internal os. This is the duct of Gartner.

## The bladder, urethra and ureter

### The bladder

The average capacity of the bladder is 400 mL. The bladder is lined with transitional epithelium. The involuntary muscle of its wall is arranged in an inner longitudinal layer, a middle circular layer and an outer longitudinal layer.

The ureters open into the base of the bladder after running medially for about 1 cm through the vesical wall. The urethra leaves the bladder in front of the ureteric orifices; the triangular area lying between the ureteric orifices and the internal meatus is known as the trigone. At the internal meatus, the middle layer of vesical muscle forms anterior and posterior loops round the neck of the bladder, some fibres of the loops being continuous with the circular muscle of the urethra.

The base of the bladder is related to the cervix, with only a thin layer of connective tissue intervening. It is separated from the anterior vaginal wall below by the pubocervical fascia, which stretches from the pubis to the cervix.

### The urethra

The female urethra is about 3.5 cm long, and has a slight posterior angulation at the junction of its lower and middle thirds. It is lined with transitional epithelium. The smooth muscle of its wall is arranged in outer longitudinal and inner circular layers. As the urethra passes through the two layers of the urogenital diaphragm (triangular ligament), it is embraced by the striated fibres of the deep transverse perineal muscle (compressor urethrae), and some of the striated fibres of this muscle form a loop on the urethra. Between the muscular coat and the epithelium is a plexus of veins. There are a number of tubular mucous glands and, in the lower part, a number of crypts, which occasionally become infected. In its upper two-thirds the urethra is separated from the symphysis by loose connective tissue, but in its lower third it is attached to the pubic ramus on each side by strong bands of fibrous tissue called the pubourethral ligaments. Posteriorly it is related to the anterior vaginal wall, to which it is firmly attached in its lower two-thirds. The upper part of the urethra is mobile, but the lower part is relatively fixed. Figure 2.11 depicts the bladder and urethra.

Medial fibres of the pubococcygeus of the levator ani muscles are inserted into the urethra and vaginal wall. When they contract, they pull the anterior vaginal wall and the upper part of the urethra forwards, forming an angle of about 100° between the posterior wall of the urethra and the bladder base. On voluntary voiding of urine, the base of the bladder and the upper part of the urethra descend and this posterior angle disappears, so that the base of the bladder and the posterior wall of the urethra come to lie in a straight line. It was formerly claimed that absence of this posterior angle was the cause of stress incontinence, but this is probably only one of a number of mechanisms responsible.

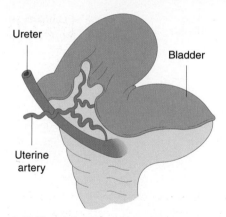

**Figure 2.12** The relationship of the uterine artery and ureter.

## The ureter

As the ureter crosses the brim of the pelvis it lies in front of the bifurcation of the common iliac artery. It runs downwards and forwards on the lateral wall of the pelvis to reach the pelvic floor, and then passes inwards and forwards, attached to the peritoneum of the back of the broad ligament, to pass beneath the uterine artery. It next passes forwards through a fibrous tunnel, the ureteric canal, in the upper part of the cardinal ligament. Finally it runs close to the lateral vaginal fornix to enter the trigone of the bladder.

The ureter's blood supply is derived from small branches of the ovarian artery, from a small vessel arising near the iliac bifurcation, from a branch of the uterine artery where it crosses beneath it, and from small branches of the vesical arteries.

Because of its close relationship to the cervix, the vault of the vagina and the uterine artery, the ureter may be damaged during hysterectomy (Fig. 2.12). Apart from being cut or tied, in radical procedures the ureter may undergo necrosis because of interference with its blood supply. It may be displaced upwards by fibromyomata or cysts that are growing between the layers of the broad ligament, and may suffer injury if its position is not noticed at operation.

## The rectum

The rectum extends from the level of the third sacral vertebra to a point about 2.5 cm in front of the coccyx, where it passes through the pelvic floor to become continuous with the anal canal. Its direction follows the curve of the sacrum and it is about 11 cm in length.

The front and sides of the upper third are covered by the peritoneum of the rectovaginal pouch; in the middle third only the front is covered by the peritoneum. In the lower third there is no peritoneal covering and the rectum is separated from the posterior wall of the vagina by the rectovaginal fascial septum. Lateral to the rectum are the two uterosacral ligaments, beside which run some of the lymphatics draining the cervix and vagina.

## The pelvic muscles, ligaments and fasciae

### The pelvic diaphragm

The pelvic diaphragm is formed by the levator ani muscles (Fig. 2.13).

*Levator ani muscles*
Each is a broad, flat muscle, the fibres of which pass downwards and inwards. The two muscles, one on either side, constitute the pelvic diaphragm. The muscle arises by a linear origin from:
- the lower part of the body of the os pubis,
- the internal surface of the parietal pelvic fascia along the white line,
- the pelvic surface of the ischial spine.
  The levator ani muscles are inserted into:
- the pre-anal raphé and the central point of the perineum where one muscle meets the other on the opposite side,

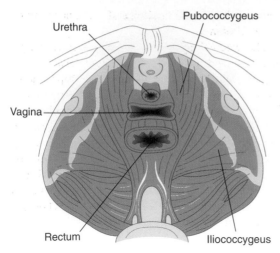

**Figure 2.13** Diagrammatic representation of the superior aspect of the pelvic floor.

- the wall of the anal canal, where the fibres blend with the deep external sphincter muscle,
- the postanal or anococcygeal raphé, where again one muscle meets the other on the opposite side,
- the lower part of the coccyx.

The muscle is described in two parts: the pubococcygeus, which arises from the pubic bone and the anterior part of the tendinous arch of the pelvic fascia (white line), and the iliococcygeus, which arises from the posterior part of the tendinous arch and the ischial spine.

The medial borders of the pubococcygeus muscles pass on either side from the pubic bone to the pre-anal raphé. They thus embrace the vagina, and on contraction have some sphincteric action. The nerve supply is from the third and fourth sacral nerves.

The pubococcygeus muscles support the pelvic and abdominal viscera, including the bladder. The medial edge passes beneath the bladder and runs laterally to the urethra, into which some of its fibres are inserted. Together with fibres from the opposite muscle, they form a loop, which maintains the angle between the posterior aspect of the urethra and the bladder base. During micturition this loop relaxes to allow the bladder neck and upper urethra to open and descend.

*Urogenital diaphragm*

The urogenital diaphragm (triangular ligament) lies below the levator ani muscles and consists of two layers of pelvic fascia, which fill the gap between the descending pubic rami. The deep transverse perineal muscle (compressor urethrae) lies between the two layers, and the diaphragm is pierced by the urethra and the vagina.

## The perineal body

This is the perineal mass of muscular tissue that lies between the anal canal and the lower third of the vagina. Its apex is at the lower end of the rectovaginal septum, at the point where the rectum and posterior vaginal walls come into contact. Its base is covered with skin and extends from the fourchette to the anus. It is the point of insertion of the superficial perineal muscles and is bounded above by the levator ani muscles where they come into contact in the midline between the posterior vaginal wall and the rectum.

## The pelvic peritoneum

The peritoneum is reflected from the lateral borders of the uterus to form, on either side, a double fold of peritoneum – the broad ligament. This is not a ligament but a peritoneal fold, and it does not support the uterus. The Fallopian tube runs in the upper free edge of the broad ligament as far as the point at which the tube opens into the peritoneal cavity. The part of the broad ligament that is lateral to the opening is called the infundibulopelvic fold, and in it the ovarian vessels and nerves pass from the side wall of the pelvis to lie between the two layers of the broad ligament. The mesosalpinx, the portion of the broad ligament which lies above the ovary, is layered; between its layers are to be seen any Wolffian remnants that may be present. Below the ovary, the base of the broad ligament widens out and contains a considerable amount of loose connective tissue, called the parametrium. The ureter is attached to the posterior leaf of the broad ligament at this point.

The ovary is attached to the posterior layer of the broad ligament by a short mesentery (the mesovarium), through which the ovarian vessels and nerves enter the hilum.

The rectovaginal pouch has already been described. It will be noted that while the vagina does not have any peritoneal covering in front, behind it is in contact with the rectovaginal pouch for about 2 cm where the vagina is separated from the abdominal cavity only by the peritoneum and thin fascia. The peritoneal cavity can be opened by posterior colpotomy at this point.

## The ovarian ligament and round ligament

The ovarian ligament lies beneath the posterior layer of the broad ligament and passes from the medial pole of the ovary to the uterus just below the point of entry of the Fallopian tube.

The round ligament is the continuation of the same structure and runs forwards under the anterior leaf of peritoneum to enter the inguinal canal, ending in the subcutaneous tissue of the labium majus. Together, the ovarian and round ligaments are analogous to the gubernaculum in the male.

## The pelvic fascia and pelvic cellular tissue

Connective tissue fills the irregular spaces between the various pelvic organs. Much of it is loose cellular tissue, but in some places it is condensed to form strong ligaments, which contain some smooth muscle fibres and which form the fascial sheaths enclosing the various viscera. The pelvic arteries, veins, lymphatics, nerves and ureters run through it.

The cellular tissue is continuous above with the extraperitoneal tissue of the abdominal wall, but below it is cut off from the ischiorectal fossa by the pelvic fascia and the levator ani muscles. There is a considerable collection of cellular tissue in the wide base of the broad ligament and at the side of the cervix and vagina, called the parametrium. The pelvic fascia may be regarded as a specialized part of this connective tissue. Anatomists describe parietal and visceral components.

The parietal pelvic fascia lines the wall of the pelvic cavity, covering the obturator internus and pyramidalis muscles. There is a thickened tendinous arch (or white line) on the side wall of the pelvis. It is here that the levator ani muscle arises and the cardinal ligament gains its lateral attachment. Where the parietal pelvic fascia encounters bone, as in the pubic region, it blends with the periosteum. It also forms the upper layer of the urogenital diaphragm (triangular ligament).

Each viscus has a fascial sheath, which is dense in the case of the vagina and cervix and at the base of the bladder, but is tenuous or absent over the body of the uterus and the dome of the bladder. Various processes of the visceral pelvic fascia pass inwards from the peripheral layer of the parietal pelvic fascia. From the point of view of the gynaecologist, certain parts of the visceral fascia are of particular importance, as follows.

The cardinal ligaments (transverse cervical ligaments) provide the essential support of the uterus and vaginal vault. These are two strong, fan-shaped, fibromuscular expansions that pass from the cervix and vaginal vault to the side wall of the pelvis on either side.

The uterosacral ligaments run from the cervix and vaginal vault to the sacrum. In the erect position they are almost vertical in direction and support the cervix.

The bladder is supported laterally by condensations of the vesical pelvic fascia one each side; there is also a sheet of pubocervical fascia which lies beneath it anteriorly.

## Arteries supplying the pelvic organs

### The ovarian artery

Because the ovary develops on the posterior abdominal wall and later migrates down into the pelvis, it derives its blood supply directly from the abdominal aorta. The ovarian artery arises from the aorta just below the renal artery and runs downwards on the anterior surface of the psoas muscle to the pelvic brim, where it crosses in front of the ureter and then passes into the infundibulopelvic fold of the broad ligament. The artery divides into branches that supply the ovary and tube and then run on to reach the uterus, where they anastomose with the terminal branches of the uterine artery.

### The internal iliac (hypogastric) artery

This vessel is about 4 cm in length and begins at the bifurcation of the common iliac artery in front of the sacroiliac joint. It soon divides into anterior and posterior divisions; the branches that supply the pelvic viscera are all from the anterior division.

The uterine artery provides the main blood supply to the uterus. The artery first runs downwards on the lateral wall of the pelvis, in the same direction as the ureter. It then turns inwards and forwards, lying in the base of the broad ligament. By this change of direction the artery crosses above the ureter, at a distance of about 2 cm from the uterus, at the level of the internal os. On reaching the wall of the uterus, the artery turns upwards to run tortuously to the upper part of the uterus, where it anastomoses with the ovarian artery. In this part of its course it sends many branches into the substance of the uterus.

The artery supplies a branch to the ureter as it crosses it, and shortly afterwards another branch is given off to supply the cervix and upper vagina.

The vaginal artery is another branch of the internal iliac artery that runs at a lower level to supply the vagina.

The vesical arteries are variable in number. They supply the bladder and terminal ureter. One usually runs in the roof of the ureteric canal.

The middle rectal artery often arises in common with the lowest vesical artery.

The pudendal artery is another branch of the internal iliac artery. It leaves the pelvic cavity through the sciatic foramen and, after winding round the ischial spine, enters the ischiorectal fossa, where it gives off the inferior rectal artery. It terminates in branches that supply the perineal and vulval structures, including the erectile tissue of the vestibular bulbs and clitoris.

## The superior rectal artery

This artery is the continuation of the inferior mesenteric artery and descends in the base of the pelvic mesocolon. It divides into two branches, which run on either side of the rectum and supply numerous branches to it.

## The pelvic veins

The veins around the bladder, uterus, vagina and rectum form plexuses which intercommunicate freely.

Venous drainage from the uterine, vaginal and vesical plexuses is chiefly into the internal iliac veins.

Venous drainage from the rectal plexus is via the superior rectal veins to the inferior mesenteric veins, and the middle and inferior rectal veins to the internal pudendal veins and so to the iliac veins.

The ovarian veins on each side begin in the pampiniform plexus that lies between the layers of the broad ligament. At first there are two veins on each side accompanying the corresponding ovarian artery. Higher up, the vein becomes single; that on the right ends in the inferior vena cava and that on the left in the left renal vein.

## The pelvic lymphatics

Lymph draining from the lower extremities and the vulval and perineal regions is all filtered through the inguinal and superficial femoral nodes before continuing along the deep pathways on the side wall of the pelvis. One deep chain passes upwards lateral to the major blood vessels, forming in turn the external iliac, common iliac and para-aortic groups of nodes.

Medially, another chain of vessels passes from the deep femoral nodes through the femoral canal to the obturator and internal iliac groups of nodes. These last nodes are interspersed among the origins of the branches of the internal iliac artery, receiving lymph directly from the organs supplied by this artery, including the upper vagina, cervix and body of the uterus.

From the internal iliac and common iliac nodes, afferent vessels pass up the para-aortic chains, and finally all the lymphatic drainage from the legs and pelvis flows into the lumbar lymphatic trunks and the cisterna chyli at the level of the second lumbar vertebra. From here, all the lymph is carried by the thoracic duct through the thorax, with no intervening nodes, to empty into the junction of the left subclavian and internal jugular veins.

Tumour cells that penetrate or bypass the pelvic and para-aortic nodes are rapidly disseminated via the great veins at the root of the neck.

## Lymphatic drainage from the genital tract

The lymphatic vessels from individual parts of the genital tract drain into this system of pelvic lymph nodes in the following manner (Fig. 2.14).

The vulva and the perineum medial to the labiocrural skin folds contain superficial lymphatics that pass upwards towards the mons pubis and then curve laterally to the superficial inguinal and femoral nodes. Drainage from these is through the fossa ovalis into the deep femoral nodes. The largest of these, lying in the upper part of the femoral canal, is known as the node of Cloquet.

The vagina: the lymphatics of the lower third follow the vulval drainage to the superficial inguinal nodes, whereas those from the upper two-thirds pass upwards to join the lymphatic vessels of the cervix.

The cervix: the lymphatics pass either laterally in the base of the broad ligament or posteriorly along

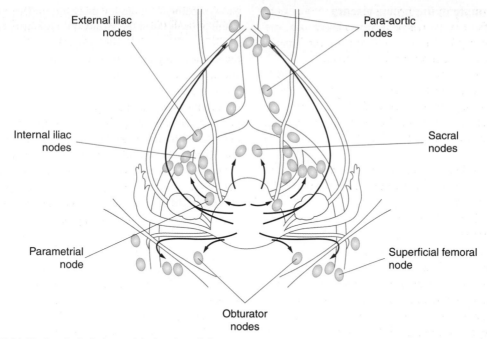

**Figure 2.14** The lymphatic drainage of the female genital organs.

the uterosacral ligaments to reach the side wall of the pelvis. Most of the vessels drain to the internal iliac, obturator and external iliac nodes, but vessels also pass directly to the common iliac and lower para-aortic nodes, so that radical surgery for carcinoma of the cervix should include removal of all these node groups on both sides of the pelvis.

The corpus uteri: nearly all the lymphatic vessels join those leaving the cervix and therefore reach similar groups of nodes.

A few vessels at the fundus follow the ovarian channels, and there is an inconsistent pathway along the round ligament to the inguinal nodes.

The ovary and Fallopian tube have a plexus of vessels that drain along the infundibulopelvic fold to the para-aortic nodes on both sides of the midline. On the left, these are found around the left renal pedicle, whereas on the right there may be only one node intervening before the lymph flows into the thoracic duct, thus accounting for the rapid early spread of metastatic carcinoma to distant sites such as the lungs.

The bladder and urethra: the drainage is to the iliac nodes, whilst the lymphatics of the lower part of the urethra follow those of the vulva.

The rectum: the lymphatics from the lower anal canal drain to the superficial inguinal nodes, and the remainder of the rectal drainage follows pararectal channels accompanying the blood vessels to both the internal iliac nodes (middle rectal artery) and the para-aortic nodes at the origin of the inferior mesenteric artery.

## Nerves of the pelvis

### Nerve supply of the vulva and perineum

The pudendal nerve arises from the second, third and fourth sacral nerves. As it passes along the outer wall of the ischiorectal fossa, it gives off an inferior rectal branch and divides into the perineal nerve and the dorsal nerve of the clitoris. The perineal nerve gives the sensory supply to the vulva; it also innervates the anterior part of the external anal sphincter and levator ani, and the superficial perineal muscles. The dorsal nerve of the clitoris is sensory.

Sensory fibres from the mons and labia also pass, in the ilioinguinal and genitofemoral nerves, to the first lumbar root. The posterior femoral cutaneous nerve carries sensation from the perineum to the small sciatic nerve, and thus to the first, second and third sacral nerves.

The main nerve supply of the levator ani muscles comes from the third and fourth sacral nerves.

## Nerve supply of the pelvic viscera

To describe what can be seen on dissection of the extensive autonomic nerve supply of the pelvic organs is one thing – to determine the physiological functions of the various parts of the system is another.

Nerve fibres of the pre-aortic plexus of the sympathetic nervous system are continuous with those of the superior hypogastric plexus, which lies in front of the last lumbar vertebra and is wrongly called the presacral nerve. Below, the superior hypogastric plexus divides, and on each side its fibres are continuous with fibres passing beside the rectum to join the uterovaginal plexus (inferior hypogastric plexus, or plexus of Frankenhäuser). This plexus lies in the loose cellular tissue posterolateral to the cervix below the uterosacral folds of peritoneum.

Parasympathetic fibres from the second, third and fourth sacral nerves join the uterovaginal plexus. Fibres from (or to) the bladder, uterus, vagina and rectum join the plexus. The uterovaginal plexus contains a few ganglion cells, so it is likely that a few motor nerves have their relay stations there and then pass onwards with the blood vessels to the viscera.

The ovary is not innervated by the nerves already described but from the ovarian plexus, which surrounds the ovarian vessels and joins the pre-aortic plexus high up.

This description has avoided any conjecture as to the particular function of the sympathetic and parasympathetic nerves, and no opinion has been expressed as to whether the various nerves carry sensory or motor impulses. Clinical facts are few. It is evident that afferent sensory impulses are often carried in the superior hypogastric plexus. If this is divided during presacral neurectomy, pain from the bladder and uterus can often be blocked. Apart from a transient pelvic hyperaemia, there is no change in the motor function of either bladder or uterus. At an ordinary hysterectomy, the uterovaginal plexus is not disturbed, but after a more extensive Wertheim operation, there may be painless atony and distension of the bladder, which is attributed to loss of bladder sensation because the sacral connections of the uterovaginal plexus have been divided.

The motor effects are even less certain than the sensory. Stimulation of the cut lower end of the hypogastric plexus seems to have no effect on the bladder or the uterus. Although it has been stated that the parasympathetic nerves are excitatory to the musculature of the body of the uterus and inhibitory to that of the cervix, and that the sympathetic nerves have the opposite effect, there is not general agreement about this.

The myometrium contains both α and β adrenergic receptors and also cholinergic receptors. In the non-pregnant uterus, the balance of their action is uncertain, but during pregnancy, strong stimulation of β-receptors with β-mimetic drugs such as isoxsuprine will inhibit myometrial activity.

### 🔑 Key Points

- The nephrogenic cord develops from the mesoderm and forms the urogenital ridge and the mesonephric duct. The paramesonephric duct, which later forms the Müllerian system, is the precursor of female genital development.
- The lower ends of the Müllerian ducts come together in the midline, fuse and develop into uterus and cervix.
- Most of the upper vagina is of Müllerian origin. The lower vagina forms from the sinovaginal bulbs.
- The primitive gonad is first evident at 5 weeks of embryonic life and forms on the medial aspect of the mesonephric ridge.
- The size and ratio of the cervix to uterus change with age and parity.
- Vaginal pH is normally acidic and has a protective role for decreasing the growth of pathogenic organisms.
- An adult uterus weighs about 70 g and consists of three layers: the peritoneum, the myometrium and the endometrium.
- The cervix is narrower than the body of the uterus and is approximately 2.5 cm in length. The ureter runs about 1 cm lateral to the supravaginal cervix.
- The epithelium of the cervix in its lower third is stratified squamous epithelium and the junction between this and the columnar epithelium is where most cervical carcinoma arises.
- The ovary is the only intraperitoneal structure not covered by peritoneum.
- The main supports to the pelvic floor are the connective tissue and levator ani muscles. The main supports of the uterus are the uterosacral ligaments, which are condensations of connective tissue.
- The ovarian arteries rise from the aorta. The right ovarian vein drains into the vena cava; the left ovarian vein usually drains into the left renal vein.
- The major nerve supply of the pelvis comes from the pudendal nerves, which arise from the second, third and fourth sacral nerves.

# Chapter 3

# Normal and abnormal sexual development and puberty

## OVERVIEW

Sexual differentiation and normal subsequent development are fundamental to the continuation of the human species. In recent years, our understanding of the control of this process has greatly increased. Following fertilization, the human embryo will differentiate into a male or female fetus, and subsequent development is genetically controlled. This chapter describes the processes involved and discusses the subsequent evolution to full maturation.

## Sexual differentiation

The means by which the embryo differentiates is controlled by the sex chromosomes. This is known as genetic sex. The normal chromosome complement is 46, including 22 autosomes derived from each parent. An embryo that contains 46 chromosomes and has the sex chromosomes XY will develop as a male. If the sex chromosomes are XX, the embryo will differentiate into a female. The resulting development of the gonad will create either a testis or an ovary. This is known as gonadal sex. Subsequent development of the internal and external genitalia gives phenotypic sex or the sex of appearance. Cerebral differentiation to a male or female orientation is known as brain sex.

## Genetic sex

In the developing embryo with a genetic complement of 46 XY, it is the presence of the Y chromosome that determines that the undifferentiated gonad will become a testis (Fig. 3.1). Absence of the Y chromosome will result in the development of an ovary. On the short arm of the Y chromosome is a region known as the *SRY* gene, which is responsible for the determination of testicular development as it produces a protein known as testicular determining factor (TDF). TDF directly influences the undifferentiated gonad to become a testis. When this process occurs, the testis also produces Müllerian inhibitor.

The undifferentiated embryo contains both Wolffian and Müllerian ducts. The Wolffian ducts have the

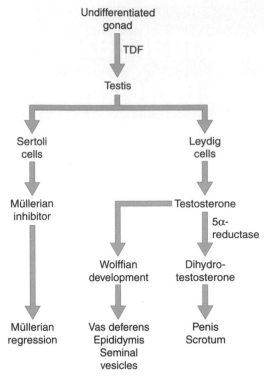

**Figure 3.1** Male differentiation. (TDF, testicular determining factor.)

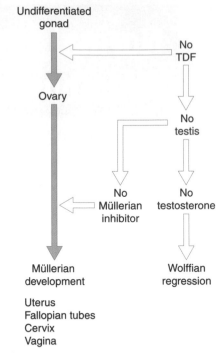

**Figure 3.2** Female differentiation. (TDF, testicular determining factor.)

potential to develop into the internal organs of the male, and the Müllerian ducts into the internal organs of the female. If the testis produces Müllerian inhibitor, the Müllerian ducts regress.

The testis differentiates into two cell types, Leydig cells and Sertoli cells. The Sertoli cells are responsible for the production of Müllerian inhibitor, which leads to Müllerian regression. The Leydig cells produce testosterone, which promotes the development of the Wolffian duct, leading to the development of vas deferens, the epididymis and the seminal vesicles. Testosterone by itself does not have a different effect on the cloaca; in order to exert its androgenic effects, it needs to be converted by the cloacal cells through the enzyme 5α-reductase to dihydrotestosterone. These androgenic effects lead to the development of the penis and the scrotum.

The absence of a Y chromosome and the presence of two X chromosomes mean that Müllerian inhibitor is not created, and the Müllerian ducts persist in the female (Fig. 3.2). The absence of testosterone means that the Wolffian ducts regress, and the failure of androgen to affect the cloaca leads to an external female phenotype.

## Abnormal development

Any aberration in development that results in an unexpected developmental sequence of events may be mediated in a number of ways.

## Chromosome abnormalities

In an embryo that loses one of its sex chromosomes, the total complement of chromosomes will be reduced to 45, leaving a fetus viable only where this is 45 XO (Turner's syndrome). Here, the absence of the second X chromosome or Y chromosome means there is no testicular development and therefore the phenotype is female (Fig. 3.3). The gonad is, however, unable to complete its development and, although it initially differentiates to be an ovary, the oogonia are unable to complete their development and at birth only the stroma of the ovary is present (streak ovaries). Thus, in Turner's syndrome, the absence of a functional ovary means that there is no oestrogen production at puberty, and secondary sexual characteristics cannot develop.

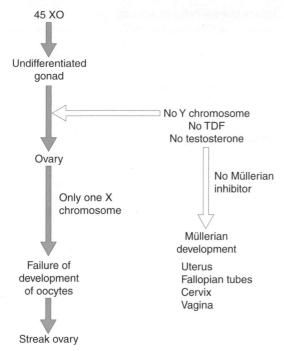

**Figure 3.3** Turner's syndrome. (TDF, testicular determining factor.)

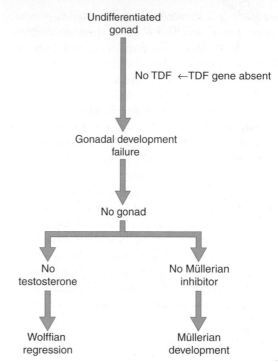

**Figure 3.4** XY gonadal agenesis. (TDF, testicular determining factor.)

As the genes involved in achieving final height are shared by the sex chromosomes, the absence of one sex chromosome will also lead to short stature.

In females who have an XY karyotype, a mutation at the site on the short arm of the Y chromosome resulting in failure of production of TDF will mean there is no testicular development (XY gonadal agenesis). The default phenotypic state is female (Fig. 3.4). In these circumstances, the absence of a testis means that the internal genitalia will persist as a result of the development of Müllerian structures, and the Wolffian ducts will regress. The external genitalia will be female.

## Gonadal abnormalities

In males, a number of gonadal abnormalities may exist. One of these is known as the vanishing testis syndrome: an XY fetus develops testes that then undergo atrophy. The reason for this remains speculative, although torsion, thrombosis and viral infections have been suggested. However, the failure of the development of the testes leads to a female default state, as above (similar to Fig. 3.4).

In Leydig cell hypoplasia, the Leydig cells responsible for the production of testosterone either completely fail to produce this or produce it in only small quantities. A range of abnormalities may result, dependent on the level of androgen produced, and therefore the phenotype may range from female through to the hypospadiac male.

In XY gonadal dysgenesis, a genetic abnormality leads to an abnormal testicular development. The testis fails to secrete androgen or Müllerian inhibitor, resulting in an XY female. If the genetic abnormality leads to an enzyme deficiency in the biosynthetic pathway to androgen, testosterone will fail to be secreted by the testis. However, some androgen may be produced, depending on which enzyme is absent in the pathway. Therefore some effect on the external genitalia may be possible and a varying degree of virilism will occur. If the biosynthetic production of Müllerian inhibitor is deficient, its absence will, of course, mean the persistence of the Müllerian duct. This is an extremely rare syndrome.

In the female, gonadal dysgenesis may occur, and in this situation (similar to Turner's syndrome) the gonad is present only as a streak. These individuals have been found to have small fragments of a Y chromosome and, as a result of this, the gonad may undergo mitotic change, which leads to the development of a gonadal tumour, e.g. a gonadoblastoma. The Müllerian structures remain and the Wolffian structures regress, because of the absence of testes. At puberty, the failure of development of the ovary will mean that there is no possibility for the production of oestradiol, and a failure of secondary sexual characteristic growth will occur.

In the rare condition known as mixed gonadal dysgenesis, there is a testis and a streak gonad in the same individual. The chromosome complement is typically 46 XX or a mosaic with a Y component. Here, strangely, the Wolffian structures develop only on the side of the testis, but all Müllerian structures regress. The external genitalia in this rare condition may be ambiguous, depending on the functional capacity of the testis.

In true hermaphrodites, the gonad may develop into either a testis or an ovary, or a combination of the two known as an ovotestis. Here, a number of permutations may occur, with either a testis and an ovary, or an ovotestis with a testis, an ovary or another ovotestis (Fig. 3.5). This usually results from a mosaic XX:XY karyotype, and the predominance of either ovarian or testicular tissue in the gonad depends on the percentage of cell lines in the mosaic. As can be seen from Figure 3.5, the combination of gonads will determine the degree of virilization: the greater the testicular component, the more virilized the resulting development and the more likely the presence of Müllerian inhibitor. Thus, in the true hermaphrodite, it is possible to get co-existent Müllerian and Wolffian structures in terms of internal development, and varying degrees of masculinization of the external genitalia, depending on the combination of gonads.

## Internal genitalia abnormalities

In males there are three fundamental changes that may lead to abnormalities of the internal genitalia. The first of these is androgen insensitivity (Fig. 3.6). In this condition the fetus fails to develop androgen receptors due to mutations in the androgen receptor gene. Failure to possess the receptor means that although the testis will be producing testosterone, the androgenic effect cannot be translated into the end organ as it is not recognized by the cell wall. The result here is that the fetus develops in the default female state, as it is unable to recognize the androgenic impact. This is the commonest type of XY female and the Wolffian ducts regress, as they also have no androgen receptor. However, the Müllerian ducts also regress because the testis is normal and produces Müllerian inhibitor. Girls with this abnormality present with primary amenorrhoea at puberty.

A further aberration in XY females also exists with a condition known as 5α-reductase deficiency (Fig. 3.7). As outlined above, this enzyme is responsible for the conversion of testosterone to dihydrotestosterone resulting in virilization of the cloaca. If this enzyme is absent, the external genitalia will be female but the internal genitalia will be male. The Müllerian ducts will regress. Here again, this female will present with primary amenorrhoea.

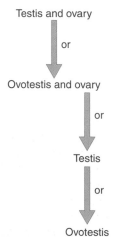

**Figure 3.5** True hermaphrodite.

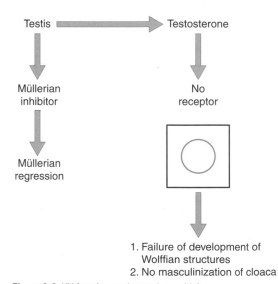

**Figure 3.6** XY female – androgen insensitivity.

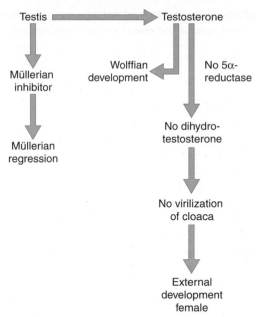

**Figure 3.7** XY female – 5α-reductase deficiency.

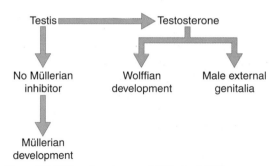

**Figure 3.8** XY female – absence of Müllerian inhibitor.

Finally, a rare condition known as Müllerian inhibitory deficiency may mean that an XY male may have persistent Müllerian structures, due to the absence of Müllerian inhibitory factor, and co-existent male and female internal structures (Fig. 3.8).

In 46 XX females, a genetic defect that results in failure of development of the uterus, cervix and vagina is known as the Rokitansky syndrome. This is the second most common cause of primary amenorrhoea in women, the first being Turner's syndrome. Here the ovaries are normal, and the external genitalia are normally female. The internal genitalia are either absent or rudimentary. Variations on this may lead to development of the vagina without development of the uterus, or development of the uterus without subsequent development of the cervix or vagina, and a

functional uterus may result. The aetiology of this developmental abnormality remains to be clarified. It is probably, however, a defect in the genes responsible for the development of the internal female genitalia. These genes, known as the homeobox genes, are likely to possess either deletions, which may be partial or complete, or point mutations and, as a consequence of these variations, the resulting structures of the internal genitalia will vary in their development. However, the overall effect of this developmental abnormality is a failure of uterine and vaginal development, leading to infertility. These patients will present at puberty with either primary amenorrhoea or, in circumstances when a small portion of uterus may be functional, with cyclical abdominal pain due to retained menstrual blood.

Two other developmental abnormalities may occur. The first of these is maldevelopment of the uterus, in which fusion defects occur from the extreme of a double uterus with a double cervix through to the normally fused uniform uterus. These abnormalities have been classified and result from the failure of fusion of the paramesonephric ducts at their lower border. A maldeveloped uterus may be associated with some degree of reproductive failure.

The development of the vagina involves a downgrowth of the vaginal plate and subsequent union of this with the cloaca and thereafter canalization. This process can also fail, leading to the second developmental abnormality, transverse vaginal septae, in which the passage of the vagina is interrupted and therefore at puberty menstrual blood is trapped in an upper vagina that does not connect to the lower vagina. In the unusual condition of a double uterus, a double vagina can also exist, and failure to develop the full double vaginal system may result in a blind hemivagina, again leading to a collection of menstrual blood at puberty.

## External genitalia abnormalities

In males, the external genitalia may fail to develop for a number of the above reasons, and the phallus may be underdeveloped, leading to hypospadias. In hypospadias, the urethra often fails to reach the end of the phallus or penis, and urine exits from the base of the penis.

In females, the external genitalia may be virilized, giving a masculine appearance. This is most commonly seen in a condition known as congenital adrenal hyperplasia. In this condition, an enzyme defect in the adrenal gland – usually 21-hydroxylase deficiency – prevents the fetal adrenal gland from producing cortisol. Failure of the production of cortisol means that the feedback mechanism on the hypothalamus leads to an elevation of adrenocorticotrophic hormone (ACTH). This in turn stimulates the adrenal gland to undergo a form of hyperplasia, and the excessive production of steroid precursors (17-hydroxyprogesterone) means that the adrenal gland produces excessive amounts of androgen. This androgen enters the fetal circulation and impacts on the developing cloaca, thereby leading to virilization. The female child is then born with a degree of phallic enlargement, and the lower part of the vagina may be obliterated by the development of a male-type perineum and hence a vaginal orifice is not apparent.

Virilization of the cloaca can also occur if the fetus is exposed to androgen in an androgenic drug ingested by the mother or, in many cases, the virilization is idiopathic. The end result in both of these circumstances is known as the intersex state. At birth, investigation of the chromosomes, the endocrine status of the infant and ultrasound of the internal organs will lead to a rapid diagnosis, revealing whether the child is a female with a virilization state, which is most likely to be congenital adrenal hyperplasia, or a male who has been under-masculinized.

## Brain sex

The sex of orientation of a human is influenced by many factors. Theories exist that this is genetically predetermined and it is most likely that our sexual orientation is in fact determined by our sexual make up. However, this may be influenced by androgen exposure in utero or by other genetic and environmental factors that impact on this function. Enormous care has to be taken before a final decision is made on the sex of rearing of those individuals who are uncertain about their sexual orientation.

## Puberty

The hypothalamo–pituitary–ovarian axis is functionally complete during the latter half of fetal life. Follicle-stimulating hormone (FSH) levels are suppressed from 20 weeks' gestation by the production of oestrogen by the placenta and by the fetus itself. At birth, the fetus is separated from its placenta and therefore the major source of oestrogen is removed. The FSH

level then rises in response to the hypo-oestrogenic state of the fetus and remains elevated for some 6–18 months after birth. During this time it is suppressed due to the central inhibition of the production of gonadotrophin-releasing hormone (GnRH), which controls the pituitary production of FSH. The mechanism by which this is achieved remains speculative, but almost certainly is controlled by a gene in the GnRH cell nucleus in the hypothalamus. It is possible that there is a relationship between the production of leptin, a peptide produced by fat cells, and the subsequent control of this gene.

During childhood, FSH pulses are almost undetectable, and at around the age of 8 or 9 years a change gradually occurs in the function of the GnRH cell. This change begins with the production of single nocturnal spikes of GnRH and subsequently FSH. These spikes of FSH increase in frequency during the night-time hours over a period of 1–2 years. Eventually, the frequency of the FSH pulses increases such that they are detectable in the daylight hours, and thereafter, after a period of 4–5 years, a fully functional production of GnRH with normal adult frequency and pulse amplitude leads to the establishment of the ovulatory menstrual cycle. Puberty therefore occurs over a total of 5–10 years, and involves five types of development (see box below).

## The physiology of puberty

The sequence of events that occur in the physical change resulting in the adult fertile female is usually the growth spurt, followed by breast development, pubic hair growth, menarche, and finally axillary hair growth. Although this is the sequence of events in 70 per cent of girls, variations often occur. The description of pubertal development is credited to Tanner. He has classified the stages of development into five stages for breast growth and pubic hair growth.

### Five stages of puberty

- Growth spurt
- Breast development
- Pubic hair growth
- Menstruation
- Axillary hair growth

The breast bud responds to the production of oestradiol by the ovary, which is itself reliant on GnRH production, as outlined above. The breast grows in phases. Initially the body of the breast grows; this is then superseded by areolar development, which leads to a pronounced areola in comparison with the rest of the breast, and at this stage the breast has reached Tanner stage 4. Finally, the breast tissue grows to become confluent with the areola and the breast has then completed its development.

Pubic hair growth begins on the labia and extends gradually up onto the mons and then into the inguinal regions. It is perfectly normal for pubic hair to extend along the midline up towards the umbilicus, but this is often misconstrued by women as being abnormal.

The growth spurt begins around the age of 11 years in girls, and the rate at which growth occurs increases from about 6 to 10 cm per year for around 2 years. Finally, the effect of oestrogen on the end-plate of the femur causes fusion, and growth ceases; by the age of 15, most girls have achieved their final height.

Menarche (the first menstrual period) occurs at any age between 9 and 17 years. As one would imagine, the hypothalamo–pituitary–ovarian axis is not fully mature at the time of menarche, and subsequent menstrual cycles are commonly irregular. Menstrual loss may also vary enormously, as a result of the immaturity of the axis. It takes between 5 and 8 years from the time of menarche for women to develop ovulatory cycles 100 per cent of the time. In understanding the menstrual difficulties that might arise during adolescent life, this piece of physiology is important to bear in mind.

## Common clinical presentations and problems (Table 3.1)

### Turner's syndrome

Patients with this condition may present at two ages in their life: either soon after birth or, more rarely, at a time of delayed puberty. The manner of presentation in infancy is variable. In the first few months of life there may be unexplained oedema of the hands and feet, loose folds of skin at the neck and occasionally unusual facies. In older children, the oedema usually disappears, although it can persist, but the main feature of the growing child is shortness of

**Table 3.1** Common clinical presentations and problems

| Conditions | Signs and symptoms | Investigations |
| --- | --- | --- |
| Turner's syndrome | Oedema of hands and feet<br>Short stature<br>Webbed neck<br>Wide carrying angle<br>Broad chest | FSH and LH<br>Karyotype 45 XO |
| XY females | Primary amenorrhoea<br>Usually normal breast development<br>Scanty/absent pubic and axillary hair<br>Absent uterus and tubes<br>Undescended/maldescended testes | Karyotype 46 XY |
| Intersex | Ambiguous genitalia at birth | Karyotype 46 XX |
| Vaginal atresia | Primary amenorrhoea<br>Normal secondary sexual characteristics<br>Absent vagina and uterus<br>Normal ovaries | |

FSH, Follicle-stimulating hormone; LH, luteinizing hormone.

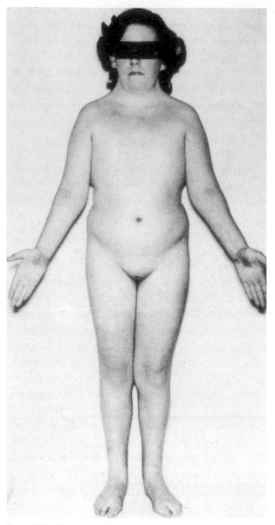

**Figure 3.9** Turner's syndrome.

stature. It is this that suggests to the clinician the possibility of a sex chromosome anomaly. As the child grows, a wide carrying angle of the arms may become apparent, the neck may become webbed in its appearance, and the chest becomes broad with widely spaced nipples. Individuals occasionally have associated features such as colour blindness, coarctation of the aorta and short metatarsals (Fig. 3.9). As these girls approach puberty, they have streak ovaries and are, therefore, incapable of producing oestradiol. The hypothalamus and pituitary function normally and therefore FSH levels and luteinizing hormone (LH) levels are elevated due to ovarian failure. As mentioned previously, the internal genitalia are otherwise normal, and investigation will reveal a karyotype that is

typically 45 XO and measurement of gonadotrophins will show markedly elevated FSH and LH.

The treatment of this condition falls into two phases. The first phase is the induction of puberty, which involves the administration of hormone replacement therapy. In order to ensure that secondary sexual characteristics appear normally, oestrogen is administered orally, beginning at an extremely low dose and gradually increasing over a number of years. As puberty itself takes 5 years to complete, the same time frame should be anticipated when puberty is induced by exogenous oestrogen. The introduction of progesterone to the regime usually occurs after 18 months to 2 years, when withdrawal bleeds from the patient's functioning uterus will occur.

The second phase of treatment is at a time when the patient desires a pregnancy. As she is deficient of oocytes, pregnancy can only be achieved with the aid of a donor egg, which, with a sperm from the patient's partner, is used to create an embryo, which is then transferred to the recipient's uterus. Pregnancy progresses normally thereafter, although childbirth may be difficult because of the short stature.

If investigations reveal a diagnosis of 46 XX gonadal dysgenesis, the gonads have a 30 per cent risk of developing a gonadoblastoma (a malignant tumour of the ovary) and therefore patients should be advised to have their gonads removed. Again, these women require induction of puberty in the same way as Turner's syndrome patients.

## XY females

These patients present at puberty with primary amenorrhoea. Patients with androgen insensitivity are phenotypically normal females with breast development because their testes have produced androgen at puberty, which is converted peripherally to oestrogen by aromatase activity in fat cells. This oestrogen then enters the circulation and induces breast growth. It is common for breast growth to be complete at the time of presentation.

However, the absence of an androgen receptor means that pubic and axillary hair is either very scanty or absent. The vagina is short and, of course, the uterus and tubes are absent. The testes may be found in the lower abdomen, groins or, rarely, in the labia majora. These girls may well have presented in childhood with inguinal herniae, which have been operated on, and the gonads will have been discovered at that stage and removed. If this has not been the case and the testes are still present, advice that they should be removed because of the risk of malignancy should be given. The clinical appearance of these patients makes the diagnosis straightforward, and only confirmation by karyotyping is necessary.

Oestrogen will need to be administered to these women in order to maintain their female body habitus, but the failure of the development of the Müllerian structures means pregnancy is impossible, except in those cases of XY gonadal agenesis or the XY female with absent Müllerian inhibitor only.

## Intersex

Ambiguous genitalia are usually diagnosed at birth when the infant is clearly neither male nor female. In these circumstances, gender assignment should be withheld until the infant can be fully evaluated. A very sensitive approach to the clinical situation must be taken. The parents will obviously be anxious to learn as swiftly as possible whether their child is male or female. Initially the most important investigation is karyotyping and, with the facilities that now exist, the karyotype can be determined within 24 hours on white blood cells taken from the infant.

The most common cause of ambiguous genitalia is congenital adrenal hyperplasia. Therefore, as we know that affected individuals are females with a masculinized vulva, ultrasound of the pelvis will reveal a normal uterus and ovaries. This, in conjunction with a karyotype of 46 XX, will almost always clinch the diagnosis. These children fail to produce cortisol and have high levels of circulating 17-hydroxyprogesterone, another investigative test that should be performed. The infants require cortisol supplementation in order to avoid an adrenal crisis. Further investigation may be required if the karyotype is 46 XY, and the possibilities for this are outlined earlier in the chapter.

## Vaginal atresia

The presentation of an adolescent with primary amenorrhoea and normal secondary sexual characteristics should raise the possibility of congenital absence of the vagina as the primary concern until proven otherwise. Here, the clinical story is a simple one, with absence of the establishment of menses. Clinical examination of the vulva will reveal a normal external appearance. However, parting the labia will reveal an absent vagina. An ultrasound examination of the pelvis will then confirm the absence of the development of the internal genitalia, but the presence of normal ovaries. The management of these patients is extremely sensitive, as their diagnosis will cause them great distress. Teenage girls are emotionally labile during puberty and adolescent development, and the news that they have no vagina and no uterus is very distressing to them and to their parents.

It is impossible currently to offer any help for the absence of the uterus. However, it is possible to create a vagina so that sexual intercourse may occur normally. This may be created in one of two ways, either non-surgically or surgically. The non-surgical technique involves the use of graduated glass dilators, which will stretch the small vagina into a fully functional vagina. This may be achieved over a period of 6–8 weeks of gradual dilatation, which is performed by the patient herself. In order for this technique to be successful, which it is in some 85 per cent of girls, motivation must be appropriate and it usually helps if the patient is in an established relationship and wishes to have sexual intercourse. For those patients for whom this cannot be successfully achieved, a surgical approach may be necessary to create a vagina. Several techniques have been described, involving various materials, including skin grafts, amnion or bowel. Again, subsequent to the surgery, dilators are required in order to maintain the surgically created neovagina.

## Obstructive outflow tract problems

Two varieties of outflow tract problems exist in the developmental abnormalities observed by gynaecologists in their female patients. The first of these is known as transverse vaginal septae. The simplest and most common is the imperforate hymen, where menstrual blood is trapped behind a thin hymenal membrane. This situation is easily resolved by a cruciate incision, which releases the menstrual blood; subsequent sexual activity is normal and there are no sequelae.

In cases where a transverse vaginal septum results from failure of canalization of the vagina, septae may

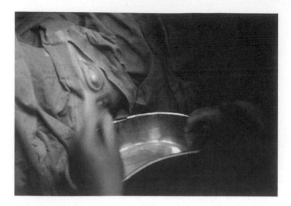

**Figure 3.10** A haematocolpos seen in the theatre just before incision.

occur at three levels: the lower third, middle third or upper third of the vagina. In all these cases, women present with cyclical abdominal pain, and the development of a pelvic mass as menstrual blood accumulates in the vagina, thereby distending it. In some cases the vagina may distend to give a mass, which may extend to the umbilicus. Investigation of these circumstances demands an ultrasound scan that will demonstrate the presence of a haematocolpos (blood in the vagina) (Fig. 3.10). Having established the anatomical defect, corrective surgery is required to excise and reconstruct the vagina, thereby creating a normal vagina, with normal menstrual drainage and normal function, both for sexual intercourse and subsequent conception.

Where there is a vertical septal defect, a midline septum persists between two hemi-vaginas, one of which has successfully developed and the other has failed to reach the perineum. In these circumstances the hemi-uterus on the blind side bleeds into the blind hemi-vagina, creating a haematocolpos. Cyclical abdominal pain occurs with increasing severity, but this time the patient does have periods because the other hemi-uterus and hemi-vagina function normally. Excision of the midline septum results in proper drainage of the menstrual flow, thereby resolving the problem.

## Menorrhagia in adolescence

Menstrual problems in adolescence are very common, and may manifest themselves in a number of ways. The periods may be irregular and very heavy and occasionally result in marked anaemia, or they may be very light and infrequent and cause equal concern. As outlined above, an understanding of the physiology of the onset of the menstrual cycle and its subsequent normal development is imperative for the clinician to manage these patients correctly.

In the former group of heavy menstrual loss, if the patient is not anaemic, it is unnecessary to offer any treatment other than reassurance. If the patient does become anaemic, some control of menstrual loss must be undertaken. This is best achieved either by progestogens or by the oral contraceptive pill. Control of the cycle will result until such time as the hypothalamo–pituitary–ovarian axis has matured.

In the group of patients who have very infrequent periods, a further investigation may be required, and this is best carried out by assessing several levels of gonadotrophins and by ultrasound of the ovary. In some circumstances, a diagnosis of polycystic ovary syndrome may be made, and these patients may require menstrual cycle control in the form of the oral contraceptive pill. They also may develop oligomenorrhoea later in life, which may contribute towards an infertility problem that may require attention. However, it is important to remember that the vast majority of these teenage girls will eventually establish a normal menstrual cycle and be fertile. The clinician is well advised to be cautious in giving advice about fertility potential, as incorrect advice may invoke unnecessary anxiety.

## Precocious puberty

Occasionally, pubertal changes may occur earlier than normal, and they have been known to occur as early as 3 or 4 years of age. Most cases of precocious puberty are idiopathic, but result from premature activation of the gene in the GnRH cell. The sequence of events that occur subsequently mimics normal puberty, and therefore ovulatory cycles may result in very young children if they are not treated. In fact, pregnancy has been known to occur in 5 and 6-year-olds in whom sexual maturity has been reached. Precocious puberty may, however, also result from abnormal situations, e.g. a granulosa cell tumour that produces oestradiol, and this will lead to pubertal development, or from pituitary or hypothalamic tumours, which lead to FSH production, e.g. craniopharyngioma.

When investigating these children, the exclusion of a serious tumour is of primary importance, and imaging techniques can be used to achieve this. As the majority of cases are idiopathic, treatment is targeted at down-regulation of the pituitary using GnRH analogues.

## New developments

Laparoscopic techniques have been developed to help form a neovagina in cases of vaginal atresia. Although more invasive than using dilators, they allow a functional vagina to be formed more quickly.

## Key Points

- Genetic sex is determined by the presence of the sex chromosomes X and Y.
- The presence of a Y chromosome determines male development; the absence of a Y chromosome leads to a female phenotype.
- In Turner's syndrome, the absence of a second X chromosome leads to streak ovaries.
- If the testis fails to develop or cannot function, the default state is female.
- True hermaphrodites have both ovarian and testicular tissue. The effect is determined by the dominant cell line.

- Congenital absence of the uterus and vagina is the second most common cause of primary amenorrhoea.
- Uterine maldevelopment does not usually result in reproductive failure.
- External genitalia in girls may be virilized by excessive androgen exposure in utero.
- Puberty is genetically determined and controlled from the hypothalamus.

## Additional reading

Edmonds DK. Normal and abnormal development of the genital tract. Gynaecological disorders of childhood and adolescence. In: Edmonds DK (ed.), *Dewhurst's textbook of obstetrics and gynaecology for postgraduates*, 6th edn. Oxford: Blackwell Science, 1999, 1–11 and 12–16.

Moore KL, Persaud TVN. *The developing human: clinically orientated embryology*, 6th edn. Philadelphia: WB Saunders, 1998.
Sanfilippo JS (ed.). *Pediatric and adolescent gynecology*, 2nd edn. Philadelphia: WB Saunders, 2001.

# The normal menstrual cycle

## OVERVIEW

Women in the Western world have around 400 menstrual cycles during the course of their lifetimes. In the UK, disorders of menstruation are one of the commonest reasons why women present to their general practitioner. An understanding of the physiology of the normal menstrual cycle is required in order to tackle subjects such as infertility and the prevention of unwanted pregnancy. This chapter aims to describe the events of the normal menstrual cycle. At each stage, the clinical relevance of menstrual cycle physiology is emphasized.

## Introduction

The most obvious manifestation of the normal menstrual cycle is the presence of regular menstrual periods. These occur as the endometrium is shed following failure of implantation or fertilization of the oocyte. Menstruation is initiated in response to changes in steroids produced by the ovaries, which themselves are controlled by the pituitary and hypothalamus.

## The ovary

Within the ovary, the menstrual cycle can be divided into three phases:
1. the follicular phase
2. ovulation
3. the luteal phase.

## Follicular phase

The development of the oocyte is the key event in the follicular phase of the menstrual cycle. The ovary contains thousands of primordial follicles that are in a continuous state of development from birth, through periods of anovulation, such as pregnancy, to the menopause. These initial stages of follicular development are independent of hormonal stimulation. In the absence of the correct hormonal stimulus, however, follicular development fails at the pre-antral stage, with ensuing follicular atresia. Development beyond the pre-antral stage is stimulated by the pituitary hormones (luteinizing hormone [LH] and follicle-stimulating hormone [FSH]), which can be considered as key regulators of oocyte development.

At the start of the menstrual cycle, FSH levels begin to rise as the pituitary is released from the negative-feedback effects of progesterone, oestrogen and inhibin.

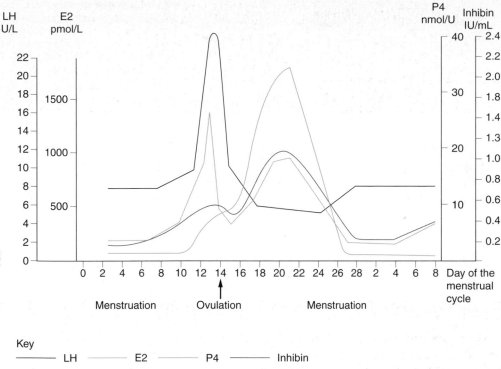

**Figure 4.1** Pituitary and ovarian hormones during the menstrual cycle: luteinizing hormone (LH), inhibin, oestradiol (E2), progesterone (P4).

Rising FSH levels rescue a cohort of follicles from atresia, and initiate steroidogenesis. Figure 4.1 shows the hormonal changes throughout the ovarian and menstrual cycles.

### Steroidogenesis

The basis of hormonal activity in pre-antral to pre-ovulatory follicles is described as the 'two cell, two gonadotrophin' hypothesis. Steroidogenesis is compartmentalized in the two cell types within the follicle: the theca and granulosa cells. The two cell, two gonadotrophin hypothesis states that these cells are responsive to the gonadotrophins LH and FSH respectively.

Within the theca cells, LH stimulates the production of androgens from cholesterol. Within the granulosa cells, FSH stimulates the conversion of thecally derived androgens to oestrogens (aromatization) (Fig. 4.2). In addition to its effects on aromatization, FSH is also responsible for the proliferation of granulosa cells. Although other mediators are now known to be important in follicular development, this hypothesis is still the cornerstone to understanding events in the ovarian follicle. The respective roles of FSH and LH in follicular development are evidenced by studies on women undergoing ovulation induction in whom endogenous gonadotrophin production has been suppressed. If pure FSH alone is used for ovulation induction, an ovulatory follicle can be produced, but oestrogen production is markedly reduced. Both FSH and LH are required to generate a normal cycle with adequate amounts of oestrogen.

Androgen production within the follicle may also regulate the development of the pre-antral follicle. Low levels of androgens enhance aromatization and therefore increase oestrogen production. In contrast, high androgen levels inhibit aromatization and produce follicular atresia. A delicate balance of FSH and LH is required for early follicular development. The ideal situation for the initial stages of follicular development is low LH levels and high FSH levels, as seen in the early menstrual cycle. If LH levels are too high, theca cells produce large amounts of androgens, causing follicular atresia.

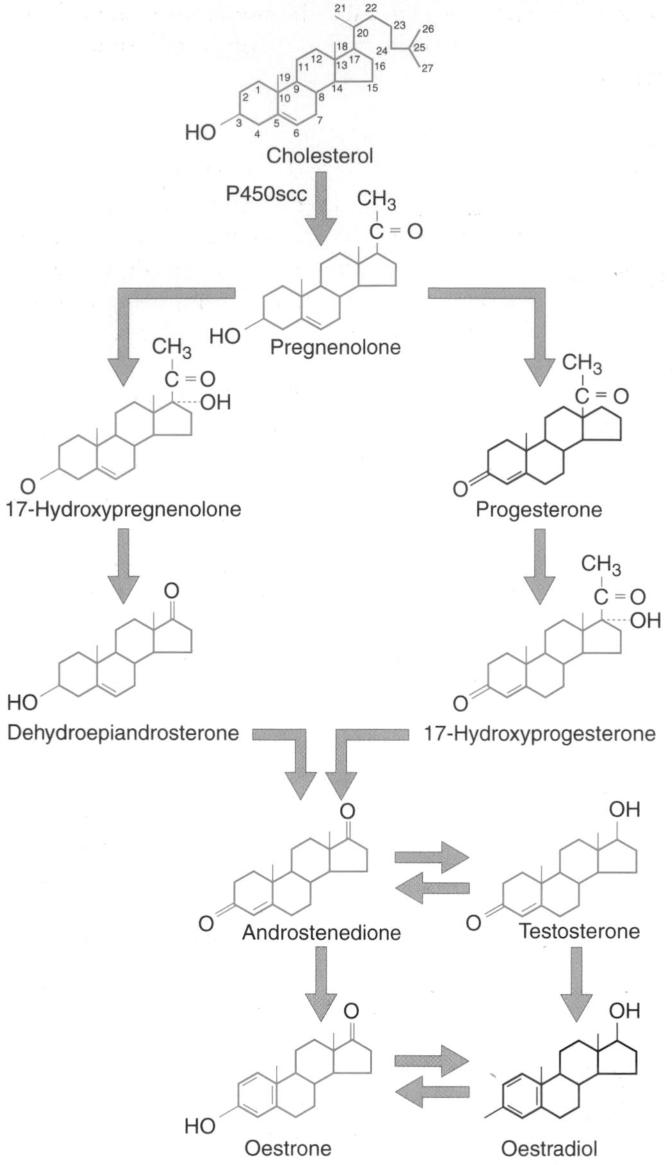

**Figure 4.2** Ovarian steroidogenesis. The ovary has the capacity to synthesize oestradiol (E2) from cholesterol. The major products of the ovary are oestradiol and progesterone (P4), although small amounts of testosterone and androstenedione are also produced.

## Selection of the dominant follicle

The developing follicle grows and produces steroid hormones under the influence of the gonadotrophins LH and FSH. These gonadotrophins rescue a cohort of pre-antral follicles from atresia. However, normally only one of these follicles is destined to grow to a pre-ovulatory follicle and be released at ovulation – the dominant follicle.

The selection of the dominant follicle is the result of complex signalling between the ovary and the pituitary. In simplistic terms, the dominant follicle is the largest and most developed follicle in the ovary at the mid-follicular phase. Such a follicle has the most efficient aromatase activity and the highest concentration of FSH-induced LH receptors. The dominant follicle therefore produces the greatest amount of oestradiol and inhibin. Inhibin further amplifies LH-induced androgen synthesis, which is used as a substrate for oestradiol synthesis. These features mean that the largest follicle therefore requires the lowest levels of FSH (and LH) for continued development. At the time of follicular selection, FSH levels are declining in response to the negative-feedback effects of oestrogen. The dominant follicle is therefore the only follicle that is capable of continued development in the face of falling FSH levels.

Ovarian–pituitary interaction is crucial to the selection of the dominant follicle, and the forced atresia of the remaining follicles. Figure 4.3 depicts the positive-feedback and negative-feedback mechanisms of the hypothalamo–pituitary–ovarian axis. When this interaction is bypassed, as in ovulation induction with the administration of exogenous gonadotrophins, many follicles continue to develop and are released at ovulation, with an ensuing multiple gestation rate of around 30 per cent. During in-vitro fertilization (IVF), the production of many ovulatory follicles is desired, as once the oocytes have been harvested, and fertilized in vitro, the number of embryos replaced can be carefully controlled. However, if such multiple follicular development occurred unchecked in the normal cycle, it would lead to the production of multiple gestations of high-order numbers, with their associated problems.

### Inhibin and activin

Although folliculogenesis, ovulation and the production of progesterone from the corpus luteum can be explained largely in terms of the interaction between pituitary gonadotrophins and sex steroids, it is becoming clear that other autocrine or paracrine mediators also play a role. One of the most important of these is inhibin.

Inhibin was originally described as a testicular product that inhibited pituitary FSH production – hence its name. However, inhibin is also produced by a variety of other cell types, including granulosa cells within the ovary. Granulosa cell inhibin production is stimulated by FSH, but in women, as in men, inhibin attenuates FSH production. Within the ovary, inhibin enhances LH-induced androgen synthesis. The production of inhibin is a further mechanism by which FSH levels are reduced below a threshold at which only the dominant follicle can respond, ensuring atresia of the remaining follicles.

Activin is a peptide that is structurally related to inhibin. It is produced both by the granulosa cells of antral follicles and by the pituitary gland. The action of activin is almost directly opposite to that of inhibin in that it augments pituitary FSH secretion and increases FSH binding to granulosa cells. Granulosa cell activin production therefore appears to amplify the effects of FSH within the ovarian follicle.

### Insulin-like growth factors

Insulin-like growth factors (IGF-I and IGF-II) act as paracrine regulators. Circulating levels do not change during the menstrual cycle, but follicular fluid levels increase towards ovulation, with the highest level found in the dominant follicle. The actions of IGF-I and IGF-II are modified by their binding proteins: insulin-like growth factor binding proteins (IGFBPs).

In the follicular phase, IGF-I is produced by theca cells under the action of LH. IGF-I receptors are present on both theca and granulosa cells. Within the theca, IGF-I augments LH-induced steroidogenesis. In granulosa cells, IGF-I augments the stimulatory effects of FSH on mitosis, aromatase activity and inhibin production. In the pre-ovulatory follicle, IGF-I enhances LH-induced progesterone production from granulosa cells. Following ovulation, IGF-II is produced from

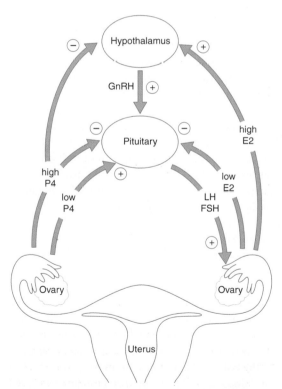

**Figure 4.3** Hypothalamo–pituitary–ovarian axis showing positive and negative feedback of hormones. It should be noted that the mechanism by which low oestrogen induces negative feedback of luteinizing hormone (LH) and follicle-stimulating hormone (FSH) production is uncertain. (GnRH, gonadotrophin-releasing hormone; P4, progesterone; E2, oestradiol.)

luteinized granulosa cells, and acts in an autocrine manner to augment LH-induced proliferation of granulosa cells.

## Ovulation

Late in the follicular phase, FSH induces LH receptors on granulosa cells. Oestrogen is an obligatory co-factor in this effect. As the dominant follicle develops further, follicular oestrogen production increases. Eventually the production of oestrogen is sufficient for it to reach the threshold required to exert a positive-feedback effect on pituitary LH secretion. Once this occurs, LH levels increase, at first quite slowly (day 8 to day 12 of the menstrual cycle) and then more rapidly (day 12 onwards). During this time, LH induces luteinization of granulosa cells in the dominant follicle, so that progesterone is produced. Progesterone further amplifies the positive-feedback effect of oestrogen on pituitary LH secretion, leading to a surge of LH. Ovulation occurs 36 hours after the onset of the LH surge. The LH surge is one of the best methods by which the time of ovulation can be determined, and is the event detected by most over-the-counter 'ovulation predictor' kits.

The peri-ovulatory FSH surge is probably induced by the positive-feedback effects of progesterone. In addition to the rise in LH, FSH and oestrogen that occurs around ovulation, a rise in serum androgen levels also occurs. These androgens are derived from the stimulatory effect of LH on theca cells, particularly those of the non-dominant follicle. This rise in androgens may have an important physiological effect in the stimulation of libido, ensuring that sexual activity is likely to occur at the time of ovulation, when the woman is at her most fertile.

Prior to the release of the oocyte at the time of ovulation, the LH surge stimulates the resumption of meiosis, a process which is completed after the sperm enters the egg. Additionally, the LH surge stimulates increased follicular expression of macrophage chemotactic protein-1 (MCP-1) and interleukin 8 (IL-8), which in turn causes an influx of macrophages and neutrophils into the pre-ovulatory follicle. Once activated, these leukocytes secrete mediators such as matrix metalloproteinases (MMPs) and prostaglandins, which cause the follicle wall to break down, releasing the oocyte at ovulation.

The crucial importance of prostaglandins and other eicosanoids in the process of ovulation is demonstrated by studies showing that inhibition of prostaglandin production may result in failure of release of the oocyte from the ovary, despite apparently normal steroidogenesis (the luteinized unruptured follicle syndrome [LUF]). Although LUF appears to be an uncommon cause of infertility, women wishing to become pregnant should be advised to avoid taking prostaglandin synthetase inhibitors such as aspirin and ibuprofen, which may inhibit oocyte release.

## Luteal phase

The luteal phase is characterized by the production of progesterone from the corpus luteum within the ovary. The corpus luteum is derived both from the granulosa cells that remain after ovulation and from some of the theca cells that differentiate to become theca lutein cells. The granulosa cells of the corpus luteum have a vacuolated appearance associated with the accumulation of a yellow pigment, lutein, from where the corpus luteum derives its name. Extensive vascularization within the corpus luteum ensures that the granulosa cells have a rich blood supply providing the precursors for steroidogenesis.

The production of progesterone from the corpus luteum is dependent on continued pituitary LH secretion. However, serum levels of progesterone are such that LH and FSH production is relatively suppressed. This effect is amplified by moderate levels of oestradiol and inhibin A, which are also produced by the corpus luteum. The low levels of gonadotrophins mean that the initiation of new follicular growth is inhibited for the duration of the luteal phase.

### Luteolysis

The duration of the luteal phase is fairly constant, being around 14 days in most women. In the absence of pregnancy and the production of human chorionic gonadotrophin (hCG) from the implanting embryo, the corpus luteum regresses at the end of the luteal phase, a process known as luteolysis. The mechanism of control of luteolysis in women remains obscure. As the corpus luteum dies, oestrogen, progesterone and inhibin A levels decline. The pituitary is released from the negative-feedback effects of these hormones, and gonadotrophins, particularly FSH, start to rise. A cohort of follicles that happen to be at the pre-antral phase is rescued from atresia and a further menstrual cycle is initiated.

## The pituitary gland

The process of follicular development, ovulation and the maintenance of the corpus luteum has been described in terms of ovarian physiology. In reality, however, the ovary, pituitary and hypothalamus act in concert (the hypothalamo–pituitary–ovarian axis) to ensure the growth and development of (ideally) one ovarian follicle, and to maintain hormonal support of the endometrium to allow implantation.

The pituitary hormones LH and FSH are, as we have seen, key regulators of folliculogenesis. The output of LH and FSH from the pituitary gland is stimulated by pulses of gonadotrophin-releasing hormone (GnRH) produced by the hypothalamus and transported to the pituitary in the portal circulation. The response of the pituitary is not constant, but is modulated by ovarian hormones, particularly oestrogen and progesterone. Thus low levels of oestrogen have an inhibitory effect on LH (negative feedback), whereas high levels of oestrogen actually stimulate pituitary LH production (positive feedback). In the late follicular phase, serum levels of oestrogen are sufficiently high that a positive feedback effect is triggered, thus generating the peri-ovulatory LH surge. In contrast, the combined contraceptive pill produces serum levels of oestrogen in the negative-feedback range, so that measured levels of gonadotrophins are low.

The mechanism of action of the positive-feedback effect of oestrogen involves an increase in GnRH receptor concentrations and an increase in GnRH production. The mechanism of the negative-feedback effect of oestrogen is uncertain.

In contrast to the effects of oestrogen, low levels of progesterone have a positive-feedback effect on pituitary LH and FSH secretion. Such levels are generated immediately prior to ovulation, and contribute to the FSH surge. High levels of progesterone, such as those seen in the luteal phase, inhibit pituitary gonadotrophin production. Negative-feedback effects of progesterone are generated both via decreased GnRH production and via decreased sensitivity to GnRH at the pituitary level. Positive-feedback effects of progesterone operate at the pituitary level only and involve increased sensitivity to GnRH. Importantly, progesterone can only have these effects if there has been prior priming by oestrogen.

As we have seen, oestrogen and progesterone are not the only hormones to have an effect on pituitary gonadotrophin secretion. The peptide hormones inhibin and activin have opposing effects on gonadotrophin production: inhibin attenuates pituitary FSH secretion, whereas activin stimulates it.

## The hypothalamus

The hypothalamus, via the pulsatile secretion of GnRH, stimulates pituitary LH and FSH secretion. Production of GnRH not only has a permissive effect on gonadotrophin production, but alterations in the amplitude and frequency of GnRH pulsation throughout the cycle are also responsible for some fine tuning of gonadotrophin production (see the section on the pituitary gland above).

The importance of GnRH secretion is seen in disorders such as anorexia nervosa and in the amenorrhoea associated with excessive exercise. In these disorders, GnRH production is suppressed, leading to anovulation and amenorrhoea. Ovulation can be restored in these women by the administration of GnRH in a pulsatile manner (although this should be approached carefully, since pregnancy is relatively contraindicated in women whose body weight is significantly below average).

It is important to remember that GnRH is produced in a pulsatile manner to exert its physiological effect. Drugs that are GnRH agonists (e.g. buserelin and goserelin) are widely used in gynaecology for the treatment of endometriosis and other disorders. Although these drugs act as GnRH agonists, they cause a decrease in pituitary LH and FSH secretion. The reason for this is that these agonists are long acting, and the continued exposure of the pituitary to moderately high levels of GnRH causes down-regulation and desensitization of the pituitary. LH and FSH production is therefore markedly decreased. Ovarian steroidogenesis is suppressed, so that serum oestrogen and progesterone fall to postmenopausal levels. Most women become amenorrhoeic whilst taking GnRH agonists. A potential disadvantage of the currently available GnRH agonists is that such down-regulation and desensitization of the pituitary take up to 3 weeks to exert their effects. The initial effect of GnRH administration is to stimulate pituitary LH and FSH production, leading to increased ovarian steroidogenesis. When a patient commences GnRH therapy, this temporary increase in ovarian steroidogenesis leads to a vaginal bleed within the first month of administration, and it is important to warn the patient of this.

## Summary of ovarian events

### Follicular phase

- LH stimulates theca cells to produce androgens.
- FSH stimulates granulosa cells to produce oestrogens.
- The most advanced follicle at mid-follicular phase becomes the dominant follicle.
- Rising oestrogen and inhibin A produced by the dominant follicle inhibit pituitary FSH production.
- Declining FSH levels cause atresia of all but the dominant follicle.

### Ovulation

- FSH induces LH receptors.
- LH surge occurs.
- Proteolytic enzymes within the follicle cause follicular wall breakdown and release of the oocyte.

### The luteal phase

- The corpus luteum is formed from granulosa and theca cells retained after ovulation.
- Progesterone produced by the corpus luteum is the dominant hormone of the luteal phase.
- In the absence of pregnancy, luteolysis occurs 14 days after ovulation.

# The endometrium

The changes in the hypothalamo–pituitary–ovarian axis during the menstrual cycle have already been described. These changes occur whether or not the uterus is still present. Menstruation, which occurs in the presence of the uterus, is the most obvious external manifestation that regular menstrual cycles are occurring. The changes in the endometrium that occur during the menstrual cycle are described below.

## Menstruation

As the corpus luteum dies at the end of the luteal phase, circulating levels of oestrogen and progesterone fall precipitously (see Fig. 4.1). In an ovulatory cycle, where the endometrium is exposed to oestrogen and then progesterone in an orderly manner, the endometrium becomes 'decidualized' during the second half of the cycle to allow implantation of the embryo. Decidualization is an irreversible process, and if implantation does not occur, programmed cell death (apoptosis) ensues. Menstruation is the shedding of the 'dead' endometrium and ceases as the endometrium regenerates.

Menstruation is initiated by the withdrawal of oestrogen and progesterone. Such an effect can be produced experimentally, and women receiving oestrogens and progestogens in the form of the combined contraceptive pill or hormone replacement therapy will experience a 'withdrawal bleed' on completion of a pack.

Withdrawal of progesterone has several main effects. First, intense spiral artery vasoconstriction is generated. Since most reports suggest that the spiral arteries do not express the progesterone receptor, it appears that the constricting effects of progesterone on the endometrial spiral arteries are indirect, and generated by locally produced prostaglandins, endothelins and angiotensin II. The other major effect of the withdrawal of progesterone, which proceeds in parallel with spiral artery vasoconstriction, is the production of pro-inflammatory cytokines such as MCP-1, IL-8 and cyclo-oxygenase-2 (which produces prostaglandins). These agents, particularly MCP-1 and IL-8, attract and activate macrophages and neutrophils, respectively, into the endometrium. Both invading leukocytes and endometrial stromal cells then release and activate MMPs, which break down extracellular matrix. The final main effect is that tissue hypoxia induced by vasoconstriction leads to the production of vascular endothelial growth factor (VEGF), which stimulates angiogenesis (important in postmenstrual tissue repair) and MMP production.

The above events lead to ischaemia (particularly of the upper endometrium) and tissue damage, shedding of the functional endometrium (the stratum compactum and stratum spongiosum) and bleeding from fragments of arterioles remaining in the basal endometrium.

Menstruation ceases as the damaged spiral arteries vasoconstrict and the endometrium regenerates. Rising oestrogen and progesterone levels inhibit MMP production. Thus, haemostasis in the endometrial vessels differs from haemostasis elsewhere in a number of important aspects. Normally, bleeding from a damaged vessel is stemmed by platelet accumulation, fibrin deposition and platelet degranulation. Such events may, however, lead to scarring. In the endometrium, scarring would significantly inhibit function (as seen in Asherman's syndrome), and an alternative system of haemostasis is therefore required. Vasoconstriction is the mechanism by which haemostasis is initially secured in the endometrium. Scarring is minimized by enhanced fibrinolysis, which breaks down blood clots. Later, repair of the endometrium and new blood vessel formation (angiogenesis) lead to the complete cessation of bleeding within 5–7 days from the start of the menstrual cycle.

Endometrial repair involves both glandular and stromal regeneration and angiogenesis. Both VEGF and fibroblast growth factor (FGF) are found within the endometrium, and both are powerful angiogenic agents. Increasing evidence suggests that oestrogen-induced glandular and stromal regeneration is mediated by epidermal growth factor (EGF). Other growth factors, such as transforming growth factors (TGFs) and IGFs, and the interleukins, particularly IL-1, may also be important.

Increased understanding of the agents involved in menstruation may improve attempts to control pathologically excessive menstruation. Prostaglandin synthetase inhibitors such as mefenamic acid (Ponstan) are widely used in the UK as a first-line treatment for menorrhagia. They are thought to increase the ratio of the vasoconstrictor prostaglandin (PG) F2α to the vasodilator prostaglandin PGE2. Although mefenamic acid does reduce menstrual loss, the mean reduction is only in the order of 20–25 per cent in women with true menorrhagia, and the search for more effective agents has therefore continued.

## The proliferative/follicular phase

Once endometrial repair is completed, usually at around day 5–6 of the cycle, menstruation ceases. Within the endometrium, the remainder of the follicular phase is characterized by glandular and stromal growth – hence the name the proliferative phase. During this time, the epithelium lining the endometrial glands changes from a single layer of low columnar cells to pseudostratified epithelium with frequent mitoses. The stromal component of the endometrium re-expands, and is infiltrated by bone marrow-derived cells. The massive development taking place in the endometrium is reflected in the increase in endometrial thickness, from 0.5 mm at menstruation to 3.5–5 mm at the end of the proliferative phase.

## The secretory/luteal phase

The postovulatory or luteal phase of the menstrual cycle is characterized by endometrial glandular secretory activity – hence the name the secretory phase. Under the action of progesterone, oestrogen-induced cellular proliferation is inhibited, and the depth of the endometrium remains fixed. Despite this, some elements continue to grow, leading to increased tortuosity of both the glands and spiral arteries in order to fit into the endometrial layer.

Shortly after ovulation, vacuoles containing subnuclear intracytoplasmic granules appear in glandular cells. These vacuoles progress to the apex of the glandular cells and their contents are released into the endometrial cavity. Peak secretory activity occurs at the time of implantation, 7 days after the gonadotrophin surge. Progesterone is essential for the induction of endometrial secretory changes and these changes are only seen after ovulation in the absence of exogenous steroid therapy. Histological examination of luteal phase endometrium used to be performed commonly to confirm that ovulation had occurred (Fig. 4.4). However, access to inexpensive, accurate steroid hormonal assays has rendered this invasive test obsolete, so that ovulation is now confirmed by serum progesterone measurements in the luteal phase.

Within the stroma, oedema is induced in the secretory phase under the influence of oestrogen and progesterone. The predominant bone marrow-derived cell within the endometrium is the large granulated lymphocyte, which has properties similar to those of

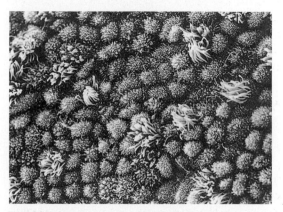

**Figure 4.4** Scanning electron micrograph of the normal endometrium at the secretory phase of the menstrual cycle. (Illustration kindly provided by Dr Gill Irvine.)

the natural killer cell and is thought to be important in regulating trophoblast invasion during implantation. In the late secretory phase, progesterone induces irreversible decidualization of the stroma. Histologically, decidualization is initiated around blood vessels. The

surrounding stromal cells display increased mitotic activity and nuclear enlargement and a basement membrane is generated (Fig. 4.5).

Immediately prior to menstruation, three distinct zones of the endometrium can be seen. The basalis is the basal 25 per cent of the endometrium, which is retained during menstruation and shows few changes during the menstrual cycle. The mid-portion is the stratum spongiosum, with oedematous stroma and exhausted glands. The superficial portion (the uppermost 25 per cent) is the stratum compactum, with prominent decidualized stromal cells. The withdrawal of oestrogen and progesterone leads to collapse of the decidualized endometrium, repeated vasoconstriction and relaxation of the spiral arterioles, and consequent shedding of the endometrium. The onset of menstruation heralds the end of one menstrual cycle and the beginning of the next.

## Summary of endometrial events

### Menstruation
- Menstruation is initiated largely by arteriolar vasoconstriction.
- The functional layer (upper 75 per cent) is shed.
- Menstruation ceases due to vasoconstriction and endometrial repair.
- Fibrinolysis inhibits scar tissue formation.

### Proliferative phase
- This phase is characterized by oestrogen-induced growth of glands and stroma.

### Luteal phase
- This phase is characterized by progesterone-induced glandular secretory activity.
- Decidualization is induced in the late secretory phase.
- Decidualization is an irreversible process and leads to endometrial apoptosis and menstruation unless pregnancy occurs.

## The normal menstrual cycle

### Clinical features

Medical students are taught that the normal menstrual cycle is 28 days long (from the start of one cycle to the start of the next) and that the usual duration of menstrual flow is 3–7 days. In fact, only 15 per cent of

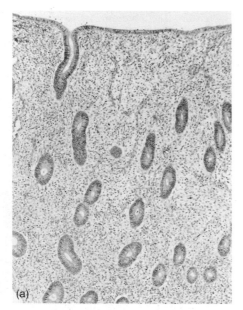
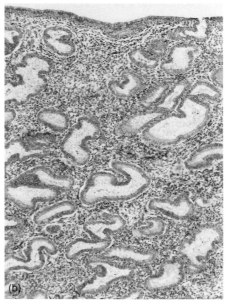

**Figure 4.5** Tissue sections of normal endometrium stained with haematoxylin and eosin during the proliferative (a) and secretory (b) phases of the menstrual cycle. (Illustration kindly provided by Dr Colin Stewart.)

women have a perfect 28-day cycle, and any cycle of between 21 and 35 days long can be regarded as normal. Menstrual cycles are longest immediately after puberty and in the 5 years leading up to the menopause, corresponding to the peak incidence of anovulatory cycles. The length of the menstrual cycle is determined by the length of the follicular phase. Once ovulation occurs, luteal phase length is fairly fixed at 14 days in almost all women.

The duration of menstrual flow also varies among women from 2 to 8 days. The amount of menstrual flow peaks on the first or second day of menstruation. The normal volume of menstrual loss is 35 mL per month. A menstrual loss of greater than 80 mL is considered to be excessive – this level is rather arbitrary and corresponds to the threshold at which iron deficiency anaemia may ensue unless treated.

## New developments

### Oocyte growth in vitro

During IVF, exogenous gonadotrophins are administered to stimulate follicular growth within the ovary. The administered dose of gonadotrophins has to be controlled carefully to achieve adequate follicular growth with minimal side effects. Ideally, many ovulatory follicles should be generated and harvested prior to ovulation. However, such a process requires intensive monitoring, which is time consuming for both the patient and physician.

At present, follicular growth can only be achieved in vivo, although in future it may be possible to culture primordial follicles in vitro from frozen ovarian biopsies. If ovulatory follicles could be generated, this would be a major advance – the adverse effects of gonadotrophin therapy could be avoided, and there would be no need for frequent hospital attendances for scans and hormone assays during ovulation induction. Moreover, ovarian biopsies could be taken (before pelvic radiotherapy, for example) and stored until required.

### GnRH antagonists

We have seen that the use of GnRH agonists is associated with an initial increase in ovarian steroidogenesis until down-regulation of the pituitary is achieved. GnRH antagonists have now been developed. GnRH antagonists inhibit the action of GnRH at the pituitary and therefore reduce LH and FSH secretion. The use of GnRH antagonists avoids the initial stimulatory effect of GnRH agonists at the pituitary gland; hence a therapeutic effect is achieved more rapidly, and some of the side effects of the GnRH agonists can be prevented.

## Clinical points

### Hormone assays

- Pituitary and ovarian hormones change constantly throughout the menstrual cycle.
- A single blood test at a random point in the menstrual cycle is of little value.
- Hormonal assays should be carefully timed to give the maximum information.

1. To determine whether a patient is ovulating:
   - measurement of serum progesterone is the most helpful test,
   - progesterone of 10 nmol/L indicates that ovulation has occurred,
   - blood should be withdrawn in the mid-luteal phase (normally day 21 of the cycle),
   - the results can only be interpreted if a menstrual period occurs around 7 days after sampling.
2. To determine whether a patient is menopausal:
   - measurement of serum gonadotrophins is the most helpful test,
   - elevated gonadotrophin levels indicate that the stock of ovarian follicles is exhausted,
   - blood should be withdrawn within 5 days after menstruation to avoid the mid-cycle surge,
   - abnormal results should be confirmed by repeat sampling.

### Ovarian cysts

- The pre-ovulatory follicle reaches a diameter of 20 mm.
- These follicles contain fluid and can be seen on ultrasound examination.
- A 'cyst' of up to 20 mm in diameter in a premenopausal women at mid-cycle is likely to be a pre-ovulatory follicle.
- In practice, single unilocular ovarian cysts of up to 50 mm in diameter are likely to be functional cysts.
- The appropriate initial management of a functional cyst is observation by serial ultrasound.

## Key Points

- An intact hypothalamo–pituitary–ovarian axis is required for normal menstruation.
- The ovary should ideally produce only one ovulatory follicle each cycle.
- Pituitary–ovarian dialogue ensures selection of the dominant follicle and atresia of the remaining follicles.
- Ovulation occurs 36 hours after the start of the mid-cycle LH surge.
- Progesterone produced by the corpus luteum induces decidualization of the endometrium.
- The embryo can only implant in the decidualized endometrium.
- In the absence of pregnancy, the lifespan of the corpus luteum is 14 days.
- Following luteolysis, steroid hormone levels fall, the endometrium dies and menstruation occurs.

## Additional reading

Cameron IT, Irvine G, Norman JE. Menstruation. In: Hillier SG, Kitchener HC, Neilson JP (eds), *Scientific essentials of reproductive medicine*. London: WB Saunders, 1996, 208–18.

McGavigan J, Lumsden MA. Menstruation and menstrual abnormality. In: Shaw R, Soutter WP, Stanton SL (eds), *Gynaecology*, 3rd edn. Edinburgh: Churchill Livingstone, 2003, 459–76.

# Disorders of the menstrual cycle

## OVERVIEW

Disorders of the menstrual cycle are one of the most common reasons for women to attend their general practitioner and, subsequently, a gynaecologist. Although rarely life threatening, menstrual disorders lead to major social and occupational disruption, and can also affect psychological well-being. Clinicians treating women with menstrual problems need not only to have a detailed understanding of normal menstrual physiology, and the various disorders that commonly present (as detailed in this chapter), but also to approach women with a presenting complaint of menstrual disorder in a compassionate and empathetic manner.

## MENORRHAGIA

### Definition

The average menstrual period lasts for 3–7 days, with a mean blood loss of 35 mL.

Menorrhagia ('heavy periods') is defined as a blood loss of greater than 80 mL per period. This definition is rather arbitrary, but represents the level of blood loss at which a fall in haemoglobin and haematocrit concentration commonly occurs.

### Prevalence

Menorrhagia is extremely common. Indeed, each year in the UK, 5 per cent of women between the ages of 30 and 49 consult their general practitioner with this complaint. Menorrhagia is the single leading cause of referral to hospital gynaecology clinics.

### Classification

Menorrhagia can be classified as:
- idiopathic, where no organic pathology can be found: idiopathic menorrhagia is otherwise known as dysfunctional uterine bleeding (DUB). The majority of women who present with menorrhagia will have DUB,
- secondary to an organic cause, such as fibroids.

### Aetiology

Despite extensive research, the aetiology of DUB remains unclear. Disordered endometrial prostaglandin production has been implicated in the aetiology of this condition, as have abnormalities of endometrial vascular development.

There are clearer reasons why many more women complain of menorrhagia now than they did a century ago. With decreasing family size, women now experience many more menstrual cycles. Additionally, the changing role of women in society and more liberated attitudes to the discussion of sexual and reproductive health mean that women are now much less likely to tolerate menstrual loss that they consider to be excessive.

## Other physiology

Menorrhagia is a feature of a number of organic conditions, which should be considered in the differential diagnosis. These include:

- von Willebrand's disease,
- other bleeding diatheses,
- fibroid uterus,
- endometrial polyp,
- thyroid disease,
- drug therapy, including intrauterine contraceptive devices (IUCDs),
- bleeding in pregnancy.

## Clinical features

### History

The hallmark of menorrhagia is the complaint of regular 'excessive' menstrual loss occurring over several consecutive cycles. This is largely a subjective definition, and it can be hard for the woman to communicate in words how much blood she is losing. Discussion of the number of towels and tampons used per day may be useful – perhaps accompanied by a menstrual pictogram in selected cases (Fig. 5.1). Of perhaps greater relevance is to determine the impact of the condition on the patient's lifestyle and quality of life. For example, the patient whose menorrhagia is so severe that she does not leave the house during her period clearly has a much greater problem (and may wish to pursue treatment further) than one to whom menorrhagia is a minor inconvenience.

### Is it relevant to determine the precise amount of menstrual loss in women complaining of menorrhagia?

This vexed question arises from the finding that only 50 per cent of women who complain of heavy periods actually have a blood loss that would fulfill the medical definition of menorrhagia. There is no single correct answer to this question and, as is often the case in medicine, each patient needs to be considered in the light of her own circumstances. The rationale for any investigation should be: 'Is this going to change the treatment I prescribe for this patient?'. In general, demonstration of the amount of blood lost during each period will not change the treatment plan. Since it is the patient's perception of loss that is important, treatment may be appropriate for all women, regardless of the actual amount of blood loss. There are a few exceptions to this rule, and there is a small proportion of women (often young at the beginning of their reproductive life) for whom the demonstration that their blood loss is in fact 'normal' may be sufficient to reassure them and make further treatment unnecessary.

It is also important to determine the duration of the current problem, and any other symptoms or factors of potential importance. The following symptoms should be enquired about specifically, as they may suggest a diagnosis other than DUB: irregular, intermenstrual or postcoital bleeding, a sudden change in symptoms, dyspareunia, pelvic pain or premenstrual pain, and excessive bleeding from other sites or in other situations (e.g. after tooth extraction).

### Clinical examination

Unless specific factors in the history alert the clinician to the presence of organic disease, clinical examination of women presenting with menorrhagia usually fails to reveal any significant signs. Despite this, it is important to perform a physical examination, including an abdominal and bimanual pelvic examination, in all women complaining of menorrhagia. A cervical smear should be performed if one is due.

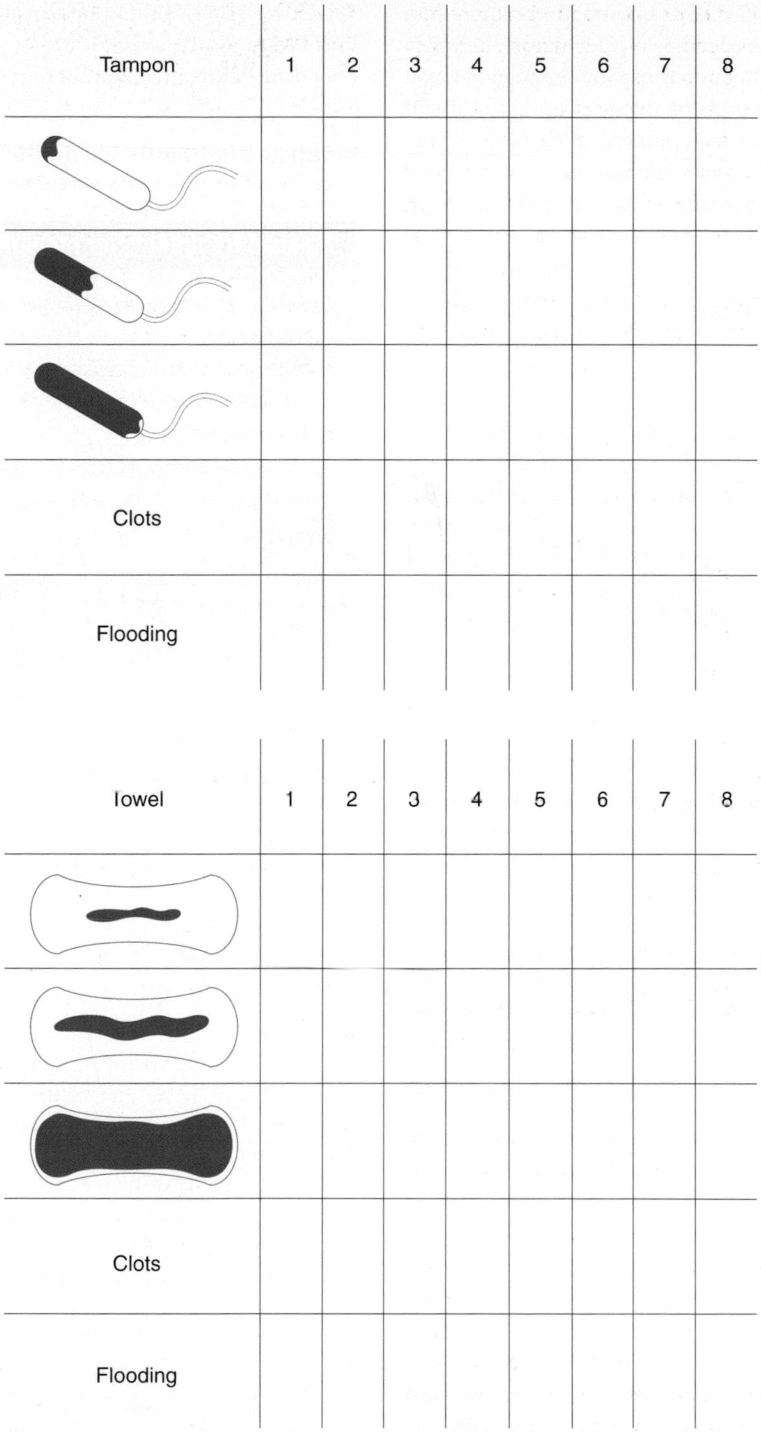

**Figure 5.1** Menstrual pictogram.

Abnormalities on clinical examination require further investigation. Depending on their nature, they may either suggest an organic cause for the menorrhagia (e.g. an enlarged uterus might suggest a diagnosis of uterine fibroids), or may point to other (coincident) pathology entirely. Investigations relevant to these conditions are discussed elsewhere in this book (Chapters 9 and 10).

## Initial investigations

### Full blood count
A full blood count (FBC) is done to ascertain the need for iron therapy.

In women in whom menorrhagia is the only relevant symptom, and in whom examination reveals no abnormalities (other than perhaps a slightly enlarged uterus, no greater than 10 weeks' gestation in size), further extensive investigation is not needed. Specifically, tests of thyroid function and endometrial assessment are *not* required routinely.

## Investigations in women who fail to respond to treatment after 3 months

- Transvaginal ultrasound, to look at the myometrium, endometrium and ovaries.
- Endometrial biopsy (with hysteroscopy *if* transvaginal ultrasound is abnormal).

## Treatments

There is a host of different treatments for menorrhagia, all of which have different efficacies and side effects. Some prevent conception on a temporary (e.g. levonorgestrel intrauterine system [LNG-IUS]) or permanent (e.g. hysterectomy) basis. Others are contraindicated in pregnancy but are not themselves effective contraceptives (e.g. danazol). Each treatment option is associated with a different array of side effects, which may be acceptable to some women but not others. For these reasons, and since menorrhagia is rarely life threatening but has an adverse impact on the woman's quality of life, it is essential that the treatment plan is determined in collaboration with the patient. The following is an outline of the medical and surgical treatment options. The *British National Formulary* (BNF) should be consulted for a detailed list of cautions, contraindications and side effects for each drug before prescription to patients.

## Medical treatments for menorrhagia

### Medical treatments for menorrhagia

*Drugs that are compatible with ongoing attempts at conception*
- Mefenamic acid and other non-steroidal anti-inflammatory drugs (NSAIDs)
- Tranexamic acid

*Drugs that are incompatible with ongoing attempts at conception but not licensed for use as contraceptives*
- Danazol

*Drugs licensed for use as contraceptives that are effective in the treatment of menorrhagia*
- Combined oral contraceptive pill
- LNG-IUS

*Second-line drugs with few advantages over the forgoing, and whose side effects limit long-term use*
- Danazol
- Gestrinone
- Gonadotrophin-releasing hormone analogues

### Drugs compatible (with caution) with ongoing attempts at conception
Mefenamic acid and other non-steroidal anti-inflammatory drugs
These agents are associated with a reduction in mean menstrual blood loss (MBL) of about 35 mL (95 per cent confidence interval (CI) 27–43 mL). This may be sufficient in some women to restore menstrual blood loss either to normal or to a level that is compatible with normal life. Their mode of action is probably in restoring imbalanced endometrial prostaglandin synthesis. An added benefit of these drugs is their pain-relieving properties; thus they are useful alone or in combination for women who complain of both menorrhagia and dysmenorrhoea.

Tranexamic acid
This agent is associated with a mean reduction in MBL of about 50–100 mL. Its mode of action is by inhibiting fibrinolysis (clot breakdown) in the

endometrium. In view of this, theoretical concerns have been raised that tranexamic acid may be associated with an increased risk of venous thrombosis. This theoretical risk is not borne out by the studies that have investigated it to date.

### Drugs incompatible with ongoing attempts at conception but not licensed for use as contraceptives

Danazol

Treatment with danazol for 2–3 months is associated with a mean reduction in MBL in the order of 100 mL. However, danazol is associated with androgenic side effects such as weight gain, acne, hirsutism and voice changes. Although the majority of these (with the exception of voice changes) are reversible on cessation of treatment, the fact that they can occur is enough to prevent most women with menorrhagia from opting for danazol treatment.

### Drugs licensed for use as contraceptives that are effective in the treatment of menorrhagia

Combined oral contraceptive pill

The combined oral contraceptive pill (COCP) is widely used for the treatment of menorrhagia, particularly by women who require contraception, and is believed to be effective. The evidence of its efficacy is, however, limited to non-randomized trials/case-control studies, which demonstrate a mean reduction in MBL of around 50 per cent. The side effects of the combined contraceptive pill are well known and, although no worse than the alternatives, many women are reluctant to take the COCP for non-contraceptive uses because of the potential adverse effects.

LNG-IUS (Fig. 5.2)

It is no exaggeration to say that the LNG-IUS has revolutionized the treatment of menorrhagia. For the first time, the LNG-IUS provides a highly effective alternative to surgical treatment for menorrhagia, with few side effects. Indeed, the Royal College of Obstetricians and Gynaecologists (RCOG) has suggested that the LNG-IUS should be considered in the majority of women as an alternative to surgical treatment. Mean reductions in MBL of around 95 per cent by 1 year after LNG-IUS insertion have been demonstrated. These results are similar to those for the surgical procedure endometrial resection, and the patient satisfaction rates for the two treatments were found to be similar in one study. Notwithstanding, the side

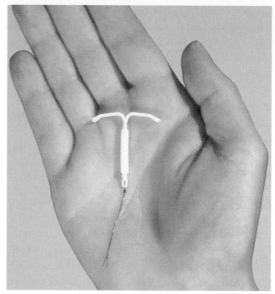

**Figure 5.2** The levonorgestrel intrauterine system.

effect of irregular menses for the first 3–6 months after insertion should be discussed in detail with the patient. Around 30 per cent of women with the LNG-IUS are amenorrhoeic by 1 year after insertion. For most women, this is a welcome side effect; however, there are a few women for whom it is not, so again, careful discussion is necessary before the LNG-IUS is inserted.

### Second-line drugs with few advantages over the forgoing and whose side effects limit long-term use

- Danazol
- Gestrinone
- Gonadotrophin-releasing hormone (GnRH) analogues.

---

**Medical and surgical treatments that are *not* effective in the treatment of menorrhagia**

- Ethamsylate
- Luteal phase progestogens
- Uterine curettage

---

## Surgical treatments for menorrhagia

Surgical treatment is normally restricted to women for whom medical treatments have failed. Women contemplating surgical treatment for menorrhagia should be certain that their family is complete. Whilst this caveat is obvious for women contemplating hysterectomy, in which the uterus will be removed, it also applies to women contemplating endometrial ablation. Women wishing to preserve their fertility for future attempts at childbearing should therefore be advised to have the LNG-IUS rather than endometrial ablation or hysterectomy.

### Endometrial ablation

All endometrial destructive procedures employ the principle that ablation of the endometrial lining of the uterus to sufficient depth prevents regeneration of the endometrium. During normal menstruation, the upper functional layer of the endometrium is shed, whilst the basal 3 mm of the endometrium is retained (see Chapter 4). At the end of menstruation and the beginning of the next cycle, the upper functional layer of the endometrium regenerates from the basal endometrium. In endometrial ablation, the basal endometrium is destroyed, and thus there is little or no remaining endometrium from which functional endometrium can regenerate.

There is a variety of methods by which endometrial ablation can be achieved, including the following.

Methods performed under direct visualization at hysteroscopy:
- Laser
- Diathermy
- Transcervical endometrial resection.

Methods performed non-hysteroscopically (i.e. without direct visualization of the endometrial cavity at the time of the procedure)
- Thermal uterine balloon therapy
- Microwave ablation
- Heated saline.

All the above operations are performed through the uterine cervix. Most take around 30–45 minutes to perform, and in the majority of cases the patient can return home that evening. The mean reduction in MBL associated with endometrial ablation is around 90 per cent.

In many units, endometrial ablation is performed using a single method and, in practice, patients may not be able to choose a particular technique for this procedure. This may not be important, as comparative studies have shown that the complication rates and the rates of patient satisfaction are similar for the available methods. There is some evidence that the rate of amenorrhoea is greater with the hysteroscopic methods, but this has to be set against the greater duration of the procedure, and the greater number of procedures needed to learn the technique, in comparison with the non-hysteroscopic methods.

The complications associated with endometrial ablation include uterine perforation, haemorrhage and fluid overload. Around 4 per cent of women have some sort of immediate complication. In 1 per cent of women, the complications arising during the procedure are sufficiently serious to prompt either laparotomy or another unplanned surgical procedure.

The majority of women who undergo this procedure are satisfied with their treatment. Five years post-treatment, approximately 60 per cent of women randomized to one study were happy with their treatment, compared with only 40 per cent randomized to medical therapy (excluding the LNG-IUS).

Some authorities have suggested that endometrial ablation is so successful that all women with DUB should be encouraged to consider it before opting for hysterectomy. Whilst there are merits to this argument, those women who, after informed discussion, still prefer hysterectomy should not be prevented from having this operation.

### Hysterectomy

Hysterectomy involves the removal of the uterus. It is an extremely common surgical procedure in the UK – indeed, 20 per cent of women will have a hysterectomy at some point in their lives.

Hysterectomy can be 'total', in which the uterine cervix is also removed, or 'subtotal', in which the cervix is retained. Hysterectomy is often accompanied by bilateral oophorectomy (removal of both ovaries). The precise choice of operation should be determined after detailed discussion between the doctor and patient. In terms of the treatment of menorrhagia, it is removal of the uterus that effects a cure, and thus removal of the cervix and/or ovaries is an 'optional extra'.

The main perceived advantage of oophorectomy is a reduced risk of ovarian cancer. Additionally, women with pelvic pain and/or severe premenstrual syndrome in addition to their menorrhagia may find that hysterectomy and bilateral salpingo-oophorectomy is more effective at treating their symptoms than hysterectomy alone. These advantages have to be set against the adverse effects of oestrogen loss on bone density for women who do not take hormone replacement therapy (HRT) after oophorectomy.

Removal of the uterus and ovaries without the woman's consent (or without her full understanding of the nature of the procedure) is a recurrent cause of litigation in gynaecology (see Appendix 2). It is essential, therefore, to obtain express consent for each part of the procedure before embarking on hysterectomy.

### Mode of hysterectomy

Total hysterectomy may be achieved using three main techniques:
* abdominal hysterectomy
* vaginal hysterectomy
* laparoscopically assisted hysterectomy.

## DYSMENORRHOEA

### Definition

Dysmenorrhoea is defined simply as painful menstruation.

### Prevalence

Dysmenorrhoea is a very common complaint, experienced by 45–95 per cent of women of reproductive age.

### Classification

Dysmenorrhoea can be classified as either primary (where there is no organic pathology) or secondary (where identifiable organic pathology such as endometriosis is likely to be responsible, at least in part, for the pain).

### Aetiology

#### Primary dysmenorrhoea

The risk factors for primary dysmenorrhoea include:
* duration of menstrual flow of >5 days,
* younger than normal age at menarche,
* cigarette smoking.

There is some evidence to support the assertion that dysmenorrhoea improves after childbirth, and it also appears to decline with increasing age.

### Secondary dysmenorrhoea

Secondary dysmenorrhoea may be a symptom of:
* endometriosis
* pelvic inflammatory disease
* adenomyosis
* Asherman's syndrome
* (rarely) cervical stenosis.

### Clinical features

Dysmenorrhoea typically consists of crampy suprapubic pain which starts at the onset of menstrual flow and lasts 8–72 hours.

### Investigations

A history alone is usually sufficient to make the diagnosis of dysmenorrhoea. If the symptoms persist, it is appropriate to examine the patient to exclude other possible pathologies. An endocervical swab for *Chlamydia trachomatis* and *Neisseria gonorrhoea* and a high vaginal swab for other pathogens should be taken at this stage. If examination is abnormal, or if an organic cause appears likely, it may be appropriate to perform pelvic ultrasound, followed, if necessary, by laparoscopy to investigate further. (If other features in the history suggest the possibility of Asherman's syndrome or cervical stenosis, hysteroscopy can be used to investigate these further. However, these conditions are infrequent causes of dysmenorrhoea, and their investigation should not be routine.)

In the absence of abnormal findings on examination, it is reasonable to try to treat the patient symptomatically without further investigation.

### Treatment

The following treatment options should be considered for women with dysmenorrhoea.
* NSAIDs, such as naproxen, ibuprofen and mefenamic acid, are reasonably effective. Aspirin

is less effective (although still more effective than placebo).

- Oral contraceptives are widely used but, surprisingly, there is little evidence.
- Nifedipine is widely used in Scandinavia, but is not licensed for this indication in the UK.
- Surgical treatments aimed at interrupting the nerve pathways from the uterus have been employed, and there is some evidence of their efficacy in the long term. Until more evidence is available, however, this should be confined to specialist centres for the treatment of women whose condition is unresponsive to other therapies.

## AMENORRHOEA/OLIGOMENORRHOEA

### Definition

Amenorrhoea is defined as the absence of menstruation. It may be classified as either primary or secondary. There are, of course, physiological situations in which amenorrhoea is normal, namely pregnancy, lactation and prior to the onset of puberty.

- Primary amenorrhoea describes the condition in which girls fail to develop secondary sexual characteristics by 14 years of age or fail to menstruate by 16 years of age.
- Secondary amenorrhoea describes the cessation of menstruation for more than 6 months in a normal female of reproductive age that is not due to pregnancy.

### Classification

Amenorrhoea is the primary complaint in a complex and often confusing array of clinical conditions (listed in the box for reference). A detailed knowledge of all the possible causes is not necessary (or possible) at undergraduate level, and students should not therefore try to commit this list to memory. They should, however, be aware that the conditions causing amenorrhoea can broadly be categorized as follows.

- Reproductive outflow tract disorders.
- Ovarian disorders.
- Pituitary disorders.
- Hypothalamic disorders.

### Causes of amenorrhoea

**Reproductive outflow tract disorders**
- Asherman's syndrome
- Müllerian agenesis
- Transverse vaginal septum
- Imperforate hymen
- Testicular feminization syndrome

**Ovarian disorders**
- Anovulation, e.g. polycystic ovarian syndrome (PCOS)
- Gonadal dysgenesis, e.g. Turner's syndrome
- Premature ovarian failure
- Resistant ovary syndrome

**Pituitary disorders**
- Adenomas such as prolactinoma
- Pituitary necrosis, e.g. Sheehan's syndrome

**Hypothalamic malfunctions**
- Resulting from excessive exercise
- Resulting from weight loss/anorexia nervosa
- Resulting from stress
- Craniopharyngioma
- Kallman's syndrome

The more common examples of these conditions are described in the following section.

### Aetiology

#### Reproductive outflow tract abnormalities

These may result from abnormal sexual development, as described in Chapter 3. An alternative diagnosis is Asherman's syndrome. This refers to the presence of intrauterine adhesions, which prevent endometrial proliferation (and thus menstruation). The commonest cause of Asherman's syndrome in developed countries is over-vigorous uterine curettage (e.g. at uterine evacuation). Tuberculosis of the uterus has similar signs and symptoms, and should be considered in the differential diagnosis in areas where the infection is endemic.

#### Ovarian disorders

Ovarian failure is the term used to describe the condition in which the stock of functional primordial follicles is exhausted and normal follicular development (as described in Chapter 4) fails to occur despite the pituitary producing increasing amounts of gonadotrophins (luteinizing hormone [LH] and follicle-stimulating hormone [FSH]). Obviously in normal women ovarian failure occurs at the menopause (at a mean age of 51 years). In some women, however, it may happen early (premature ovarian failure), possibly as a result of chemotherapy or radiotherapy, or in association with autoimmune disease.

It has recently become clear that some women present with symptoms, signs and blood results identical to those of ovarian failure but that they do in fact have viable follicles in the ovary. These follicles are unresponsive to elevated gonadotrophin levels, giving rise to the term resistant ovary syndrome. Women with the resistant ovary syndrome may occasionally ovulate and conceive. It is not normally possible to differentiate between the resistant ovary syndrome and ovarian failure without performing a full-thickness ovarian biopsy. Since this biopsy might itself remove any remaining viable follicles, it is not normally indicated.

The last relatively common diagnosis in women with ovarian failure is that of gonadal dysgenesis (see Chapter 3). In this condition, ovarian development is rudimentary. The stock of primordial follicles is either exhausted in early childhood, leading to lack of ovarian oestrogen production and failure of development of the secondary sexual characteristics, or exhausted in early adulthood, leading to premature ovarian failure. One of the commonest chromosomal disorders seen in association with gonadal dysgenesis is Turner's syndrome (XO chromosomal complement).

The other common ovarian disorder leading to anovulation and amenorrhoea is PCOS (see below).

## Pituitary disorders

The commonest form of pituitary disease seen in association with amenorrhoea is a pituitary adenoma. The commonest of these, the prolactinoma, secretes prolactin. This causes the symptom of galactorrhoea and inhibits gonadotrophin activity, leading to oligomenorrhoea or amenorrhoea. Prolactinomas normally respond very well to treatment with bromocriptine or to newer drugs such as cabergoline. Large prolactinomas may press on the optic chiasm, causing the classic sign of bitemporal hemianopia.

Women with significantly elevated prolactin levels (>1000 pmol/L) should therefore be further investigated with computerized tomography (CT) scanning or magnetic resonance imaging (MRI) to visualize the pituitary.

Prolactin levels may alternatively be elevated as a side effect of some drug treatments (e.g. phenothiazines), and thus is it worth reviewing the drug history in any patient with hyperprolactinaemia.

## Hypothalamic disorders

Excessive weight loss (to 15–20 per cent below ideal body weight) and/or excessive exercise can lead to amenorrhoea by switching off hypothalamic stimulation of the pituitary (hypogondotrophic hypogonadism). Such women will have low (or normal) gonadotrophin levels. Presumably this is a protective mechanism by which the body avoids pregnancy in what it perceives to be an unsuitable environment. Stress may also induce amenorrhoea via this mechanism.

## Clinical features of oligomenorrhoea/amenorrhoea

A detailed history may help determine a correct diagnosis in a patient with amenorrhoea. Pregnancy should be excluded as early as possible. Although clearly primary and secondary amenorrhoea may have mutually exclusive causes, in practice it is best to keep an open mind at the outset and consider possible causes of both in any woman presenting with amenorrhoea. A comprehensive history will include:
- developmental history,
- age of onset of menarche,
- presence or absence of cyclical symptoms,
- history of chronic illness,
- excessive weight loss/presence of an eating disorder,
- excessive exercise,
- history or family history of anosmia,
- menstrual/contraceptive and reproductive history,
- past medical and surgical histories,
- presence of menopausal symptoms,
- current medications,
- family history of premature menopause,

- development of any virilizing signs or galactorrhoea (milk discharge from breasts),
- psychological history,
- recent stressful events (past or present history of depression or an eating disorder).

## Clinical examination

In addition to a general examination, particular emphasis should be placed on the following areas of clinical examination.

- Height: an abnormality in appropriate height for age may reflect an underlying chromosomal disorder (patients with Turner's syndrome are often short, whereas patients with androgen insensitivity are often tall).
- Development of secondary sexual characteristics or any evidence of abnormal virilization.
- Visual field disturbance or papilloedema may imply a pituitary lesion.
- Pelvic examination may detect a structural outflow abnormality. Also look for evidence of atrophic effects of hypo-oestrogenism within the lower genital tract. (In women who have never been sexually active, it may be appropriate to defer pelvic examination until initial investigations have been carried out.)

## Investigations

Since there are many causes of amenorrhoea, it is inappropriate to focus on a specific diagnosis at the outset. The following scheme of investigation will allow the physician to exclude or confirm the cause to be one of the four categories described above. Thereafter, more detailed investigation (and/or referral to a sub-specialist in this area) will enable the precise cause to be determined.

## Step 1

*Initial hormone tests*
- Pregnancy test
- Prolactin
- Thyroid function
- LH and FSH
- Testosterone

*Progesterone withdrawal test*

This involves giving a progesterone (such as medroxyprogesterone acetate 10 mg) for 5 days, and then stopping. If the outflow tract (uterus and vagina) is normal, and there is sufficient endogenous oestrogen to induce endometrial proliferation, progesterone will decidualize the endometrium. On withdrawing the progesterone, the decidualized endometrium will break down, and menstruation will ensue.

- Abnormal prolactin or thyroid function will suggest a possible diagnosis of a prolactinoma or thyroid disease.
- Testosterone levels >5 nmol/L should prompt a search for a testosterone-secreting tumour.
- If the hormone levels are normal and the patient fails to menstruate in response to progesterone, the possible options are either that there is an outflow tract disorder or that endogenous oestrogen levels are low.
- If the hormone tests are normal (or show mildly elevated testosterone), and there is a positive progesterone withdrawal test, the likely diagnosis is anovulation, often secondary to PCOS. Further investigation is not necessary.

## Step 2

If the patient does not bleed in response to progesterone, she should be given orally active oestrogen (e.g. oestradiol 2 mg) for 21 days, followed by progesterone as above.

- If the patient still fails to bleed in response to this treatment, the diagnosis is one of an outflow tract abnormality.
- If bleeding does occur in response to sequential oestrogen and progesterone, this indicates the problem is in the hypothalamo–pituitary–ovarian axis.

## Step 3

Having excluded an outflow tract disorder, measurement of the LH and FSH levels should be repeated. Ideally, this should be done 6 weeks after the initial tests were performed, and 2 weeks after administration of either oestrogen or progesterone. Elevated LH and FSH levels (>40 IU/L and 30 IU/L, respectively) on two or more occasions at least 6 weeks apart and in the absence of menstruation suggest ovarian failure. If LH and FSH levels are not elevated, and the above scheme of investigation has been followed, the disorder can be reliably localized to the hypothalamus. This is commonly due to stress or weight loss (including weight loss due to anorexia nervosa), but may also be seen in severe systemic illness. Typically, the serum LH and FSH levels in these conditions will be <5 IU/L.

The above schedule of investigation should determine in which compartment the cause of the amenorrhoea lies. Depending on the result, further investigations may be appropriate (e.g. karyotyping may help in the diagnosis of Turner's syndrome).

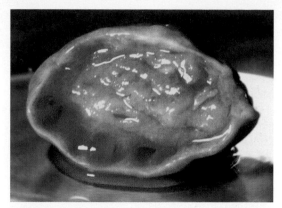

**Figure 5.3** Gross appearance of polycystic ovary. (Image courtesy of Dr Sladkevicius.)

## Treatment

The treatment of amenorrhoea depends somewhat on the cause. Some specific causes (e.g. prolactinoma) can be readily treated with appropriate therapy. In women in whom endogenous oestrogen levels are low (e.g. ovarian failure or hypogonadotrophic hypogonadism), oestrogen and progesterone replacement (e.g. in the form of HRT) can be given. Oestrogen replacement is important to prevent bone loss. If oestrogen and progesterone are given cyclically, normal menstrual rhythm will be restored. In young women, oestrogen replacement may be given in the form of the oral contraceptive pill. This has the added advantage of preventing pregnancy should spontaneous resolution of the cause of the amenorrhoea occur.

The treatment of anovulatory women with normal or high oestrogen levels is as described for PCOS below.

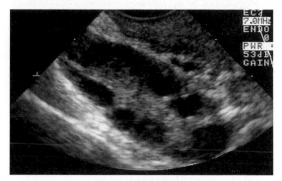

**Figure 5.4** Ultrasound picture of polycystic ovary. (Image courtesy of Dr Sladkevicius.)

ovary) is sufficient for clinical diagnosis. Its clinical manifestations may include menstrual irregularities, signs of androgen excess and obesity. Insulin resistance and elevated serum LH levels are also common features in PCOS. PCOS is associated with an increased risk of type 2 diabetes and cardiovascular events.

## POLYCYSTIC OVARIAN SYNDROME

## Prevalence

Polycystic ovarian syndrome affects around 5–10 per cent of women of reproductive age. The prevalence of polycystic ovaries seen on ultrasound is much higher – around 25 per cent (Fig. 5.4).

## Definition

The best current definition of PCOS is that generated at the 2003 Rotterdam ESHRE/ASRM-Sponsored PCOS Consensus Workshop on PCOS, which concluded that PCOS is a syndrome of ovarian dysfunction along with the cardinal features of hyperandrogenism and polycystic ovary morphology (Fig. 5.3). PCOS remains a syndrome, and as such no single diagnostic criterion (such as hyperandrogenism or polycystic

## Aetiology

The aetiology of PCOS remains unclear. Women with this syndrome have increased ovarian androgen production, due partly to disordered ovarian cytochrome P450 activity and partly to increased LH stimulation. Additionally, increasing evidence suggests a role for (peripheral) insulin resistance in the pathophysiology of PCOS, with the resulting hyperinsulinaemia also promoting ovarian androgen production.

Polycystic ovarian syndrome appears to cluster in families, and it seems likely that there is a gene or collection of genes that are important in its development. Work is ongoing to identify these genes.

## Clinical features

The clinical features of PCOS are as follows.
- Oligomenorrhoea/amenorrhoea: this occurs in up to 65–75 per cent of patients with PCOS and is predominantly related to chronic anovulation.
- Hirsutism: this occurs in 30–70 per cent of women.
- Subfertility: up to 75 per cent of women with PCOS who try to conceive have difficulty doing so.
- Obesity: at least 40 per cent of patients with PCOS are clinically obese.
- Recurrent miscarriage: PCOS is seen in around 50–60 per cent of women with more than three early pregnancy losses.
- Acanthosis nigricans: areas of increased skin pigmentation that are velvety in texture and occur in the axillae and other flexures occur in around 2 per cent of women with PCOS.

## Diagnosis

No single test is diagnostic of PCOS. The definition above emphasizes the importance of considering other conditions before a diagnosis of PCOS can be confidently made, and it is often a diagnosis of exclusion. In women with PCOS symptoms, and in whom the other conditions described above have been excluded, the following findings on investigation are supportive of a diagnosis of PCOS.

### Laboratory tests

- Elevated testosterone levels.
- Decreased sex hormone binding globulin (SHBG) levels.
- Elevated LH levels.
- Elevated LH:FSH ratio.
- Increased fasting insulin levels.

It is important to note that total testosterone levels may be only marginally elevated (or even normal) in women with PCOS. Free testosterone is higher than normal, since SHBG levels are low. Testosterone levels of >5 nmol/L should prompt a search for an androgen-secreting tumour.

### Ultrasound

The ultrasound criteria for the diagnosis of a polycystic ovary are eight or more subcapsular follicular cysts ≤10 mm in diameter and increased ovarian stroma. Whilst these findings support a diagnosis of PCOS, they are not by themselves sufficient to identify the syndrome.

## Treatment

There is no treatment for PCOS as such. Treatment should be directed at the symptoms that the patient complains of, as follows.

### Oligomenorrhoea/amenorrhoea

Women with PCOS tend to be anovulatory, but to have normal or high oestrogen levels. Without treatment, there is a theoretical risk that unopposed oestrogenic stimulation of the endometrium may increase the risk of endometrial cancer. Additionally, oligomenorrhoeic women with PCOS tend to have infrequent but heavy bleeds, as the endometrium that develops under the influence of oestrogen eventually becomes unsustainable and sheds. For these reasons, cyclical progesterone is often useful in the treatment of women with PCOS, in order to induce regular menstruation and to protect the endometrium. Oral progesterone should be given for at least 10 days in each month (e.g. medroxyprogesterone acetate 10 mg daily for 10 days). The woman will normally bleed a few days after progesterone treatment stops. The bleeding should be similar in amount to that of a normal period.

An alternative treatment for women who do not wish to conceive is the oral contraceptive pill.

Since PCOS is driven in part by insulin resistance, it is not surprising that metformin, a drug that increases insulin sensitivity, is partially effective in its treatment. Unfortunately, many of the studies using metformin have been uncontrolled. In controlled studies, metformin has been shown to increase ovulation rates (and therefore frequency of menses) by around once every 5 months.

## Hirsutism

Hirsutism arises from the growth-promoting effects of androgen at the hair follicle. Some of these growth-promoting effects are irreversible, even when androgen levels fall. Thus treatments aimed at reducing testosterone levels will not restore the hair to its pre-PCOS pattern. However, lowering free androgen levels will slow the rate of hair growth, which most patients see as a benefit. The possible treatment options include the following.

- Eflornithine cream, applied topically.
- Cyproterone acetate: an anti-androgen that competitively inhibits the androgen receptor. It may be given either as a low dose (in the form of the contraceptive pill Dianette™, which consists of cyproterone acetate 2 mg and 35 mcg of ethinylestradiol), or at a higher dose of 50–100 mg daily. If the higher dose is chosen, it is usual to give it for the first 10 days of each month, initially in combination with oestrogen, and then followed by oestrogen alone for a further 11 days – the 'reverse sequential regimen'. A low-dose oral contraceptive may be given as an alternative to oestrogen in this regimen.
- Metformin: a recent study showed metformin and Dianette™ to have similar efficacies on both subjective and objective measures of hirsutism in women with PCOS.
- GnRH analogues with low-dose HRT: this regime should be reserved for women intolerant to other therapies, or for short-term treatment, since bone loss is an inevitable side effect.
- Surgical treatments aimed at destroying the hair follicle, such as laser or electrolysis: surgical treatments are effective permanent methods of hair removal. They are not, however, widely available within the National Health Service (NHS), and some, such as electrolysis, are associated with side effects such as scarring.

## Subfertility

The anovulation often seen in association with PCOS may respond to treatment either with clomiphene or (if this is unsuccessful) with gonadotrophin therapy (see Chapter 7). Again, there is some evidence that metformin may increase ovulation rates, either alone or when used in combination with clomiphene, but more evidence is needed.

## Obesity

Obesity is common in women with PCOS. Weight reduction is notoriously difficult to achieve, even with pharmacological support. There is some evidence that the metabolism of women with PCOS does appear to be different, so that women with PCOS do find it more difficult to lose weight than others. The usual array of dietary modifications (with or without drugs such as orlistat) may be considered. Additionally, there is some evidence that metformin may be associated with a small reduction in body mass index (BMI) in women with PCOS.

## Long-term sequleae

Emerging evidence suggests that women with PCOS are at increased risk of developing diabetes and cardiovascular disease later in life. However, at present there is no evidence that they would benefit from any pharmacological intervention prior to the development of established disease. Clearly, however, lifestyle advice (such as dietary modification and increasing exercise) is appropriate.

## POSTMENOPAUSAL BLEEDING

### Definition

Postmenopausal bleeding (PMB) is defined as vaginal bleeding after the menopause. In women who are not taking HRT, any bleeding is abnormal. In women on combined cyclical HRT, bleeding in the progesterone-free period is normal. Unscheduled bleeding refers to bleeding at other times, and this is abnormal and should be investigated.

## Aetiology

The majority of women with PMB will be found to have atrophic vaginitis, whereby the vaginal epithelium thins and breaks down in response to low oestrogen levels. This is a benign condition, which is relatively easily treated with topical oestrogens. However, around 10 per cent of women with PMB will be found to have endometrial cancer, the risk of which is greater for those who are not currently taking HRT, and progressively increases with increasing age.

## Clinical features

In postmenopausal women who are not taking HRT, any bleeding is abnormal. In women taking HRT, bleeding should be regarded as abnormal if it is unscheduled in timing or abnormal in amount.

## Differential diagnosis

The differential diagnosis in women with PMB includes:
- endometrial carcinoma
- endometrial hyperplasia
- endometrial polyps
- cervical malignancy
- atrophic vaginitis.

## Investigations

A full history should be taken for women with PMB and they should undergo a pelvic examination and cervical smear. Thereafter, an ultrasound scan may be used to determine which women require further investigation and which do not. Women with an endometrial thickness of 3 mm or less on ultrasound (or 5 mm or less for women on HRT) can be reassured that the likelihood of endometrial carcinoma is extremely low. For those with an endometrial thickness greater than 3 mm (5 mm for those on HRT), further endometrial assessment is warranted. This is usually endometrial biopsy, with or without hysteroscopy,

which can be done under local anaesthetic in most patients.

## Treatment

The treatment of PMB depends on the cause. If investigation reveals no underlying pathology, hypo-oestrogenic atrophic changes are the most likely cause, and can be treated with systemic or local hormonal replacement.

## PREMENSTRUAL SYNDROME

## Definition

Premenstrual syndrome (PMS) is the occurrence of cyclical somatic, psychological and emotional symptoms that occur in the luteal (premenstrual) phase of the menstrual cycle and resolve by the time menstruation ceases.

## Prevalence

Premenstrual symptoms occur in almost all women of reproductive age, but in only about 5 per cent are they sufficiently severe to cause significant problems.

## Aetiology

The aetiology of PMS is unknown, although it clearly arises from variations in sex steroid levels, and low serotonin levels may also play a role.

## Clinical features

The symptoms of PMS may include any of the following:
- bloating
- cyclical weight gain
- mastalgia
- abdominal cramps
- fatigue
- headache

- depresssion
- irritability.

## Differential diagnosis

Premenstrual syndrome should be distinguished from any underlying psychiatric disorders. The cyclical nature of PMS is the cornerstone of the diagnosis. A symptom chart, to be filled in by the patient prospectively, may help in this regard.

## Treatment

The following therapies have been shown to have some efficacy in the treatment of PMS.
- Selective serotonin reuptake inhibitors (SSRIs) such as fluoxetine significantly improve PMS, although patients should be warned about the adverse effects associated with them.

- Diuretics are helpful for the treatment of bloating and breast tenderness.
- NSAIDs may be effective in the treatment of physical symptoms.

### Key Points

- Most women with menorrhagia do not have an organic cause for their condition.
- Measurement of menstrual loss in menorrhagia is not normally helpful.
- The LNG-IUS is highly effective in the treatment of menorrhagia and should be considered before surgical therapies are undertaken.
- Careful investigation of oligomenorrhoea/amenorrhoea should reveal the likely cause.
- Insulin-sensitizing agents are increasingly used for the treatment of PCOS symptoms, and may be effective in inducing ovulation and reducing hirsutism.
- A complaint of unscheduled postmenopausal bleeding should always be investigated.

## C A S E   H I S T O R Y

Ms S, a 20-year-old nursing student, presents with a 5-year history of irregular periods and worsening facial hair.

Her menarche occurred at the age of 14 years and her cycle has always been irregular, usually with only three to four periods per year. She is not currently using any contraception.

Her mother had a hysterectomy at the age of 39 years for 'heavy periods'; her father has non-insulin-dependent diabetes. There is no other history of note.

Clinical examination reveals a BMI of 36, blood pressure of 110/65 mmHg, a moderate degree of facial hirsutism and prominent facial acne. Abdominal and pelvic examinations were normal.

### What is the most likely diagnosis?
Given the history of irregular menstrual periods and the presence of hyperandrogenic symptoms (hirsutism and acne), the most likely diagnosis would be PCOS.

### What investigations would help confirm the diagnosis?
- Serum androgen levels (which may be marginally elevated) and SHBG (which may be reduced).
- A blood test for gonadotrophins (which may show an elevated LH:FSH ratio).

- Transvaginal ultrasound may demonstrate the classical appearances of polycystic ovaries, i.e. multiple peripheral ovarian cysts and increased ovarian stromal volume.

### What treatment options should be discussed with the patient?
The patient should be encouraged to lose weight, as her symptoms may improve with weight loss alone.

Her menstrual irregularity may be controlled with either cyclic progestogens or the combined oral contraceptive pill. The use of a contraceptive pill containing cyproterone actetate may help control the hyperandrogenic features of hirsutism and acne. She should be advised that an improvement in hirsutism might not be seen for several months.

Metformin may be considered as a second-line treatment.

### What other health issues should be discussed with the patient?
The patient should be counselled regarding the long-term health implications of PCOS: she should be informed of her increased risk of diabetes and coronary heart disease. In addition, the long-term effects of chronic anovulation on the endometrium and fertility issues (see Chapter 7) also need to be discussed.

## Additional reading

Duckitt K. Menorrhagia. In: *Clinical evidence*. London: BMJ Publishing Group. <www.clinicalevidence.com>.

Farquhar C, Proctor M. Dysmenorrhoea (search date October 2001) *Clinical evidence*. London: BMJ Publishing Group, 2002. <www.clinicalevidence.com>.

*Investigation of post menopausal bleeding*. Guideline No. 61. Edinburgh: Scottish Intercollegiate Guideline Network, 2002. <www.sign.ac.uk>.

Revised 2003 consensus on diagnostic criteria and long-term health risks related to polycystic ovary syndrome. *Fertil steril* 2004; **81**: 19–25.

RCOG Guidelines. *Initial management of menorrhagia* (1998) and *The management of menorrhagia in secondary care* (1999). National Evidence Based Clinical Guidelines. London: Royal College of Obstetricians and Gynaecologists. <www.rcog.org.uk>.

Wyatt K. Premenstrual syndrome (search date February 2002). *Clinical evidence*. London: BMJ Publishing Group. <www.clinicalevidence.com>.

# Fertility control

## OVERVIEW

Most individuals at some time in their lives will use contraception. The worldwide trend towards delayed onset of childbearing and smaller families means that many women will need to use contraception for up to 30 years. Women will use different methods at different stages of their lives, and when they no longer wish to conceive, a sterilization method may be appropriate. Even when contraception is widely available, unplanned pregnancies will occur, and some women may consider termination of pregnancy, either medical or surgical.

## CONTRACEPTION

Men and women have used contraception, in one form or another, for thousands of years. There is no one method that will suit everyone, and individuals will use different types of contraception at different stages in their lives. The characteristics of the ideal contraceptive method are:

- highly effective
- no side effects
- cheap
- independent of intercourse
- rapidly reversible
- widespread availability
- acceptable to all cultures and religions
- easily distributed
- can be administered by non-healthcare personnel.

There is enormous variation in the uptake and use of methods of contraception in different countries worldwide. More than 95 per cent of women in the UK who do not want to become pregnant will use contraception; details of the methods currently available are given in Table 6.1. Some couples may use more than one method at the same time, such as taking the oral contraceptive pill in conjunction with using condoms. Some methods of contraception can only be prescribed by a doctor, whereas others can be used without ever having to seek medical advice.

Virtually all methods of contraception occasionally fail and some are much more effective than others. Failure rates are traditionally expressed as the number of failures per 100 woman-years (HWY), i.e. the number of pregnancies if 100 women were to use the method for 1 year. Failure rates for some methods vary considerably, largely because of the potential for failure caused by imperfect use (user failure) rather than an intrinsic

**Table 6.1**   Use of contraception in the UK

| Method of contraception | Use (%) |
| --- | --- |
| Combined oral contraceptive pill | 36 |
| Condoms | 20 |
| Diaphragms | 2 |
| Intrauterine devices (IUDs) | 6 |
| Natural family planning | 1.5 |
| Vasectomy | 16 |
| Female sterilization | 10 |

**Table 6.2**   Efficacy of methods of contraception

| Contraceptive method | Failure rate per 100 women-years |
| --- | --- |
| Combined oral contraceptive pill | 0.1–1 |
| Progestogen-only pill | 1–3 |
| Depo-Provera | 0.1–2 |
| Implanon | 0 |
| Copper-bearing IUD | 1–2 |
| Levonorgestrel-releasing IUD | 0.5 |
| Male condom | 2–5 |
| Female diaphragm | 1–15 |
| Persona | 6 |
| Natural family planning | 2–3 |
| Vasectomy | 0.02 |
| Female sterilization | 0.13 |

IUD, intrauterine device.

## Classification

**Hormonal contraception**
- Combined oral contraceptive pills
- Combined hormonal patches
- Progestogen-only preparations
  - Progestogen-only pills
  - Injectables
  - Subdermal implants

**Intrauterine contraception**
- Copper intrauterine device (IUD)
- Hormone-releasing intrauterine system (IUS)

**Barrier methods**
- Condoms
- Female barriers

**Coitus interruptus**

**Natural family planning**

**Emergency contraception**

**Sterilization**
- Female sterilization
- Vasectomy

failure of the method itself. The efficacy rates of the various contraceptive methods are listed in Table 6.2.

## Hormonal contraception

## Combined oral contraceptive pills

Combined oral contraception (COC) – 'the pill' – was first licensed in the UK in 1961. It contains a combination of two hormones: a synthetic oestrogen and a progestogen (a synthetic derivative of progesterone). Since COC was first introduced, the doses of both oestrogen and progestogen have been reduced dramatically, which has considerably improved its safety profile. It is estimated that at least 200 million women worldwide have taken COC since it was first marketed, and there are currently around 3 million users in the UK alone.

Combined oral contraception is easy to use and offers a very high degree of protection against pregnancy, with many other beneficial effects. It is mainly used by young, healthy women who wish a method of contraception that is independent of intercourse.

### Formulations

There are many different formulations and brands of COC (Fig. 6.1). Most modern preparations contain the oestrogen ethinyl oestradiol in a daily dose of between 20 and 35 µg. Those containing lower dosages are associated with slightly poorer cycle control. Those containing a higher daily dosages, e.g. 50 µg ethinyl oestradiol, are generally now only prescribed in special situations, discussed below. Higher dosages of oestrogen are strongly linked to increased risks of

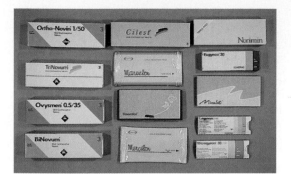

**Figure 6.1** Combined oral contraceptive pill preparations.

---

**Table 6.3** Hormonal content of commonly used monophasic combined oral contraceptive (COC) preparations

| Oestrogens | Progestogens |
|---|---|
| Ethinyloestradiol: 20, 30, 35 and 50 µg<br>Mestranol 50 µg | Second generation:<br>    norethisterone acetate 0.5, 1.0 and 1.5 mg<br>    levonorgestrel 0.15, 0.25 mg<br>Third generation:<br>    gestodene 0.075 mg<br>    desogestrel 0.15 mg<br>    norgestimate 0.25 mg<br>Anti-mineralocorticoid and anti-androgenic:<br>    drospirenone 3 mg |

both arterial and venous thrombosis (see below). Most COC contains progestogens that are classed as second or third generation. Commonly prescribed formulations are listed in Table 6.3.

Monophasic pills contain standard daily dosages of oestrogen and progestogen. Biphasic or triphasic preparations have two or three incremental variations in hormone dose. Current thinking is that biphasic and triphasic preparations are more complicated for women to use and have few real advantages.

Most brands contain 21 pills; one pill to be taken daily, followed by a 7-day pill-free interval. There are also some every-day (ED) preparations that include seven placebo pills that are taken instead of having a pill-free interval. For maximum effectiveness, COC should always be taken regularly at roughly the same time each day.

## Mode of action
Combined oral contraception acts both centrally and peripherally.
- Inhibition of ovulation is by far the most important effect. Both oestrogen and progestogen suppress the release of pituitary follicle-stimulating hormone (FSH) and luteinizing hormone (LH), which prevents follicular development within the ovary and therefore ovulation.
- Peripheral effects include making the endometrium atrophic and hostile to an implanting embryo and altering cervical mucus to prevent sperm ascending into the uterine cavity.

## Contraindications and complications
There are very lengthy lists of both absolute and relative contraindications to COC (the most important are summarized in the box below). Most of these can be worked out quite logically and are mainly related to the side effects of sex steroid hormones on the cardiovascular and hepatic systems. Women should ideally discontinue COC at least 2 months before any elective pelvic or leg surgery.

### Contraindications to COC

**Absolute contraindications**
- Circulatory diseases:
  - ischaemic heart disease
  - cerebrovascular accident
  - significant hypertension
  - arterial or venous thrombosis
  - any acquired or inherited pro-thrombotic tendency
  - any significant risk factors for cardiovascular disease
- Acute or severe liver disease
- Oestrogen-dependent neoplasms, particularly breast cancer
- Focal migraine

**Relative contraindications**
- Generalized migraine
- Long-term immobilization
- Irregular vaginal bleeding (until a diagnosis has been made)
- Less severe risk factors for cardiovascular disease, e.g. obesity, heavy smoking, diabetes

## Side effects

The vast majority of women tolerate COC well, with few problems. However, a large number of potential side effects exists, the most important relating to cardiovascular disease. Other side effects are listed in Table 6.4. Many minor side effects will settle within a few months of starting COC.

### Venous thromboembolism

Oestrogens alter blood clotting and coagulation in a way that induces a pro-thrombotic tendency, although the exact mechanism of this is poorly understood. The higher the dose of oestrogen within COC, the greater the risk of venous thromboembolism (VTE). Type of progestogen also affects the risk of VTE, with users of COC containing third-generation progestogens being twice as likely to sustain a VTE.

The risks of VTE are:

- 5 per 100 000 for normal population,
- 15 per 100 000 for users of second-generation COC,
- 30 per 100 000 for users of third-generation COC,
- 60 per 100 000 for pregnant women.

**Table 6.4**  Other potential side effects of combined oral contraceptive (COC) preparations

| | |
|---|---|
| Central nervous system | Depression |
| | Headaches |
| | Loss of libido |
| Gastrointestinal | Nausea and vomiting |
| | Weight gain |
| | Bloatedness |
| | Gall-stones |
| | Cholestatic jaundice |
| Genitourinary system | Cystitis |
| | Irregular bleeding |
| | Vaginal discharge |
| | Growth of fibroids |
| Breast | Breast pain |
| | Increased risk of breast cancer |
| Miscellaneous | Chloasma (facial pigmentation) |
| | Leg cramps |

### Arterial disease

The risk of myocardial infarction and thrombotic stroke in young, healthy women using low-dose COC is extremely small. Cigarette smoking will, however, increase the risk, and any woman who smokes must be advised to stop COC at the age of 35 years. Around 1 per cent of women taking COC will become significantly hypertensive and they should be advised to stop taking COC.

### Breast cancer

Advising women about the association between breast cancer and COC is very difficult. Most data do show a slight increase in the risk of developing breast cancer among current COC users (relative risk around 1.24). This is not of great significance to young women, as the background rate of breast cancer is very low at their age. However, for a woman in her forties, these are more relevant data, as the background rate of breast cancer is higher. The same data also showed that beyond 10 years after stopping COC there was no increase in breast cancer risk for former COC users (Collaborative Group, 1996).

### Drug interaction

This can occur with enzyme-inducing agents such as some anti-epileptic drugs. Higher dose oestrogen pills containing 50 μg ethinyl oestradiol may need to be prescribed (see Table 6.3). Some broad-spectrum antibiotics can alter intestinal absorption of COC and reduce its efficacy. Additional contraceptive measures should therefore be recommended during antibiotic therapy and for 1 week thereafter.

## Positive health benefits

Not all side effects of COC are undesirable. COC users generally have light, pain-free, regular bleeds and therefore COC can be used to treat heavy or painful periods. It will also improve premenstrual syndrome (PMS) and reduce the risk of pelvic inflammatory disease (PID). COC offers long-term protection against both ovarian and endometrial cancers. It can also be used as a treatment for acne.

## Patient management

For a woman to take COC successfully, there must be careful teaching and explanation of the method, supplemented by information leaflets. Before COC is prescribed, a detailed past medical and family history should be taken and blood pressure checked (Fig. 6.2). Routine weighing, breast and pelvic examinations are not mandatory and should not be forced on young women requesting COC. Most women are given a 3-month supply of COC in the first instance, and 6-monthly reviews thereafter. Woman need clear advice about what to do if they miss taking their pills (Fig. 6.3).

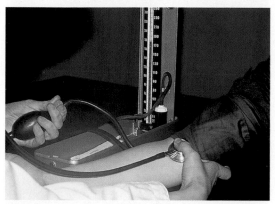

**Figure 6.2** Monitoring blood pressure in a woman taking the combined oral contraceptive pill.

## Combined hormonal patches

A contraceptive transdermal patch containing oestrogen and progestogen has been developed and releases norelgestromin 150 µg and ethinylestradiol 20 µg per 24 hours. Patches are applied weekly for 3 weeks, after which there is a patch-free week. Contraceptive patches have the same risks and benefits as COC and, although they are relatively more expensive, may have better compliance.

## Progestogen-only contraception

All other types of hormonal contraception in current use in the UK are progestogen-only and share many similar features in terms of mode of action and side effects. Because they do not contain oestrogen, they are extremely safe and can be used if a woman has

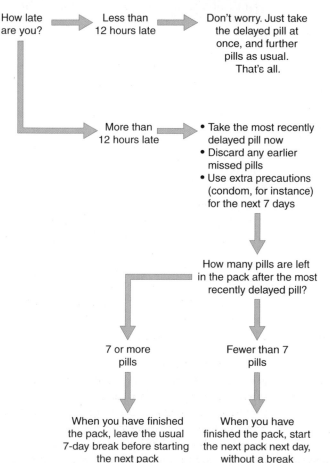

**Figure 6.3** Management of missed pills (algorithm). (Reprinted from *Handbook of family planning and reproductive health care*, 3rd edn, Loudon N, Glasier A, Gebbie A (eds), copyright 2000, with permission from Elsevier.)

How late are you? → Less than 12 hours late → Don't worry. Just take the delayed pill at once, and further pills as usual. That's all.

More than 12 hours late →
• Take the most recently delayed pill now
• Discard any earlier missed pills
• Use extra precautions (condom, for instance) for the next 7 days

How many pills are left in the pack after the most recently delayed pill?

7 or more pills

Fewer than 7 pills

When you have finished the pack, leave the usual 7-day break before starting the next pack

When you have finished the pack, start the next pack next day, without a break cardiovascular risk factors. The dose of progestogen within them varies from very low to high.

The current methods of progestogen-only contraception are:

- progestogen-only pill, or 'mini-pill'
- subdermal implant Implanon®
- injectables
- hormone-releasing intrauterine system (see 'Intrauterine contraception' below).

All progestogen-only methods work by a local effect on cervical mucus (making it hostile to ascending sperm) and on the endometrium (making it thin and atrophic), thereby preventing implantation and sperm transport. Higher dose progestogen-only methods will also act centrally and inhibit ovulation.

The common side effects of progestogen-only methods include:

- erratic or absent menstrual bleeding
- functional ovarian cysts
- breast tenderness
- acne.

### Progestogen-only pills

The progestogen-only pill (POP) is ideal for women who like the convenience of pill taking but cannot take COC. Although the failure rate of the POP is greater than that of COC (see Table 6.2), it is ideal for women at times of lower fertility. If the POP fails, there is a slightly higher risk of ectopic pregnancy. There is a small selection of brands on the market (Fig. 6.4) and they contain the second-generation progestogen norethisterone or norgestrel (or their derivatives) and the third-generation progestogen desogestrel. The POP is taken every day without a break.

Particular indications for the POP include:

- breastfeeding
- older age
- cardiovascular risk factors
- diabetes.

### Injectable progestogens

Two injectable progestogens are marketed.

- Depot medroxyprogesterone acetate 150 mg (Depo-Provera or DMPA).
- Norethisterone enanthate 200 mg (Noristerat).

Most women choose Depo-Provera and each injection lasts around 12–13 weeks. Norethisterone enanthate only lasts for 8 weeks and is not nearly so widely used.

Depo-Provera is a highly effective method of contraception and it is given by deep intramuscular

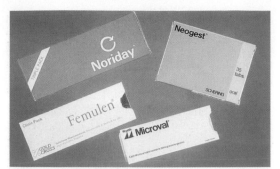

**Figure 6.4** Progestogen-only pill preparations.

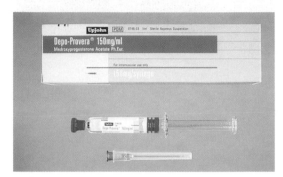

**Figure 6.5** Injection of Depo-Provera.

injection (Fig. 6.5). Most women who use it develop very light or absent menstruation. Depo-Provera will improve PMS and can be used to treat menstrual problems such as painful or heavy periods. It is particulary useful for women who have difficulty remembering to take a pill.

Particular side effects of Depo-Provera include:

- weight gain of around 3 kg in the first year,
- delay in return of fertility – it may take around 6 months longer to conceive compared to a woman who stops COC,
- persistent menstrual irregularity,
- very long-term use may slightly increase the risk of osteoporosis (because of low oestrogen levels).

### Subdermal implants

Implanon consists of a single silastic rod (Fig. 6.6) that is inserted subdermally under local anaesthetic into the upper arm. It releases the progestogen etonogestrel 25–70 µg daily (the dose released decreases with time), which is metabolized to the third-generation progestogen desogestrel. Implanon was introduced into the UK in the late 1990s and has superseded the six-rod implant Norplant, which was withdrawn from the market. It is highly effective and, to date, there have been no genuine failures reported with it.

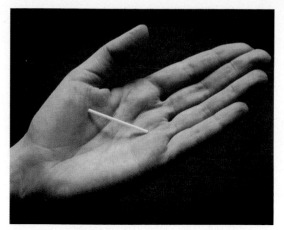

**Figure 6.6** Implanon.

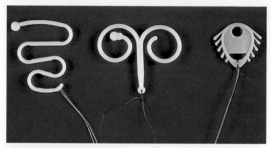

**Figure 6.7** Plastic intrauterine devices: Lippes Loop, Saf-T coil, Dalkon shield.

It lasts for 3 years and thereafter can be easily removed or a further implant inserted.

Implanon is particularly useful for women who have difficulty remembering to take a pill and who want highly effective long-term contraception. There is a rapid return of fertility when it is removed.

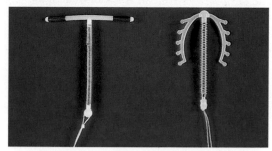

**Figure 6.8** Copper-bearing intrauterine devices: Multiload, Copper T 380.

## Intrauterine contraception

Modern IUDs are highly effective methods of contraception but are not widely used in the UK. Fitting of an IUD should be performed by trained healthcare personnel only and is a brief procedure associated with mild to moderate discomfort. A fine thread is left protruding from the cervix into the vagina and the IUD can be removed in due course by traction on this thread. An IUD is ideal for women who want a long-term method of contraception independent of intercourse and where regular compliance is not required. IUDs protect against both intrauterine and ectopic pregnancy, but if pregnancy occurs, there is a higher chance than normal that it will be ectopic.

## Types

The original IUDs were large plastic inert devices (Lippes Loop or Saf-T coil), which often caused significantly heavier and more painful menstrual periods (Fig. 6.7). These are no longer available, although some women may still have them in situ. Once fitted, they could be left until the menopause.

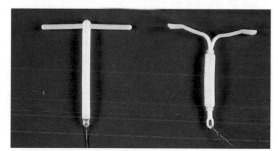

**Figure 6.9** Hormone-releasing intrauterine devices: progesterone-releasing IUD, levonorgestrel-releasing IUD.

Most women nowadays will use the smaller copper-bearing IUDs, which are available in various shapes and sizes (Fig. 6.8). They cause much less menstrual disruption than the older plastic devices. Most copper-bearing IUDs are licensed for between 3 and 5 years of use, but many will last longer, possibly up to 10 years. The more copper wire a device has, the more effective it is, and some IUDs have silver-cored copper for added efficacy. An IUD without a frame which consists of six copper beads on a prolene thread has been developed and is anchored into the uterine fundus with a knot (GyneFix).

Hormone-releasing devices have also been developed (Fig. 6.9). The levonorgestrel-releasing intrauterine

**Table 6.5** Levonorgestrel-releasing intrauterine system

| Advantages | Disadvantages |
| --- | --- |
| Highly effective | Persistent spotting and irregular bleeding in first few months of use |
| Dramatic reduction in menstrual blood loss | Progestogenic side effects, e.g. acne, breast tenderness |
| Protection against pelvic inflammatory disease | |

system (IUS) has the advantages (and disadvantages) of both hormonal and intrauterine contraception (Table 6.5). It is associated with a dramatic reduction in menstrual blood loss and is licensed for contraception and the treatment of menorrhagia.

## Mode of action

All IUDs induce an inflammatory response in the endometrium which prevents implantation. However, copper-bearing IUDs work primarily by a toxic effect on sperm which prevents fertilization. The IUS prevents pregnancy primarily by a local hormonal effect on the cervical mucus and endometrium.

## Contraindications

- Previous PID.
- Previous ectopic pregnancy.
- Known malformation of the uterus.
- Copper allergy (but could use an IUS).

## Side effects of copper-bearing IUDs

- Increased menstrual blood loss.
- Increased dysmenorrhoea.
- Increased risk of pelvic infection in the first few weeks following insertion.

## Pelvic infection and IUDs

Although IUDs increase the risk of PID in the first few weeks after insertion, the long-term risk is similar to that of women who are not using any method of contraception. In a mutually monogamous relationship, an IUD user has no increased risk of PID. If an IUD user has a partner with a sexually transmitted infection such as *Chlamydia* or gonorrhoea, the IUD will not protect against these infections, in contrast to condoms or the use of a hormonal method of contraception, which do.

## Barrier methods of contraception

### Condoms

Male condoms are usually made of latex rubber. They are cheap and are widely available for purchase or free from many clinics. They have been heavily promoted in the Safe Sex campaign to prevent the spread of sexually transmitted diseases (STDs), particularly human immunodeficiency virus (HIV) and acquired immunodeficiency syndrome (AIDS). Condoms of varying sizes and shapes are available. It is important to use condoms that reach European Union standards and are within their sell-by date. Couples using condoms should be aware of the availability of emergency contraception in the event of a condom bursting or slipping off during intercourse. Some men and women may be allergic to latex condoms or spermicide, and hypoallergenic latex condoms and plastic male condoms are available. Men must be instructed to apply condoms before any genital contact and to withdraw the erect penis from the vagina immediately after ejaculation.

### Female barriers

The diaphragm, or Dutch cap, is the female barrier used most commonly in the UK (Fig. 6.10). Other female barriers include cervical caps, vault caps and vimules. They should all be used in conjunction with a spermicidal cream or gel. Diaphragms are inserted

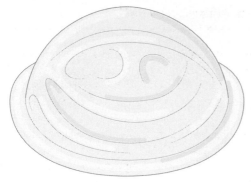

**Figure 6.10** Diaphragm.

immediately prior to intercourse and should be removed no earlier than 6 hours later. The effective use of a diaphragm requires careful teaching and fitting. Female barriers offer protection against ascending pelvic infection but can increase the risk of urinary tract infection and vaginal irritation.

Female condoms made of plastic are also available (Femidom). They offer particularly good protection against infection, as they cover the whole of the vagina and vulva and, being plastic, are less likely to burst. However, many couples find them unaesthetic and they have not achieved widespread popularity.

Although a range of spermicidal agents used to be manufactured, only gels and pessaries are still available in the UK. Spermicidal agents should not be used as a contraceptive method on their own: their main role is to make barrier methods more effective.

## Coitus interruptus

Coitus interruptus, or withdrawal, is widely practised and obviously does not require any medical supervision. It involves removal of the penis from the vagina immediately before ejaculation takes place. Unfortunately, it is not reliable, as pre-ejaculatory secretions may contain millions of sperm and young men often find it hard to judge the timing of withdrawal. The use of emergency contraception should be considered if coitus interruptus has taken place (see below).

## Natural family planning

This is an extremely important method of contraception worldwide and may be the only one acceptable to some couples for cultural and religious reasons. It involves abstaining from intercourse during the fertile period of the month.

The fertile period is calculated by various techniques such as:
- changes in basal body temperature,
- changes in cervical mucus,
- changes in the cervix,
- multiple indices.

Some commercially available kits are available, such as Persona, and use complex technology to define fertile periods when abstinence is required. The failure rates of natural methods of family planning are quite high, largely because couples find it difficult to abstain from intercourse when required.

The lactational amenorrhoea method (LAM) is used by fully breastfeeding mothers. During the first 6 months of infant life, full breastfeeding gives more than 98 per cent contraceptive protection.

## Emergency contraception

The terms 'morning-after pill' and 'postcoital contraception' have now been replaced simply by the term 'emergency contraception' (EC). EC is a method that is used after intercourse has taken place and before implantation has occurred. There is considerable interest in increasing the provision and uptake of EC, particularly in young women, as it is thought to have significant potential to reduce the rate of unplanned pregnancies. EC should be considered if unprotected intercourse has occurred, if there has been failure of a barrier method, e.g. a burst condom, or if COC has been forgotten. There are two types of EC in general use.

### Hormonal emergency contraception

Levonorgestrel, in a single dose of 1.5 mg (Levonelle), has become the main hormonal method of EC in the UK. It has to be taken within 72 hours of an episode of unprotected intercourse and is more effective the earlier it is taken. There are no real contraindications to its use. The original hormonal EC was a combination of oestrogen and progestogen, but nausea and vomiting were common side effects. Hormonal EC is not 100 per cent effective but will prevent around three-quarters of pregnancies that would otherwise have occurred. It is available on prescription from a doctor or over the counter in pharmacies, although it is relatively expensive to purchase. It can be used on more than one occasion in a short space of time, but women should consider other more effective methods if they are using EC repeatedly. The precise mechanism of action is not known but probably involves disruption of ovulation or corpus luteal function, depending on the time in the cycle when hormonal EC is taken.

## An IUD for emergency contraception

A copper-bearing IUD can be inserted for EC. It is effective for up to 5 days following the anticipated day of ovulation and can be used to cover multiple episodes of intercourse in the same menstrual cycle. The IUD prevents implantation and the copper ions exert an embryo-toxic effect. The normal contraindications to an IUD apply and, if there is a risk of sexually transmitted infection, antibiotic cover should be given. The hormone-releasing IUS has not been shown to be effective for EC and should not be used in this situation.

## Sterilization

Female sterilization and male vasectomy are permanent methods of contraception and are highly effective. They are generally chosen by relatively older couples who are sure that they have completed their families. Occasionally, however, individuals who have no children or who, for example, carry a genetic disorder may choose to be sterilized. The uptake of female sterilization and vasectomy in the UK is relatively high compared to many other European countries, with around 50 per cent of couples over the age of 40 years relying on one or other permanent method. Both female sterilization and vasectomy can be reversed, with subsequent pregnancy rates of about 25 per cent, but reversals are not available on the National Health Service (NHS) in many parts of the UK.

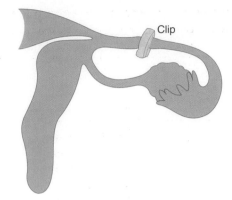

**Figure 6.11** Female sterilization.

## Consent

It is of vital importance that individuals are very carefully counselled (ideally with their partner) before sterilization and give written consent to having the procedure performed. Nowadays, consent forms do not ask for the partner's written consent. The consent form should clearly indicate that it is a permanent procedure but also acknowledge that occasionally it can fail. The failure of sterilization and vasectomy is a major area of medical litigation.

## Female sterilization

This involves the mechanical blockage of both Fallopian tubes to prevent sperm reaching and fertilizing the oocyte (Fig. 6.11). It can also be achieved by hysterectomy or total removal of both Fallopian tubes. Female sterilization should not alter the subsequent menstrual pattern per se, but if a woman stops the combined pill to be sterilized, she may find that her subsequent menstrual periods are heavier. Alternatively, if she has an IUD removed at the time of sterilization, she may find her subsequent menstrual periods are lighter.

Sterilization in the UK is most commonly performed by laparoscopy under general anaesthesia, which enables women to be admitted to hospital as a day case. Alternative techniques are mini-laparotomy with a small transverse suprapubic incision or through the posterior vaginal fornix (colpotomy). Mini-laparotomy is the technique of choice when the procedure is done postnatally (the uterus is enlarged and more

**Table 6.6** Techniques of female sterilization and their special features

| Technique of tubal occlusion | Special features |
| --- | --- |
| Ligation | Suitable for postpartum mini-laparotomy<br>Has a relatively higher failure rate |
| Electrocautery/ diathermy | May damage surrounding structures, e.g. bowel and bladder<br>Relatively higher late failure rate |
| Fallope rings | Easy to apply<br>Damages 2–3 cm of tube, thereby making subsequent reversal more difficult |
| Clips | Technique of choice<br>Simple to use<br>Occasionally may not occlude whole of Fallopian tube |
| Laser | Not widely used<br>Very expensive technique |

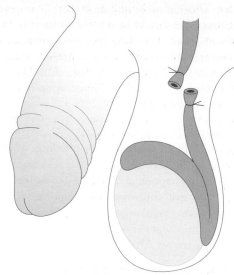

**Figure 6.12** Vasectomy.

**Table 6.7** Techniques of vasectomy and their special features

| Techniques of vasectomy | Special features |
| --- | --- |
| Ligation or clips<br>Unipolar diathermy | Most common techniques |
| Excision | Allows histological confirmation |
| No-scalpel vasectomy | Widely used in China<br>Special instruments used that puncture the skin<br>Low incidence of complications |
| Silicone plugs/sclerosing agents | Also used in China<br>Avoids a skin incision |

vascular) and in developing countries where laparoscopic equipment is not available. Different ways of occluding the Fallopian tubes are described in Table 6.6.

### Complications of female sterilization

Very occasionally, a woman may experience anaesthetic problems or there may be damage to intra-abdominal organs during the procedure. Sometimes it is not possible to visualize the pelvic organs at laparscopy due to adhesions or obesity; it may then be necessary to proceed to mini-laparotomy.

Female sterilization is highly effective. Ectopic pregnancy can be a late complication and any sterilized woman who misses her period and has symptoms of pregnancy should seek immediate medical advice.

## Vasectomy

Vasectomy involves the division of the vas deferens on each side to prevent the release of sperm during ejaculation (Fig. 6.12). It is technically an easier, more straightforward and quicker procedure than female sterilization and is usually performed under local anaesthesia. Various techniques exist to block the vas, and their effectiveness is related primarily to the skill and experience of the operator (Table 6.7).

Vasectomy differs from female sterilization in that it is not effective immediately. Sperm will still be present higher in the genital tract and azoospermia is therefore achieved more quickly if there is frequent intercourse. Men should be advised to hand in two samples of semen at 12 and 16 weeks to see if any sperm are still present. If two consecutive samples are free of sperm, the vasectomy can be considered complete. An alternative form of contraception must be used until that time.

### Complications

Immediate complications such as bleeding, wound infection and haematoma may occur. Occasionally, small lumps may appear at the cut end of the vas as a result of a local inflammatory response. These so-called 'sperm granulomas' may need surgical excision. Some men will develop anti-sperm antibodies following vasectomy. These do not cause symptoms, but if the vasectomy is reversed, pregnancy may not occur because the autoantibodies inactivate sperm.

Concerns have been raised for many years about a possible association between vasectomy and the development of both prostate and testicular cancers. Although this issue has received widespread media interest, there is currently insufficient evidence to support an association and change current practice.

## ABORTION

For centuries, women have attempted to end unplanned pregnancies by a variety of methods, and illegal abortion has been the source of considerable morbidity and mortality. Abortion is a subject that attracts very strong opinions and there is a widespread divergence of views on the subject, mainly related to religious and cultural backgrounds.

The UK Abortion Act was passed in 1967. This allowed the lawful termination of pregnancies under certain criteria, which are very widely interpreted. As a result, illegal abortion in the UK has virtually disappeared. Under the terms of the 1967 Abortion Act, a woman may have a termination of pregnancy performed if two medical practitioners acting in good faith are willing to certify to one of the following criteria.

- The continuance of the pregnancy would involve risk to the life of the pregnant woman greater than if the pregnancy were terminated.
- The termination is necessary to prevent grave permanent injury to the physical or mental health of the pregnant woman.

- The pregnancy has not exceeded its 24th week and continuance of the pregnancy would involve risk, greater than if the pregnancy were terminated, of injury to the physical or mental health of the pregnant woman.
- The pregnancy has not exceeded its 24th week and continuance of the pregnancy would involve risk, greater than if the pregnancy were terminated, of injury to the physical or mental health of any existing child(ren) of the family of the pregnant woman.
- There is a substantial risk that if the child were born, it would suffer from such physical or mental abnormalities as to be seriously handicapped.

The form must be signed by both medical practitioners prior to the abortion being performed and posted to the Chief Medical Officer of the Department of Health or of the Scottish Executive (Fig. 6.13).

Any medical practitioner who has an objection to abortion is not required to participate in abortion services unless the treatment is necessary to save the life of the pregnant woman. However, a medical practitioner who consciously objects to abortion should still be prepared to refer a woman seeking abortion to a colleague who would be willing to consider her request sympathetically and arrange termination if appropriate.

### Incidence of legal abortion

Approximately 190 000 abortions are carried out each year in England, Wales and Scotland. Abortion is only permitted in Northern Ireland when it is undertaken to save the life of the pregnant woman. The current abortion rate is around 9–14 per 1000 women aged 15–45 years, which represents a lifetime chance of abortion of around 1 in 40. The number of abortions cited for the UK includes women who travel from other countries where abortion is illegal, particularly from the Republic of Ireland. The UK has a significantly lower abortion rate than the USA, but it is still considerably higher than in some western European countries such as the Netherlands.

### Provision of abortion services

In the UK, abortions are carried out within NHS hospitals or in private hospitals and clinics run by

IN CONFIDENCE                                                                              Certificate A

Not to be destroyed within three
years of the date of the operation

ABORTION ACT 1967
Certificate to be completed in relation to an abortion
under Section 1(1) of the Act

I     ---------------------------------------------------------------------------------------------------
                                    *(Name and qualifications of practitioner: in Block Capitals)*

of    ---------------------------------------------------------------------------------------------------

      ---------------------------------------------------------------------------------------------------
                                    *(Full address of practitioner)*

Have/have not* seen/examined* the pregnant woman to whom this certificate relates at

*(\*delete as
appropriate)*
      ---------------------------------------------------------------------------------------------------

      ---------------------------------------------------------------------------------------------------
                          *(Full address of place at which patient was seen or examined)*

on    ---------------------------------------------------------------------------------------------------

and I ---------------------------------------------------------------------------------------------------
                                    *(Name and qualifications of practitioner: in Block Capitals)*

of    ---------------------------------------------------------------------------------------------------

      ---------------------------------------------------------------------------------------------------
                                    *(Full address of practitioner)*

Have/have not* seen/and examined* the pregnant woman to whom this certificate relates at

      ---------------------------------------------------------------------------------------------------

      ---------------------------------------------------------------------------------------------------
                          *(Full address of place at which patient was seen or examined)*

on    ---------------------------------------------------------------------------------------------------
      We hereby certify that we are of the opinion formed in good faith, that in the case of

      ---------------------------------------------------------------------------------------------------
                                    *(Full name of pregnant woman: in Block Capitals)*

of    ---------------------------------------------------------------------------------------------------

      ---------------------------------------------------------------------------------------------------
                          *(Usual place of residence of pregnant woman: in Block Capitals)*

☐  A  the continuance of the pregnancy would involve risk to the life of the pregnant woman
      greater than if the pregnancy were terminated.

☐  B  the termination is necessary to prevent grave permanent injury to the physical of mental
      health of the pregnant woman.

*Tick
appropriate
box*

☐  C  the pregnancy has NOT exceeded its 24th week and that the continuance of the pregnancy
      would involve risk, greater than if the pregnancy were terminated, of injury to the physical or
      mental health of the pregnant woman.

☐  D  the pregnancy has NOT exceeded its 24th week and that the continuance of the pregnancy
      would involve risk, greater than if the pregnancy were terminated, of injury to the physical or
      mental health of the existing child(ren) of the family of the pregnant woman.

☐  E  there is a substantial risk that if the child were born it would suffer from such physical or mental
      abnormalities as to be seriously handicapped.

This certificate of opinion is given before the commencement of treatment for the termination of pregnancy to which it refers.

Signed ------------------------------------------------------------------------    Date ----------------
Signed ------------------------------------------------------------------------    Date ----------------

**Figure 6.13** UK Abortion Act form.

charitable organizations. Many NHS regions have set up abortion services to allow rapid referral and the efficient management of women seeking abortion, staffed by individuals who are particularly sensitive and sympathetic. It is particularly important that women seeking abortion should not be subject to unnecessary delays in their referral, as increasing gestation increases the risks and complexity of the abortion procedure.

## Assessment and counselling

Prior to an abortion, a woman should have the following assessments.
- Confirmation of the pregnancy by a pregnancy test.
- Assessment of the gestation: the date of the last menstrual period should be documented. Abdominal and pelvice examination should be performed. If the gestation is uncertain, the woman should be referred for an ultrasound scan.
- Infection screen: all women should be screened for *Chlamydia*. Consider the need for further STD screening (including HIV and hepatitis B) if the woman has vaginal discharge, is a rape victim or is in a high-risk category.
- Haemoglobin and blood grouping: give anti-D immunoglobulin at the time of the procedure if the woman is rhesus negative.
- Cervical smear if this is due.
- Medical history to determine if there is any contraindication to surgery or anaesthetic or a history of allergies or drug reactions.
  Pre-abortion counselling is extremely important. It should be non-judgemental and offer adequate information and explanation to allow the woman to make an informed choice. Obtaining the partner's consent should be encouraged but is not mandatory. The following areas should be discussed in the counselling process.
- Alternatives to abortion: continuing the pregnancy and either keeping the baby or having it adopted.
- The type of abortion that will be performed.
- The risks of the procedure.
- The woman's relationship with her partner and his attitude to the pregnancy.
- Ensuring the woman has adequate support both before and after the abortion.
- Offering post-termination support counselling.

- Contraception to be used after the abortion.
- Arrangements for follow-up.

## Abortion techniques

The technique of inducing abortion is determined primarily by gestation. Most centres will now offer women a choice of either a surgical or medical procedure when the pregnancy is less than 9 weeks' gestation. Ideally, an abortion should always be performed at the earliest possible gestation, as both morbidity and mortality rates rise with increasing gestation. The risk of death from an early surgical termination of pregnancy is less than 1 per 100 000, which is substantially lower than the maternal mortality associated with a full-term pregnancy.

### First trimester

#### *Surgical*
The contents of the uterus are removed by suction using a small catheter inserted through the cervix and attached to an electrical pump. A general anaesthetic is almost always given. Dilatation of the cervix is required to allow the curette to pass into the uterine cavity, and the greater the gestation of the pregnancy, the greater the amount of dilatation required. Priming of the cervix with agents such as prostaglandin (given 3 hours prior to surgery) reduces the risk of cervical trauma and haemorrhage.

#### *Medical*
The discovery in 1980 of the antiprogestogenic agent mifepristone (or RU 486) has made early medical abortion possible. The action of RU 486 blocks progestogen receptors in the uterus, resulting in induction of abortion. RU 486 on its own will only induce complete abortion in around 60 per cent of women, although when given in combination with the administration of prostaglandin, the rate of complete abortion increases to more than 95 per cent. The commonly used schedule is to give 600 mg of oral RU 486, followed 48 hours later by insertion of 1 mg gemeprost vaginal pessary. Lower-dose regimens may be equally effective. The woman stays in hospital for 4–6 hours after insertion of the pessary, during which time most women will abort the pregnancy.

The medical and surgical methods of early termination are compared in Table 6.8.

**Table 6.8** Early medical and surgical abortion

|  | Surgical | Medical |
| --- | --- | --- |
| Anaesthesia/analgesia | General anaesthetic | Oral or intramuscular analgesia may be required |
| Average blood loss | 80 mL | 80 mL |
| Completeness | 95% | 95% |
| Number of visits required for procedure | 1 | 2 |
| Availability in the UK | Widespread | Regional variation, so may not be available locally |
| Contraindications | Nil | Asthma, cardiac disease |
| Patient preference | Equal | Equal |
| Reason for choice | Unaware of events | In control of situation |
| Gestation | Up to 14 weeks | Up to 9 weeks |

## Mid-trimester (14 weeks)

Although only about 10–15 per cent of all abortions in the UK are done at this stage, mid-trimester abortions are associated with many more complications. Major fetal abnormalities detected on ultrasound may necessitate a termination at a very late stage. Not infrequently, the women who present for abortion at advanced gestations are very young, or older women who attribute amenorrhoea to being menopausal.

### Surgical

Surgical techniques involve dilatation of the cervix and evacuation of the uterus (D&E) under general anaesthetic. D&E is widely performed in the USA and although often preferred by women, this procedure is generally disliked by many members of staff, as fetal parts may have to be removed piecemeal from the uterus.

### Medical

Most mid-trimester terminations in the UK involve the pre-treatment administration of RU 486, followed 36 hours later by vaginal prostaglandin pessaries. A gemeprost pessary is inserted into the vagina every 3–6 hours until the fetus is aborted. Opiate analgesia is usually required, and around 10 per cent of women need a subsequent surgical evacuation of the uterus. Older techniques involved the intra-amniotic injection of urea or hypertonic saline combined with intravenous infusions of oxytocin or prostaglandins.

These older methods were relatively inefficient, and it often took women many days to abort. The combination of RU 486 and prostaglandins used currently significantly shortens the time taken to abort the pregnancy to around 6–8 hours.

## Complications of abortion

### Incomplete abortion

Placental and/or fetal tissue may remain in the uterus after both medical and surgical abortion. Many women will spontaneously pass the remaining tissue with time, but surgical evacuation of the uterus may be required if there is heavy bleeding or the cervix is still dilated. Very occasionally, the entire pregnancy remains within the uterus after an abortion technique and the pregnancy is still ongoing.

### Infection and subfertility

Pelvic infection following an abortion will present with a febrile illness, an offensive vaginal discharge, lower abdominal pain and tenderness of the pelvic organs on vaginal examination. Antibiotic therapy should be instituted as soon as possible. Post-abortion infection may cause tubal damage and subsequent subfertility. With modern abortion techniques and screening for pelvic infection such as *Chlamydia* and gonorrhoea in high-risk women, the risk of subsequent subfertility is very low.

## Traumatic injuries

The risk of trauma to the genital tract during an abortion is minimal where there is a high standard of gynaecological practice. During surgical abortion, perforation of the uterus can occur or there may be damage to the cervix, which can predispose to the risk of preterm labour in subsequent pregnancies (cervical incompetence).

## Psychological problems

These can be minimized if the woman has been well counselled prior to the abortion. Many women feel emotionally vulnerable in the weeks following an abortion, although for many it is an enormous relief to have the ordeal over. It is quite normal for women to experience feelings of regret and guilt after an abortion, although there is no evidence of an increase in serious psychiatric disease. Many abortion units offer a post-termination support service that women may refer themselves to in the months and even years following an abortion.

## Follow-up

All women who have had an abortion should be seen for follow-up around 2 weeks following the procedure. Most hospitals do not arrange follow-up visits, so this should be done in the general practice setting or family planning clinic. This visit is essential to:
- ensure that the abortion is complete,
- exclude an ongoing pregnancy – the woman should always be examined vaginally,
- check for possible pelvic infection,
- offer advice on contraception and sexual health,
- assess the woman's emotional state.

## Contraception

Ovulation may occur within a few weeks of an abortion. It is therefore very important that contraception is discussed prior to an abortion and instituted immediately after the procedure to avoid the chance of a further unplanned pregnancy.

Combined oral contraception, the POP or Depo-Provera should be started on the day of the abortion. An IUD can be inserted at the time or, preferably, at the follow-up visit. Barrier methods of contraception can be used immediately, although it may be necessary to check and refit a new size of diaphragm. Female sterilization is usually performed 6–8 weeks after an abortion, as it has a higher failure rate when undertaken at the time of surgical abortion.

### New developments

**Contraception for women**
- Hormone-releasing vaginal rings
- Contraceptive vaccines (anti-hCG, anti-zona pellucida)
- Once-a-month RU 486
- Low-dose continuous RU 486

**Contraception for men**
- Contraceptive vaccines (anti-sperm)
- Long-acting hormonal contraception (combinations of testosterone and progestogens are under trial)

### Key Points

- There has been a significant rise in the use of contraception worldwide over the last 40 years.
- The combined pill is a method primarily used by young, healthy women and it is estimated that there are around 3 million current users in the UK.
- Progestogen-only contraception can be used by women with cardiovascular disease and is ideal for breastfeeding or older women.
- The modern copper-bearing IUDs are highly effective and their main mode of action is a toxic effect on the gametes.
- Condoms should always be recommended in new relationships for personal protection against sexually transmitted infections.
- Natural family planning is an extremely important method worldwide and, for cultural or religious reasons, may be the only method acceptable to some couples.
- Emergency contraception can prevent unplanned pregnancy and there is considerable interest in making it more available and accessible, particularly to teenagers.
- Before sterilization, men and women should give written consent to the procedure, which states that they are aware it is permanent and also that it has a very small failure rate.
- Vasectomy is generally an easier, quicker and safer procedure than female sterilization and is usually performed under local anaesthetic.

## CASE HISTORY

Miss X is aged 17 years and single. She smokes 10 cigarettes a day. Her only previous pregnancy resulted from conception when a condom burst; she had a recent termination at 14 weeks. Her GP prescribed the combined pill for her in the past, but she thought it made her gain weight and kept forgetting to take it. She has had several partners and now has a new boyfriend. She has no past medical history of note, but was found to have an asymptomatic *Chlamydia* infection when she had her termination.

As compliance seems to be an important issue here, the injectable progestogen Depo-Provera or subdermal implant Implanon would be options to consider with Miss X. She would need to be warned about possible erratic bleeding with both methods and slight weight gain with Depo-Provera.

A low-dose combined pill could also be prescribed, with reassurance that weight gain is rarely a significant problem with it. Alternatively, the weekly combined hormonal patches could be considered, as she may find compliance easier with them. Spending time with a counselling nurse would be valuable for Miss X, and back-up leaflets on all the methods would be helpful.

As she is in a new relationship, the use of condoms should be encouraged for personal protection against infection, in combination with a hormonal method. How to use condoms effectively can be demonstrated on a model, if necessary. If Miss X decides to use condoms alone, she must be given information about the use and availability of emergency contraception.

## Reference

Collaborative Group on Hormonal Factors in Breast Cancer. Breast cancer and hormonal contraceptives: collaborative reanalysis of individual data etc. *Lancet* 1996; **347**: 1713–27.

## Additional reading

Glasier A, Gebbie A (eds). *The handbook of family planning*, 4th edn. Edinburgh: Churchill Livingstone, 2000.
Guillebaud J. *Contraception – your questions answered*, 3rd edn. Edinburgh: Churchill Livingstone, 1999.

Killick S (ed.). *Contraception in practice.* London: Martin Dunitz, 2000.

# Subfertility

## OVERVIEW

Fifteen per cent of couples who want a baby experience an unwanted delay in conception. Although there has been no change in the prevalence of fertility problems, more couples seek help than did previously. The causes of fertility problems include disorders of ovulation, sperm and the Fallopian tube, although no identifiable cause is found in a third of couples trying for a baby. In 39 per cent of couples, a problem will be found in both partners. Fertility treatment may be medical, surgical or involve assisted conception whereby the egg and sperm are brought into close proximity to facilitate fertilization.

## Definition

Subfertility is defined as the failure to conceive within 1 year of unprotected regular sexual intercourse. For couples who have had no previous conception, the subfertility is defined as primary, while couples who have had a previous conception and have then not conceived again are defined as having secondary subfertility.

## Epidemiology

Approximately 50 per cent of couples will conceive after receiving advice and simple treatment, but the remainder require more complex assisted conception techniques, and 4 per cent of couples will remain involuntarily childless. The chance of a spontaneous conception over the first 6 months of unprotected

intercourse is approximately 60 per cent. At the end of 1 year, 85 per cent of couples will have conceived.

The single most important factor in determining fertility is the age of the female partner, with fertility reducing rapidly in women over 35 years of age (Fig. 7.1). Factors that reduce the chance of a spontaneous

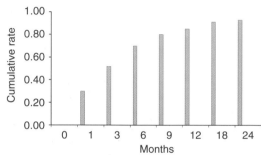

**Figure 7.1** Cumulative conception rate over first 2 years of trying to conceive. (Source: *ABC of Subfertility — Extent of the problem*. Taylor, A. Copyright 2003, BMJ.)

conception include more than 3 years of trying to con- ceive, low coital frequency and inappropriate timing of intercourse to ovulation, no previous pregnancy, smoking and a body mass index (BMI) outside the range 20–30 (weight (kg)/height (m)$^2$) in the woman. Factors affecting fertility are listed in Table 7.1. All couples trying to conceive should be given general pre- conception advice on ways to improve the chances of conception and to reduce the risk of pregnancy com- plications for the mother or fetus (Table 7.2).

**Table 7.1** Factors adversely affecting conception rates

| Female factors | Male factors | Combined factors |
| --- | --- | --- |
| Age (>37 years) | Low numbers of motile, healthy sperm | Duration of infertility (>2 years) |
| Menstrual FSH level (>10 u/L) | Drug intake | No previous conception in current relationship |

FSH, follicle-stimulating hormone.

**Table 7.2** Preconception advice

| Lifestyle | Medical |
| --- | --- |
| Stop smoking | Optimize management of medical problems |
| Stop recreational drugs | Eliminate drugs not safe for pregnancy |
| | Optimize body weight to a body mass index of 20–30 |
| | Eliminate drugs not safe for pregnancy |
| Regular sexual intercourse, 2–3 times a week | Prepregnancy assessment by an obstetric physician |
| | Commence folic acid supplements |
| | Ensure immunity to rubella |

Fertility investigations are usually commenced after 1 year of unprotected intercourse, but it is advisable to start investigations after 6 months of unprotected intercourse in women over 35 years of age. Initial management and investigations may be commenced by the general practitioner, who is also able to offer advice and support to couples requiring referral for more specialist investigations.

## Causes of female subfertility

The main causes of subfertility are ovulation dis- orders, male factors, tubal damage, unexplained, and other causes such as endometriosis and fibroids. The proportion of each type of subfertility varies in different studies and in different populations. Tubal subfertility is more common in those with secondary subfertility and in populations with a higher prevalence of sexually transmitted disease.

### P   Understanding the pathophysiology

**Oogenesis and ovulation**

The formation and maturation of an oocyte is known as oogenesis (Fig. 7.2). It starts with the growth of a primordial follicle to form a pre-antral follicle and ends with the final maturation of a pre-ovulation follicle. The formation of the pre-antral follicle takes 85 days in a human, while the final maturation stage (the follicular phase of the menstrual cycle) from the pre-antral follicle to the pre-ovulatory follicle takes 14 days to complete. Figure 7.3 shows a pre-ovulatory follicle with its blood flow.

An intact hypothalamo–pituitary–ovarian axis is essential for normal ovarian function. Gonadotrophin-releasing hormone (GnRH) is released in a pulsatile manner to control the pituitary and the release of follicle-stimulating hormone (FSH) and luteinizing hormone (LH). These hormones stimulate the development of the follicles, while a mid-cycle surge of LH (Fig. 7.4) causes rupture of the dominant follicle and release of the oocyte (ovulation).

## Ovulation problems

Ovulation problems can arise as a result of defects in the hypothalamus, the pituitary or the ovary. Factors that disrupt the normal pulsatile release of GnRH will lead to disordered ovulation. These factors include

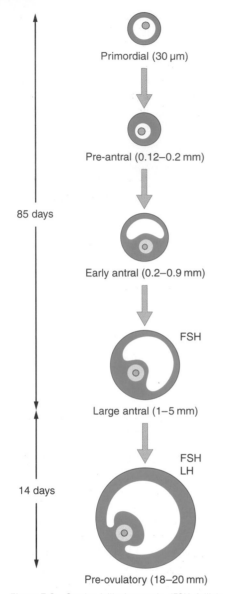

Primordial (30 μm)

Pre-antral (0.12–0.2 mm)

85 days

Early antral (0.2–0.9 mm)

FSH

Large antral (1–5 mm)

FSH
LH

14 days

Pre-ovulatory (18–20 mm)

**Figure 7.2**   Ovarian folliculogenesis. (FSH, follicle-stimulating hormone; LH, luteinizing hormone.)

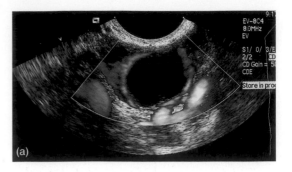

(a)

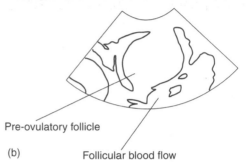

Pre-ovulatory follicle

(b)                    Follicular blood flow

**Figure 7.3**   (a) Ultrasound of a pre-ovulatory follicle with blood flow. (b) Schematic representation.

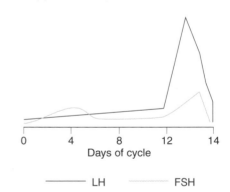

Days of cycle

———— LH        ———— FSH

**Figure 7.4**   The luteinizing hormone (LH) surge that precedes ovulation. (FSH, follicle-stimulating hormone.)

stress, psychological disturbances, weight change and systemic diseases as well as tumours and structural lesions in the hypothalamus. Both hyperthyroidism and hypothyroidism may result in ovulatory failure and will if severe lead to anovulation and amenorrhoea. Hyperprolactinaemia (as seen in women with a prolactinoma), renal failure, hepatic dysfunction and phenothiazine medication impair the pulsatile release of GnRH, leading to anovulation.

The commonest cause of anovulatory subfertility is polycystic ovary syndrome (PCOS). Women affected by this condition have a range of symptoms that may occur singly or in combination and include menstrual cycle disturbances, obesity, hirsutism, acne and subfertility. The diagnosis is based on the biochemical abnormalities (low sex hormone-binding globulin concentrations and high androgen concentrations) and the ultrasound appearance of the ovaries (an enlarged ovary with multiple subcapsular follicles and a dense stroma; Fig. 7.5).

Premature ovarian failure is a condition in which there is total failure of the ovaries in women under the age of 40 years. It is characterized by amenorrhoea and raised FSH and low oestradiol concentrations. The

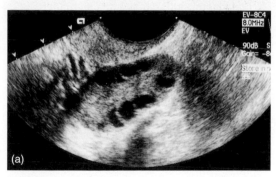
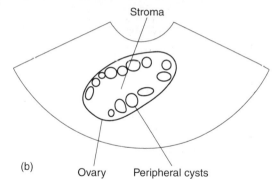

**Figure 7.5**    (a) Ultrasound of a polycystic ovary showing dense stroma and peripheral cysts. (b) Schematic representation.

condition is seen in 1 per cent of the female population. The aetiology is often not determined but can be linked to genetic causes, especially if ovarian failure occurs before puberty. In these cases a sex chromosome abnormality, such as Turner's syndrome or XY gonadal dysgenesis, is usually present. Acquired aetiologies include damage by viruses and toxins, while iatrogenic causes include pelvic surgery, irradiation and cytotoxic treatment. In some women an autoimmune problem may be detected with serum autoantibodies to steroid-producing cells including the ovary, adrenal and thyroid, resulting in degenerative changes within the ovary.

## Tubal dysfunction

Tubal damage may arise following a pelvic infection, endometriosis or pelvic surgery. The resulting damage may lead to impaired oocyte pick-up mechanisms by the fimbriae or to damaged tubal epithelium. Sexually transmitted disease caused by *Chlamydia trachomatis*, gonococci or other microorganisms most commonly leads to tubal damage, but pelvic sepsis following appendicitis or peritonitis is also a common cause.

## Disorders of implantation

Other causes of female subfertility include disorders of implantation with known defects related to endometrial development or the production of growth and adhesion molecules. Submucous fibroids may distort the endometrial cavity and impair implantation. Smoking is known to reduce fertility by two-thirds, but other environmental and psychological factors can also have an impact on conception.

### 🔑 Key Points: causes of female subfertility

- Disorders of ovulation
- Impaired oocyte production (oocyte factors)
- Tubal dysfunction
- Disorders of implantation

## Causes of male subfertility

### P  Understanding the pathophysiology

Spermatogenesis is controlled by pituitary FSH and the androgens produced by the LH-stimulated Leydig cells in the testes. Sertoli cells are embedded within the terminal epithelium of the seminiferous tubules and secrete inhibin, which controls FSH release from the pituitary with negative feedback (Fig 7.6). Mitotic division of the spermatogonia followed by meiotic division of the spermatocytes is known as spermatogenesis, while the transformation of spermatogonia into spermatozoa is called spermiogenesis. Genes involved in spermatogenesis are located on the Y chromosome.

Spermatozoa released into the lumen of the seminiferous tubules are immotile and do not acquire motility until they reach the ampulla of the vas deferens. During ejaculation the semen is released by adrenergically mediated contractions of the distal epididymis and vas deferens. Secretions from the prostate seminal vesicles and the accessory glands are subsequently added to the spermatozoa during transport along the male genital tract.

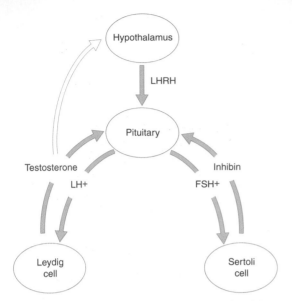

**Figure 7.6** Flow diagram illustrating the relationships of the hypothalamo–pituitary–testicular axis. (LH, luteinizing hormone; FSH, follicle-stimulating hormone; LHRH, luteinizing hormone-releasing hormone.)

Disorders of spermatogenesis may arise when the scrotal temperature rises as a result of undescended testes, varicocele, hot baths or tight underwear. Chromosomal abnormalities including microdeletions of the Y chromosome may also lead to impaired spermatogenesis. In addition sperm production and sexual function are impaired by psychotropic drugs, anti-epileptic medication, antihypertensive medication, antibiotics and chemotherapeutic agents.

Disorders of sperm transport are seen in men with congenital malformations of the epididymis or vas deferens as well as obstruction due to inflammation, infection or deliberate blockage of the outflow tract by vasectomy. Ejaculatory dysfunction can be drug-induced, idiopathic or caused by metabolic and systemic diseases such as diabetes and multiple sclerosis.

### 🔑 Key Points: causes of male subfertility

- Disorders of spermatogenesis
- Impaired sperm transport
- Ejaculatory dysfunction
- Immunological and infective factors

### Nomenclature for some semen variables

- Normozoospermia: normal ejaculate as defined by the reference value.
- Oligozoospermia: sperm concentration less than the reference value.
- Asthenozoospermia: less than the reference value for motility.
- Teratozoospermia: less than the reference value for morphology.
- Oligoasthenoterato-zoospermia: signifies disturbance of all three variables (combinations of only two prefixes may also be used).
- Azoospermia: no spermatozoa in the ejaculate.
- Aspermia: no ejaculate.

## History and examination

A full medical and surgical history should be obtained from both the male and the female partner. This should include details of drug history, family history and lifestyle, including the use of alcohol, smoking and recreational drugs. Details of coital frequency and any difficulties with coitus should be recorded. For the woman a gynaecological history should be taken, with details of the menstrual cycle including menstrual frequency. In women with irregular menstruation, direct questioning for symptoms of PCOS, thyroid disorders and hyperprolactinaemia is recommended to determine any endocrine disturbance. Assessment of the woman's general health, including a cervical smear, rubella status, body weight and blood pressure, should also be performed.

An examination of both partners is essential to ensure normal reproductive organs. In the male the examination must assess testicular size as well as excluding testicular masses, congenital absence of the vas deferens and varicocele. Small testes may be associated with primary testicular failure. In the woman a full general and pelvic examination should be carried out to check for any endocrine and gynaecological abnormalities. Ideally, each partner should be examined separately so that a confidential history regarding sexually transmitted diseases or previous pregnancies can be elicited.

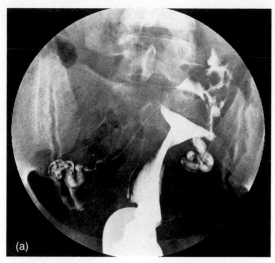

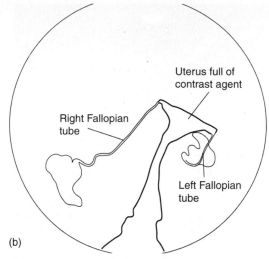

**Figure 7.7** (a) Hysterosalpingogram confirming tubal patency; there is bilateral peritoneal spill. (b) Schematic representation.

## Investigations

Investigations must be tailored to the circumstances of individual couples. Modern evidence-based investigations are cost effective and likely to achieve the best results. Investigations should include assessment of the hypothalamo–pituitary–ovarian axis, ovulation, and Fallopian tube patency. An early follicular phase (day 2–5 of the menstrual cycle) measurement of the gonadotrophins (LH and FSH) assesses the ovarian reserve of oocytes. Analysis of the mid-luteal progesterone level can be used to confirm ovulation, but correct timing of the assessment is crucial. The sample ideally needs to be taken 7 days prior to the subsequent menses. Alternatively, serial follicle-tracking scans can be used in the middle of the menstrual cycle to confirm ovulation. In women with irregular menstrual cycles, thyroid function, prolactin level and androgen levels should be analysed to look for any underlying endocrine abnormalities.

## Assessment of tubal patency

Tests of Fallopian tube patency all rely on the visualization of solutions passing through the tubes into the abdominal cavity. The three commonly used techniques of visualization are ultrasound scan, X-ray and direct visualization at laparoscopy. It is no longer justifiable to use laparoscopy routinely in the investigation of all subfertile women, but it is appropriate for the further evaluation of women with pelvic pain and those with inconclusive findings on hysterosalpingography or hysterocontrast synography (HyCoSy), in whom it can be used simultaneously for therapeutic intervention (e.g. adhesiolysis or ovarian cystectomy).

Hysterosalpingograms (Fig. 7.7) are used in women with no history of pelvic damage or infection. The test is usually performed during the follicular phase of the menstrual cycle prior to ovulation in order to avoid the risk of inducing an ectopic pregnancy or inadvertently exposing an early embryo to ionizing radiation. The procedure involves the instillation of a radio-opaque dye, through a small catheter placed in the cervical canal, into the uterine cavity. The X-ray image obtained shows the uterine cavity, the outline of the Fallopian tubes and the presence or absence of dye in the abdominal cavity. When dye is seen to flow freely into the abdominal cavity, tubal patency is confirmed. However, if the dye spill appears to be loculated or the tube appears to be in an abnormal position, peri-tubal adhesions are likely to be present. Uterine adhesions and submucous fibroids appear as filling defects on the X-ray image and require further assessment by hysteroscopy.

The technique of HyCoSy (Fig. 7.8) involves the use of ultrasound to image the uterus and Fallopian tubes and avoids exposure to X-rays. Contrast medium, either saline or Echovist, is instilled into the cavity through a cervical catheter. Saline is used to outline the uterine cavity and delineate any filling defects such

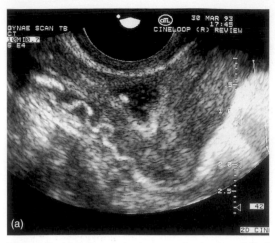 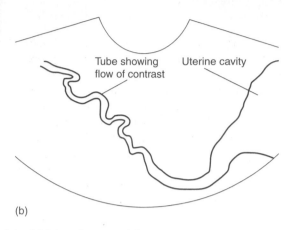

**Figure 7.8** (a) Hysterocontrast synography showing a Fallopian tube. (b) Schematic representation.

as submucous fibroids or polyps. The patency of the Fallopian tubes is confirmed by visualizing the flow of Echovist contrast medium along the tube and into the abdominal cavity. It is important to time the procedure to the pre-ovulatory phase of the menstrual cycle to avoid the risk of inducing an ectopic pregnancy.

Laparoscopy and dye intubation necessitates a general anaesthetic and direct visualization of the pelvic organs. Tubal patency is then tested by instilling methylene blue through the cervix and observing the spillage of the dye from the fimbrial ends.

## Semen analysis

Analysis of the sperm should be carried out on a sample produced after 3–5 days of sexual abstinence. If the semen parameters are not satisfactory, a second sample should be analysed. The potential of the sperm to fertilize is indicated by its progressive motility, morphology and agglutination. The presence of antisperm antibodies should be determined in men with low progressive motility. In men with very low sperm counts, an endocrine profile (including LH, FSH, testosterone and prolactin) and a chromosome analysis may be required. Screening for cystic fibrosis should also be performed in cases of azoospermia.

## Postcoital test

The postcoital test has limited prognostic value and is rarely used today. It involves an assessment of the peri-ovulatory cervical mucus and sperm in a sample obtained from the female partner 6–10 hours after coitus. Unless the sample is accurately timed to the correct phase of the menstrual cycle, it is impossible to interpret the results.

## Treatment of male and female subfertility

Specialist fertility units treating couples with subfertility should individualize the treatment to each couple's chances of success. There are many factors influencing conception rates, including the female partner's age, the baseline FSH level, previous conception and sperm function. Counselling is an essential part of subfertility management and may be beneficial to both men and women. Men with sperm abnormalities tend to suffer from low self-esteem, while women often blame themselves, with 5 per cent having suicidal tendencies. Advice regarding adoption and gamete donation should be available in subfertility clinics and given to couples when appropriate.

---

**Semen analysis** (World Health Organization reference values)

- Volume: 2–5mL
- Liquification time: within 30 minutes
- Sperm concentration: 20 million/mL
- Sperm motility: >50% progressive motility
- Sperm morphology: >30% normal forms
- White blood cells: <1 million/mL

## Ovulation problems

Ovulatory disorders should be managed by addressing the underlying cause first; ovulation induction should be considered only if regular menstruation does not resume. Women with a hypothalamic disorder caused by excessive weight gain or low body weight should optimize their weight, while those experiencing stress should address lifestyle issues. Women with hyperprolactinaemia need full investigation to exclude a medical or physiological cause. If a tumour is detected, it may require surgery or may shrink if a dopaminergic agonist is used. In women with PCOS, insulin-sensitizing drugs such as metformin may lead to a resumption of normal ovulatory cycles. Alternatively, ovarian drilling, in which a diathermy needle is used laparoscopically to make multiple small holes in the surface of the ovary, can be an effective treatment for anovulation linked to PCOS.

Ovulation induction can be performed using antioestrogen medication, including clomiphene citrate and tamoxifen or exogenous gonadotrophin, to stimulate the development of one or more mature follicles. The most appropriate treatment method is selected after identifying the location of the defect in the hypothalamo–pituitary axis. Clomiphene citrate is administered during the follicular phase of the menstrual cycle. It is thought to act by increasing gonadotrophin release from the pituitary, leading to enhanced follicular recruitment and growth. It is effective at inducing ovulation in 85 per cent of women and can be used for a maximum of a year. It is recommended that treatment cycles are monitored with serial ultrasound scans to minimize the multiple pregnancy rate and risk of ovarian hyperstimulation.

Ovulation can also be induced with exogenous gonadotrophins given by daily injection from the beginning of the cycle. The dose is titrated against the individual response and is monitored by an ultrasound assessment of follicular number and size. Ovulation is usually triggered with an injection of human chorionic gonadotrophin (hCG, which binds to the LH receptor) when 1–3 follicles are 18 mm in diameter. If more than three follicles are mature, the couple are asked to avoid sexual intercourse and hCG is withheld.

## Tubal disease

The treatment of tubal disease aims to restore normal anatomy, but the chance of success depends on the severity and location of the damage as well as on the skills of the surgeon. In-vitro fertilization (IVF) is an alternative to surgery and would be recommended if there were extensive damage or intrafallopian tubal damage, or if surgery failed to restore patency. If peritubal or peri-ovarian adhesions are present, they can be removed by a laparoscopic adhesiolysis. When the fimbriae are also involved, a fimbrioplasty to remove the fimbrial adhesions and repair the fimbrial disease can be successful. Although at least 5 per cent of the resulting conceptions will be ectopic, intrauterine pregnancy rates of 50 per cent can be seen after 6 months. Reversal of sterilization can produce good conception rates as the mucosal damage is limited and the woman has proven fertility. If the tubal damage has resulted in hydrosalpinges, it is advisable to remove the affected Fallopian tubes prior to IVF treatment as they are thought to affect implantation adversely.

## Male subfertility

Male fertility depends on sperm quality rather than the absolute number of sperm present. Men with hypogonadotrophic hypogonadism are treated with exogenous gonadotrophins and hCG to restore testicular volume and spermatogenesis. Hormonal therapy is, however, ineffective at restoring sperm production or function in men with idiopathic oligospermia. In these men intrauterine insemination with ovarian stimulation may be an appropriate treatment. Alternatively, couples may choose to proceed to IVF with intracytoplasmic sperm injection (ICSI; Fig. 7.9), or, if sperm parameters are very low, they may choose to

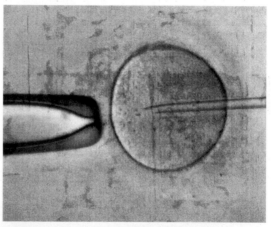

**Figure 7.9** Intracytoplasmic sperm injection.

use donor sperm. Men with obstructive azoospermia can be offered sperm aspiration followed by IVF with ICSI treatment. Although 25 per cent of men with abnormal sperm parameters have a varicocele, there is no evidence that surgical ligation improves fertility.

## Assisted conception

Assisted conception techniques have, since their introduction in the late 1970s, enabled more than a million babies to be conceived. These conceptions have depended on the development of laboratory, clinical and pharmaceutical advancements that have simplified and improved the treatment of subfertility. All the techniques rely on the basic concept of placing the egg and sperm in close proximity to facilitate fertilization. Today, the commonly used techniques of intrauterine insemination, IVF and ICSI are widely used throughout the world to assist conception.

### Abbreviations used in assisted conception

- IVF     In-vitro fertilization
- DI     Donor insemination
- GIFT     Gamete intrafallopian transfer
- ZIFT     Zygote intrafallopian transfer
- SUZI     Subzonal insemination
- ICSI     Intracytoplasmic sperm injection
- TESA     Testicular sperm aspiration
- PESA     Percutaneous sperm aspiration
- MESA     Micro-epididymal sperm aspiration

### A typical IVF–embryo transfer cycle

- Initial consultation
- Pituitary down-regulation
- Superovulation ovarian stimulation
- Ovulation trigger with hCG trigger
- Oocyte collection
- Insemination of oocytes
- Embryo transfer
- Luteal support
- Pregnancy test

### Initial consultation

Initial consultation involves a detailed history and provides an opportunity to assess the cause of subfertility and the most appropriate treatment technique. Prior to commencing IVF, a recent baseline FSH level, semen analysis and pelvic ultrasound are assessed. Forms relating to the welfare of the child will be completed, counselling provided and infection screens analysed.

### Pituitary down-regulation

Pituitary down-regulation is essential to prevent a natural LH surge during follicular stimulation as this would result in follicular rupture prior to egg retrieval. Treatment with GnRH analogues, given by daily injection, implant or nasal spray, prevents the natural LH surge and is continued throughout the treatment cycle. Alternatively, GnRH antagonists can be administered during the mid- and late follicular phases of a superovulation cycle to prevent the LH surge. A low serum oestradiol level (<100 u/L) or thin endometrium on ultrasound scan are used to confirm down-regulation of the pituitary.

### Ovarian stimulation

Ovarian stimulation is achieved by daily injections of gonadotrophins (either recombinant or urinary). The injections are continued for 11–14 days until the lead follicles are 18 mm in diameter on transvaginal ultrasound scan (Fig. 7.10).

### Ovulation trigger with hCG

In the stage of ovulation trigger with hCG, hCG is used in place of LH to trigger ovulation. The oocytes are retrieved 34–38 hours after the injection.

### Oocyte collection

Oocyte collection is normally an outpatient procedure carried out under transvaginal ultrasound guidance with the woman under intravenous sedation. The follicular fluid is aspirated from each follicle using a controlled pressure vacuum pump (Fig. 7.11). Using a microscope, the embryologist identifies the oocytes removed in the follicular fluid and then transfers these to culture medium in an incubator.

During sperm preparation, the sperm sample is washed to remove seminal plasma, leukocytes and bacteria. A laboratory process that allows the sperm to mature and undergo capacitation is performed, and the motile sperm can then be selected for use in the insemination process.

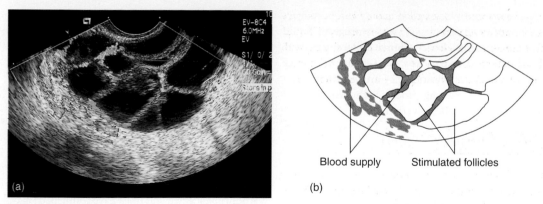

Blood supply          Stimulated follicles

**Figure 7.10**   (a) Ultrasound showing stimulated ovary with multiple follicles and associated blood supply. (b) Schematic representation.

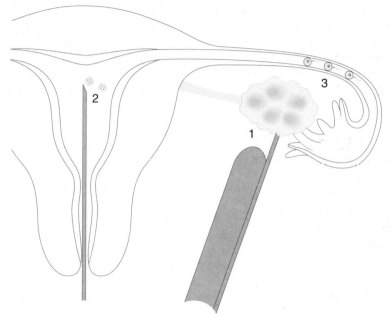

**Figure 7.11**   Techniques used in assisted conception. (1) Transvaginal oocyte collection. (2) Embryo transfer. (3) Gamete intrafallopian transfer.

## Insemination

In insemination the prepared sperm is mixed with the oocytes 4–6 hours after collection and incubated. For ICSI the eggs require an additional step to remove the surrounding cumulus cells prior to the injection of a single sperm into the cytoplasm of each oocyte. Whatever the process of insemination, the next stage involves incubating the oocytes with the sperm for 16–18 hours.

Next is fertilization and embryo cleavage. The oocytes are examined for fertilization on the day after oocyte retrieval. The presence of two pronuclei and two polar bodies indicates normal fertilization. After 48 hours in culture, the embryos are examined for cleavage, and any cleaved embryos are assessed for quality. An embryo with minimal fragmentation will be graded more highly than one with many fragments.

## Embryo transfer

In embryo transfer, the embryos are transferred into the uterus using a transcervical catheter on the second or third day of culture. In the UK regulations permit only two embryos to be transferred, except in exceptional circumstances.

Any spare embryos of good quality can be subject to embryo cryopreservation, with storage in liquid nitrogen for use in a frozen embryo replacement cycle in the future. The embryos can remain in storage without deterioration until they are required. They then undergo a thawing process with two-thirds of embryos surviving the procedure.

### Luteal support and establishment of pregnancy

Luteal support can be provided by progesterone supplements in the form of vaginal pessaries, suppositories or injections. Alternatively, low-dose hCG injections are used to stimulate progesterone production by the ovary. Pregnancy is detected by a urinary pregnancy test or by analysis of the serum β-hCG 14 days after embryo transfer.

## Intrauterine insemination

Intrauterine insemination involves the placement of a sample of purified sperm in the uterus at the time of ovulation. It is most successful if it is combined with ovarian stimulation to produce up to three mature follicles. Close monitoring of the treatment is essential as there is a high risk of multiple pregnancy if treatment continues when more than three follicles have formed. It is used to treat mild male factor subfertility as well as unexplained subfertility. Although the success rate varies between assisted conception units, approximately 10–15 per cent of couples manage to conceive by this method.

## Intracytoplasmic sperm injection

In the technique of gamete intrafallopian transfer (GIFT), a laparoscope is used to transfer the eggs and sperm to the fimbrial part of the Fallopian tube. This allows fertilization to occur in the natural location and has the advantage of requiring minimal laboratory facilities. However, GIFT has the disadvantage of requiring a general anaesthetic and laparoscopy. The treatment still requires controlled ovarian stimulation, but egg retrieval may be by a laparoscopic technique or by the more usual ultrasound-assisted transvaginal method. GIFT is infrequently performed in the UK now that IVF has become more successful and straightforward.

## Donor insemination

For couples with male factor subfertility caused by azoospermia or severe oligospermia, insemination with donor sperm may be indicated as an alternative to ICSI. It may also be used in couples where there is a risk of transmitting a genetic disorder via the male partner or for women who do not have a male partner. The treatment is undertaken by clinics licensed by the Human Fertilization and Embryology Authority (HFEA). For donor insemination, the female partner is fully investigated and must have confirmed Fallopian tube patency and the capacity to ovulate either spontaneously or with stimulation. The sperm is provided by screened healthy donors who are recruited by sperm banks. The clinics match the characteristics of the donor to those of the recipient couple. Insemination with the prepared sperm is timed to ovulation. A live birth rate of 10 per cent per treatment cycle can be expected. The regulatory authority for donor insemination, the HFEA, permits the creation of ten pregnancies from an individual sperm donor. Subsequently, that donor's sperm can only be used to make siblings for the ten babies conceived.

## Donor eggs

Oocyte donation is used in women with genetic conditions involving the X chromosomes such as fragile X and Turner's syndromes, and for women who have undergone a natural or iatrogenic premature ovarian failure. The donors may be undergoing parallel assisted conception treatment or may be altruistic but must undergo a full cycle of controlled ovarian stimulation with egg retrieval. Donors are fully counselled and are required to have a full infection, health and genetic assessment before donating oocytes. The recipients must in turn undergo detailed counselling and infection screening.

## Preimplantation diagnosis of genetic disease

For couples at risk of a child with an inherited genetic disease, the preimplantation diagnosis of genetic disease offers the opportunity to select unaffected embryos for transfer. It involves the creation of embryos by IVF followed by the removal and subsequent genetic testing of one or two of the cells. Alternatively, the sex of the embryos can be determined for sex-linked disorders. Unaffected embryos are then transferred back to the uterus.

## Regulation of fertility treatment

All assisted conception centres in the UK involved in treatment, research or the storage of human embryos must be licensed by the HFEA. The centres are legally obliged to inform the HFEA of all treatments and the outcome of those treatments. In addition the centres must ensure that the welfare of any children born as a result of the treatment or any children who will be affected by the birth of this child is adequately considered.

## Complications of assisted conception

Complications of assisted conception include the development of ovarian hyperstimulation syndrome, ectopic pregnancy and multiple pregnancy.

### Ovarian hyperstimulation syndrome
Ovarian hyperstimulation syndrome develops in women who have had an exaggerated response to the exogenous gonadotrophins or gonadotrophin analogues used for superovulation. Women who develop 20 or more follicles or have PCOS are more likely to develop the condition. It occurs after the administration of exogenous hCG or after the natural rise in hCG with conception. Patients present with abdominal pain and distension, nausea, bowel disturbance, shortness of breath and poor urinary output. These patients may require inpatient care by a specialist team.

### Ectopic pregnancy
Four per cent of pregnancies arising from IVF treatment will be ectopic, with an increased risk in women with known tubal damage. The embryos may migrate to the Fallopian tubes or are inadvertently placed there during the embryo transfer procedure.

### Multiple pregnancy
Assisted conception often results in a twin or higher-order pregnancy. HFEA regulations prevent the transfer of more than two embryos except in exceptional circumstances, when three may be transferred. In stimulated intrauterine cycles or in ovulation induction with gonadotrophins or anti-oestrogens, careful monitoring is paramount in avoiding multiple pregnancies. Multiple pregnancies have increased morbidity and mortality for both the mother and the babies, with enormous healthcare costs. Evidence for the benefits of a single embryo transfer for families and society is becoming increasingly apparent from work being undertaken in Scandinavia.

## CASE HISTORY

Mrs JD is a 25-year-old aerobics teacher. She has irregular periods and has a low BMI of 17. She exercises for 4–5 hours a day. She is otherwise well and has no significant past medical or surgical history. Her husband, Mr MD, works as a computer programmer. He is well and has no significant past medical or surgical history. They are both non-smokers and neither of them drinks alcohol.

### Investigations
Mrs JD: FSH, LH, thyroid function, prolactin level, rubella status, pelvic ultrasound examination.
Mr MD: semen analysis.

### Results
Mrs JD: rubella immune; pelvic ultrasound scan normal; FSH, 4.3u/L; LH, 3.0u/L; prolactin and thyroid function normal.

Mr MD: sperm count 53 million/mL; 45 per cent motile with good progressive motility; morphology – 65 per cent abnormality.

Mrs JD was advised to reduce the duration and frequency of exercise and to gain weight to a BMI of 19–20. The couple were reassured that all investigations were normal. Within 6 months Mrs JD had increased her weight and reduced her exercise. Subsequently, her periods became more frequent. Three months later she conceived spontaneously and proceeded to deliver a healthy male infant at term.

## CASE HISTORY

Miss EC is a 31-year-old catering assistant. She has a normal BMI, does not smoke and drinks 4 units of alcohol a week. She has a regular menstrual cycle and no gynaecological problems. She had a ruptured appendix as a child and required surgery to divide adhesions at the age of 25. Her partner, Mr DF, is a mechanic. He has two children from his previous marriage and underwent a vasectomy 6 years ago.

### Investigations

Miss EC: pelvic ultrasound scan, hysterosalpingogram.

### Results

The pelvic ultrasound was normal, but the hysterosalpingogram showed partial filling of both Fallopian tubes and no spill of dye into the abdominal cavity. Tubal blockage was therefore diagnosed.

The couple were advised that IVF would be required with percutaneous sperm aspiration to obtain the sperm from Mr DF. They would require ICSI to obtain fertilization. They proceeded to a treatment cycle of IVF with ICSI following the aspiration of the sperm. Miss EC conceived in her first cycle of treatment.

### Key Points

- History, examination, investigations and counselling must include both partners.
- The couple should be given advice regarding the effects of smoking, alcohol and lifestyle, and information concerning spontaneous conception rates.
- Treatment should be initiated taking into account the duration of infertility, the female partner's age, previous conception history and success rates.
- Women aged 35 years and above and those with irregular cycles should be referred to specialist clinics.
- Total motile, normal sperm population is more important than the sperm count, but sperm morphology is a more stable indicator of fertilization than motility.
- Men with abnormal sperm analysis should have endocrine assessment; those with low (<5 million/mL) or no sperm must be offered chromosomal analyses.
- Couples must be given written information regarding the risks of ovarian hyperstimulation syndrome, multiple gestation and ovarian tumours.
- FSH and human menopausal gonadotrophin should be used in low dose in clomiphene-resistant women; clomiphene is an effective treatment in anovulatory women.
- All ovulation induction cycles should be monitored.
- The welfare of the child born as a result of treatment, and of any existing children, must be taken into account.

# Chapter 8

# Disorders of early pregnancy

## OVERVIEW

Early pregnancy disorders currently account for approximately three-quarters of emergency gynaecological admissions in Europe and are an important cause of maternal morbidity and mortality throughout the world.

Pregnancy loss may have a profound effect on a woman and, in addition to the medical management, appropriate counselling and support should be made available.

## Introduction

The three main categories of early pregnancy disorders are:
1. spontaneous miscarriages
2. ectopic pregnancies
3. gestational trophoblastic disorders (GTDs).

Gynaecological complications, such as cervical or vaginal cancer and infections, may present with similar symptoms and should be considered in the differential diagnosis.

## The normal early pregnancy

Implantation and subsequent placental development in the human require complex adaptive changes of the uterine wall constituents.

## Development of the blastocyst

At the beginning of the 4th week after the last menstrual period, the implanted blastocyst is composed, from outside to inside, of the trophoblastic ring, the extra-embryonic mesoderm and the amniotic cavity and the primary yolk sac, separated by the bilaminar embryonic disk (Fig. 8.1). The extra-embryonic mesoderm progressively increases, and 12 days after ovulation (around the 26th menstrual day) it contains isolated spaces that rapidly fuse to form the extra-embryonic coelom. As the latter forms, the primary yolk sac decreases in size and the secondary yolk sac arises from cells growing from the embryonic disk inside the primary yolk sac.

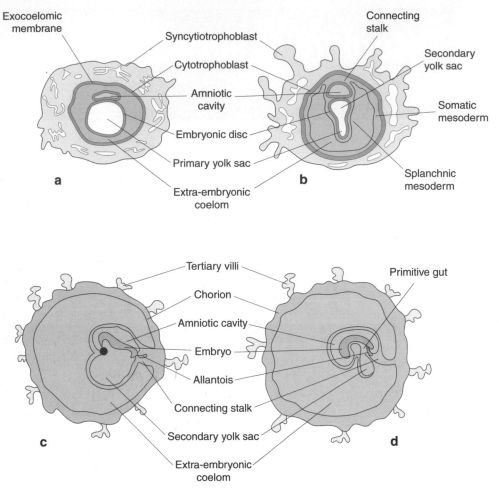

**Figure 8.1** Schematic representations of human pregnancies at the beginning (a) and at the end (b) of the 4th menstrual week and during the 5th (c) and 6th (d) menstrual weeks.

## Formation of the placenta

Primary chorionic villi develop between 13 and 15 days after ovulation (end of 4th week of gestation). Simultaneously, blood vessels start to develop in the extra-embryonic mesoderm of the yolk sac, the connecting stalk and the chorion. The primary villi are composed of a central mass of cytotrophoblast surrounded by a thick layer of syncytiotrophoblast. During the 5th week of gestation, they acquire a central mesenchymal core from the extra-embryonic mesoderm and become branched, forming the secondary villi. The appearance of embryonic blood vessels within their mesenchymal cores transforms the secondary villi into tertiary villi. Up to 10 weeks' gestation, which corresponds to the last week of the embryonic period (stages 19 to 23), villi cover the entire surface of the chorionic sac (see Fig. 8.1).

As the gestational sac grows during fetal life, the villi associated with the decidua capsularis surrounding the amniotic sac become compressed and degenerate, forming an avascular shell known as the chorion laeve, or smooth chorion. Conversely, the villi associated with the decidua basalis proliferate, forming the chorion frondosum or definitive placenta.

## Normal placentation

As soon as the blastocyst has hatched, the tropho-ectoderm layer attaches to the cell surface of the endometrium and, by simple displacement, early

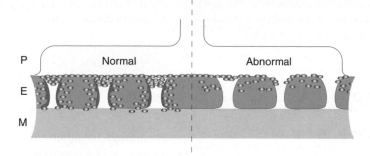

**Figure 8.2** Diagram comparing the histological features of the placental bed (P, placenta; E, endometrium; M, myometrium) in normal and abnormal pregnancies. In normal pregnancies, the extravillous trophoblast infiltrates the endometrium down to the myometrium and forms a continuous shell obliterating the tip of the transformed spiral arteries. In spontaneous abortions, there is a reduced trophoblastic infiltration, a fragmented or absent trophoblastic shell and defective transformation of the spiral arteries.

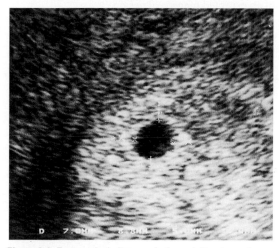

**Figure 8.3** Transvaginal ultrasound of a gestational sac at 4 weeks' gestation.

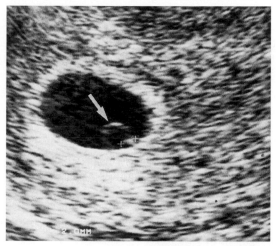

**Figure 8.4** Transvaginal ultrasound of a normal 5-week pregnancy showing, from outside to inside, the placental echogenic ring, the chorionic or exocoelomic cavity, the embryo (crown–rump length [CRL] = 2 mm) and the secondary yolk sac (arrow).

trophoblastic penetration within the endometrial stroma occurs. Progressively, the entire blastocyst will sink into maternal decidua and the migrating trophoblastic cells will encounter venous channels of increasing size, then superficial arterioles and, during the 4th week, the spiral arteries (Fig. 8.2). The trophoblastic cells infiltrate deep into the decidua and reach the deciduo-myometrial junction at between 8 and 12 weeks' gestation. This extravillous trophoblast penetrates the inner third of the myometrium via the interstitial ground substance and affects its mechanical and electrophysiological properties by increasing its expansile capacity. The trophoblastic infiltration of the myometrium is progressive and achieved before 18 weeks' gestation in normal pregnancies.

## Ultrasound imaging

The gestational sac representing the deciduo-placental interface and the chorionic cavity are the first sonographic evidence of a pregnancy (Fig. 8.3). The gestational sac can be visualized with transvaginal ultrasound around 4.4–4.6 weeks (32–34 days) following the onset of the last menstruation, when it reaches a size of 2–4 mm. By contrast, the gestational sac can only be observed by means of abdominal ultrasound imaging during the 5th week post-menstruation.

The first embryonic structure that becomes visible inside the chorionic cavity is the secondary yolk sac, when the gestational sac reaches 8 mm. Demonstration of the yolk sac (Fig. 8.4) reliably indicates that an intrauterine fluid collection represents a true gestational sac, thus excluding the possibility of a pseudosac or an ectopic pregnancy (see previous page).

## Symptomatology

The classical symptom triad for early pregnancy disorders is amenorrhoea, pelvic or low abdominal pain and vaginal bleeding. Pregnancy symptoms are often non-specific and many women of reproductive age have irregular menstrual cycles. The first test to confirm the existence of pregnancy is for the detection of human chorionic gonadotrophin (hCG) in the patient's urine or plasma.

## Pregnancy tests

Human chorionic gonadotrophin is a placental-derived glycoprotein, composed of two subunits, alpha and beta, which maintains the corpus luteum for the first 7 weeks of gestation. Extremely small quantities of hCG are produced by the pituitary gland and thus plasma hCG is almost exclusively produced by the placenta. Human chorionic gonadotrophin has a half-life of 6–24 hours and rises to a peak in pregnancy at 9–11 weeks' gestation.

### Urine testing

It is possible to detect low levels of hCG in urine by rapid (1–2 min) dipstick tests. The sensitivity of these tests is high (detection limit of around 50 iu/L) and they produce positive results around 14 days after ovulation.

### Plasma testing

Measurement of hCG in plasma is more accurate (detection limit around 0.1–0.3 iu/L) and is able to detect a pregnancy 6–7 days after ovulation, which corresponds to the time of implantation. Measurement of hCG levels may help to diagnose ectopic pregnancy

and is of pivotal importance in the follow-up of some pregnancy disorders.

## Miscarriage

### Definition

The miscarriage of an early pregnancy is the commonest medical complication in humans, with one in two conceptions lost before the end of the first trimester. Most conceptions are lost during the first month after the last menstrual period and are often undetected, particularly if they occur around the time of an expected menstrual period.

### Epidemiology and risk factors

The rate of clinical pregnancy loss is known to decrease with gestational age, from 25 per cent at 5–6 weeks to 2 per cent after 14 weeks (Table 8.1).

**Table 8.1**  Epidemiology of early pregnancy disorders

| Variable | Percentage |
| --- | --- |
| Total loss of conception | 50–70 |
| Total rate of clinical miscarriage | 25–30 |
| Before 6 weeks | 18 |
| Between 6 and 9 weeks | 4 |
| After 9 weeks | 3 |
| After 14 weeks | 2 |
| Rate of chromosomal defect in miscarriage | 50–70 |
| Rate of miscarriage in primigravidae aged <40 years | 6–10 |
| Rate of miscarriage in primigravidae aged 40+ years | 30–40 |
| Rate of recurrent miscarriages | 1–2 |
| Risk of recurrent miscarriage after three miscarriages | 25–30 |
| Ectopic pregnancies per live births | 2 |
| Complete hydatidiform mole | 0.1 |

## Chromosomal abnormalities and maternal age

The incidence of chromosomal abnormality increases with maternal age. Approximately 50–60 per cent of chromosomal abnormalities are associated with a chromosomal defect of the conceptus, and the frequency of abnormal chromosomal complement increases when embryonic demise occurs earlier in gestation (up to 90 per cent). The risk of pregnancy loss also increases with maternal age, i.e. a 40-year-old woman carries twice the risk of a 20-year-old woman. The past obstetric history also influences the risk. The pregnancy loss rate among primigravidae is 6–10 per cent, whereas the recurrent rate after three or more losses is 25–30 per cent (Table 8.1).

Autosomal trisomies are the most common, with an incidence of 30–35 per cent, followed by triploidies and monosomies X. Triploidy and tetraploidy are common but extremely lethal chromosomal abnormalities and are therefore rarely found in late abortuses. Structural chromosomal rearrangements such as translocations or inversions are present in only 1.5 per cent of abortuses in the general population but are a significant cause of recurrent miscarriages.

## Rare causes of miscarriage

The other causes of miscarriage include endocrine diseases, anatomical abnormalities of the female genital tract, infections, immune factors, chemical agents, hereditary disorders, trauma, maternal diseases and psychological factors (Table 8.2). Prospective epidemiological surveys suggest that the attributable risk of most of these factors to first trimester spontaneous

**Table 8.2**   Aetiological factors of early pregnancy disorders

**Miscarriages**

| | |
|---|---|
| Chromosomal abnormalities (Maternal age >35 years) | Trisomies (Down's syndrome) |
| | Triploidies and tetraploidies |
| | Monosomy X (Turner's syndrome) |
| | Translocation (hereditary) |
| Endocrine disorders | Diabetes, hypothyroidism, luteal phase deficiency, polycystic ovarian syndrome |
| Abnormalities of the uterus | Uterine septa (bicornuate uterus) |
| | Endometrial adhesions (post-curettage or Asherman's syndrome) |
| Infections | *Salmonella typhi*, malaria, cytomegalovirus, *Brucella*, toxoplasmosis, *Mycoplasma hominis*, *Chlamydia trachomatis*, *Ureaplasma urealyticum* |
| Chemical agents | Tobacco, anaesthetic gases, arsenic, benzene, solvents, ethylene oxide, formaldehyde, pesticides, lead, mercury, cadmium |
| Psychological disorders | |
| Immunological disorders | Antiphospholipid syndrome |
| | Thrombophilia (hereditary) |

**Ectopic pregnancies**

| | |
|---|---|
| Maternal age | >35 years |
| Contraception | Intrauterine device |
| Pelvic inflammatory disease | Gonorrhoea, *Chlamydia* |
| Pelvic surgery | Tubal surgery, myomectomy, Caesarean section |

**Complete hydatidiform mole**

| | |
|---|---|
| Maternal age | >35 years |
| Racial/dietary factor | Asia |

abortion is small. Aetiologies such as exposure to certain toxins are rare in the general population but may become an important issue in the context of ecological disasters. Some other causes, such as translocations or thrombophilia, may be found more frequently in cases of recurrent miscarriages.

Müllerian tract fusion and cervical abnormalities are well-accepted causes of second trimester losses, but are not associated with a higher rate of first trimester miscarriages.

## Differential diagnosis

There are four different clinical forms of miscarriages.

### Threatened miscarriage

A threatened miscarriage is defined as painless vaginal bleeding occurring any time between implantation and 24 weeks' gestation. Probably one-quarter of all pregnancies are complicated by threatened miscarriage, although many patients may be unaware of their pregnancy when they present with vaginal bleeding.

Threatened miscarriage is one of the most common indications (together with suspected ectopic pregnancy) for emergency referral of young women to a casualty department. The bleeding may resolve spontaneously in a few days, never to recur, or it may continue, or stop and start over several days or weeks. It is only when abdominal cramps supervene that the process may become inevitable, in particular if the

---

**P** | **Understanding the pathophysiology**

**Disturbance of placentation**

In most cases of early pregnancy failure there is an inadequate placentation. In particular, there is a defective transformation of the spiral arteries and a reduced trophoblastic penetration into the decidua and into the spiral arteries (see Fig. 8.2). This defect of placentation is more pronounced in chromosomal abnormalities.

In pregnancies complicated by hypertension, there is a probable relationship between the severity of the disease and the degree of inadequate placentation. If this concept is extrapolated to the first trimester, some forms of recurrent, early spontaneous abortions related to medical disorders associated with a defect of placentation, such as systemic lupus erythematosus, could represent the earliest manifestation of this phenomenon.

---

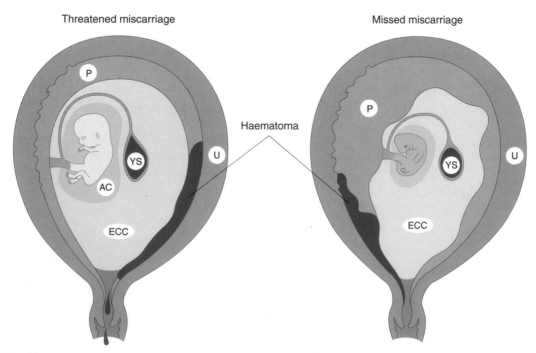

**Figure 8.5** Diagram showing the different types of miscarriage. (P, placenta; U, uterus; AC, amniotic cavity; YS, yolk sac; ECC, extra-coloemic cavity.)

cervix opens. The bleeding usually occurs between 6 and 9 weeks' gestation when the definitive placenta forms (Fig. 8.5).

The diagnosis is usually based on clinical examination. The role of ultrasound and endocrinology in predicting this type of early pregnancy complication remains controversial. Nevertheless, the evaluation of the size of the gestational sac or the embryo and demonstration of embryonic heart action are important in the management of this common pregnancy complication. Within this context, ultrasound probably plays its most important role in reassuring the patient that the fetus is alive and developing normally.

### Missed miscarriage

A missed miscarriage is a gestational sac containing a dead embryo/fetus before 20 weeks' gestation without clinical symptoms of expulsion. The diagnosis is usually made by failure to identify a fetal heart beat on ultrasound (Fig. 8.5). Within this context, the mother often complains of chronic but light vaginal bleeding. With the introduction of transvaginal ultrasound, the diagnosis can now be made from as early as 6 weeks' gestation. When the gestational sac is more than 25 mm in diameter and no embryonic/fetal part can be seen, the terms 'blighted ovum' and 'anembryonic pregnancy' are often used by pathologists and more commonly by obstetricians, suggesting wrongly that the sac may have developed without an embryo. The explanation for this feature is the early death and resorption of the embryo with persistence of the placental tissue rather than a pregnancy originally without an embryo.

### Inevitable miscarriage

An inevitable miscarriage can be complete or incomplete, depending on whether or not all fetal and placental tissues have been expelled from the uterus (Fig. 8.5). The typical features of incomplete abortion are heavy, sometimes intermittent, bleeding with passage of clots and tissue, together with lower abdominal cramps. If these symptoms improve spontaneously, a complete abortion is more likely. Ultrasound examination is important in determining the absence or persistence of conception products inside the uterine cavity.

### Recurrent miscarriage

Recurrent miscarriage is defined as three or more consecutive spontaneous abortions. The aetiologies of recurrent pregnancy failure are diverse and not well understood. They may present clinically as any of the previously described forms of miscarriages.

## Clinical features

### History

A history of amenorrhoea followed by vaginal bleeding with low abdominal pain and a positive pregnancy test is fundamental. Other factors pertinent to the history are maternal age, medical disorders and a previous history of miscarriage.

### General examination

This must include a record of pulse rate and blood pressure, and assessment of hand palm and conjunctival colour will give an idea about secondary anaemia.

### Speculum examination

When a patient is seen during the first trimester with vaginal bleeding, a history of abdominal pain and passage of clots or tissue through an open cervix, the diagnosis of abortion is usually conspicuous. When the cervix is closed and the bleeding is not heavy, however, distinguishing between complete or incomplete miscarriage and threatened or missed abortion can be difficult on clinical findings only.

### Ultrasound examination

Ultrasound will confirm the intrauterine location of the gestational sac and establish the viability of the pregnancy. If the gestational sac is smaller than expected for gestational age, the possibility of incorrect dates should always be considered, especially in the absence of clinical features suggestive of threatened abortion. Under these circumstances a repeat scan should be arranged after a period of at least 7 days and be performed by an experienced operator.

### Laboratory investigations

These must include a full blood count and blood group. Patients who are Rhesus negative must systematically receive a dose of anti-D in case of bleeding during pregnancy.

Human chorionic gonadotrophin, progesterone and other placental hormones are of limited use in predicting a miscarriage. The correlations of ultrasound and circulating placental protein measurements indicate that the diagnostic value of ultrasound in threatened miscarriage is often better than that of biochemical tests. As a clinical predictive tool, measurement of placental proteins is often unnecessary if fetal life can be demonstrated by ultrasound.

## Management

### Surgical

The mechanical dilatation and curettage of the uterus for the evacuation of retained products of conception is usually a simple procedure. Complications are uncommon and include cervical tears, uterine perforation and the creation of false passage. Some of these complications can be prevented by cervical preparation, using prostaglandins.

### Medical

This includes surveillance, drug therapy and psychological support. Women with minimal residual tissue in the uterine cavity on ultrasound can be safely treated

**Table 8.3**   Diagnosis and management of early pregnancy disorders

| | Features |
|---|---|
| **Miscarriage** | |
| Threatened miscarriage | Normal hCG for gestational age |
| | Intrauterine gestational sac |
| | Embryonic/fetal heart activity |
| | Intrauterine bleeding/haematoma |
| Management → Clinical surveillance including weekly ultrasound examination | |
| Missed miscarriage | Low hCG for gestational age |
| | Intrauterine gestational sac (>20 mm in diameter) with no embryo or with 6 mm embryo with no heart activity on TVS |
| Management → Surgical evacuation (ERPC) or medical induction (RU486 + Pgs) | |
| Incomplete miscarriage | Persistence of conception products inside the uterine cavity on TVS |
| Management → Surgical evacuation (ERPC) or medical induction (RU486 + Pgs) | |
| **Ectopic pregnancies** | Normal to low hCG for gestational age (discriminatory level) |
| | Small uterus for gestational age with no gestational sac or small pseudosac (decidual reaction) on TVS |
| | Adnexal gestational sac or mass with or without pelvic fluid on TVS |
| Management → Salpingectomy (removal of the tube and gestational sac) or salpingotomy (opening of the tube and removal of the gestational sac only) via laparoscopy or laparotomy | |
| **Complete hydatidiform mole** | Very high hCG for gestational age |
| | Uterine enlargement greater than expected for gestational age |
| | Uterine cavity filled with multiple sonolucent areas of varying size and shape without associated embryo/fetus |
| Management → Surgical evacuation (ERPC) and weekly hCG level monitoring until undetectable, followed by monthly monitoring for 6–24 months | |

hCG, human chorionic gonadotrophin; TVS, transvaginal ultrasound; ERPC, evacuation of retained products of conception; RU486 + Pgs, prostaglandins.

expectantly. Prostaglandin analogues have been used within the context of missed abortion but so far the results have been disappointing. This is because when they are administered vaginally, complete evacuation of the uterus is achieved in only half the cases because of the long interval required. Mifepristone (RU 486) is a progesterone competitive antagonist, which, used in combination with prostaglandin analogues, has been shown to be effective in about 90 per cent of cases.

### Follow-up

Although the majority of miscarriages are not treatable, the prognosis for future pregnancies is directly dependent on the type of abnormality and on whether the mother or her partner carries it. Counselling the parents regarding the diagnostic evaluation processes, treatments required, prognosis and risks for future pregnancies should always be offered in cases of early pregnancy failure.

For couples with recurrent miscarriages (more than three consecutive miscarriages) investigation should include parental and fetal karyotype to exclude a translocation, gynaecological examination to exclude a uterine abnormality, and blood tests (glucose level, thyroid function tests, antiphospholipid and anticardiolipin antibodies, lupus anticoagulant) (Table 8.3).

## Ectopic pregnancy

## Definition

An ectopic pregnancy occurs when the conceptus implants either outside the uterus (Fallopian tube, ovary or abdominal cavity) or in an abnormal position within the uterus (cornua, cervix). Combined tubal and uterine (heterotopic) pregnancies are uncommon.

## Epidemiology and risk factors

The incidence of ectopic pregnancy is 22 per 1000 live births and 16 per 1000 pregnancies. A dramatic increase in incidence over time has been reported in several countries. During the period 1970–1992 in the USA, the overall increase was almost fivefold, from 4 to 19 per 1000 pregnancies. Between 95 and 98 per cent of ectopic pregnancies occur in the Fallopian tube. More than 50 per cent of tubal pregnancies are situated in the ampulla, approximately 20 per cent occur in the isthmus, around 12 per cent are fimbrial and approximately 10 per cent are interstitial (Fig. 8.6).

### Risk factors

The risk of ectopic pregnancy increases with maternal age, number of sexual partners, the use of an intrauterine device, after proven pelvic inflammatory disease (gonorrhoea, *Chlamydia*) and after pelvic surgery. The risk of recurrence is around 10 per cent and is increased in those who have had a previous miscarriage or who have suffered tubal damage.

### Mortality rate

In England and Wales, the mortality rate due to ectopic pregnancy fell from 17 per million deliveries in 1961–63 to 4 per million in 1982–84. Despite this decline in case-fatality rates, mortality from ectopic pregnancy remains high, representing 13 per cent of all maternal deaths in 1989. The fatality rate of ectopic pregnancy is about four times that of childbirth.

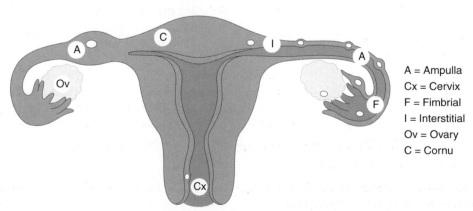

A = Ampulla
Cx = Cervix
F = Fimbrial
I = Interstitial
Ov = Ovary
C = Cornu

**Figure 8.6** Diagram showing the different possible locations of an ectopic pregnancy.

## P  Understanding the pathophysiology

### Ectopic pregnancy

In theory, any mechanical or functional factors that prevent or interfere with the passage of the fertilized egg to the uterine cavity may be aetiological factors for an ectopic pregnancy.

It is believed that the main cause for a tubal implantation of the gestational sac is a low-grade infection, as approximately 50 per cent of women operated on for an ectopic pregnancy have evidence of chronic pelvic inflammatory disease. A high proportion of women with a tubal pregnancy miscarry during the early stages of gestation. The products of conception may persist for a considerable period of time within the tube as one form of 'chronic ectopic pregnancy', or they may be gradually absorbed.

If implantation occurs into a site of the tube that offers a sufficient area for placentation, the process is very similar to that of an intrauterine pregnancy, for the conceptus penetrates the tubal mucosa and becomes embedded in the tissues of the tubal wall (Fig. 8.6). The extravillous trophoblast will penetrate the full thickness of the muscular layer of the tube to reach the subserosa and the tubo-ovarian circulation. Due to its limited distensibility, the tube will rupture. Although this event is usually accompanied by fetal death, occasionally following the rupture the fetus retains sufficient attachment to its blood supply to maintain viability and secondary abdominal pregnancy can proceed to term.

In an ectopic pregnancy, the uterine endometrium usually responds to the hormonal changes of pregnancy and undergoes focal decidua changes (Arias–Stella reaction). If the ectopic pregnancy miscarries, the uterine decidua may slough off as a cast, but more commonly as fragments mixed with small blood clots.

## Clinical features

Compared to the other forms of early pregnancy disorders, there is no pathognomonic pain or findings on clinical examination that are diagnostic of a developing extrauterine pregnancy. Vaginal bleeding (usually old blood in small amounts) and chronic pelvic pain (iliac fossa, sometimes bilateral) are the most commonly reported symptoms.

### General examination

This must include a record of pulse rate and blood pressure. Shoulder pain, which may occur secondary to blood irritating the diaphragm and vascular instability characterized by low blood pressure, fainting, dizziness and rapid heart rate may be noted. These symptoms are present in about 59 per cent of patients and are most typical of patients whose ectopic pregnancy has ruptured (intra-abdominal bleeding).

### Gynaecological examination

Speculum or bimanual examination must be performed in an environment where facilities for resuscitation are available, as this examination may provoke the rupture of the tube.

### Laparoscopy and uterine curettage

These have traditionally been the gold standard by which to establish the diagnosis of extrauterine pregnancy. The mere absence of placental villi in the curettage does not necessarily indicate an ectopic pregnancy. Conversely, the presence of placental villi in the curettage does not completely exclude a diagnosis of ectopic pregnancy because an ectopic pregnancy in a tube, cornu or the cervix may partially abort.

### Culdocentesis

Culdocentesis to exclude haemoperitoneum has also been a routine investigation in the emergency room to rule out ectopic pregnancy. Because this test is based on late development in the natural history of the ectopic pregnancy, it is obviously not going to be useful in detecting an early ectopic pregnancy.

### Human chorionic gonadotrophin and transvaginal ultrasound

Screening algorithms incorporating plasma hCG and transvaginal sonography have allowed for a less invasive evaluation of the patient with a suspected ectopic pregnancy. The hCG levels and ultrasound findings must be interpreted together. One of the most important parameters is the discriminatory hCG level above which the gestational sac of an intrauterine pregnancy should be detectable by ultrasonography (usually 1000 iu/L).

The presence or absence of an intrauterine gestational sac is the principal point of distinction between intrauterine and tubal pregnancy. The sonographic finding of an extrauterine sac with an embryo or embryonic remnants is the most reliable diagnosis of ectopic pregnancy. An empty ectopic sac or a hetero-geneous adnexal mass is a more common ultrasound feature. The presence of fluid in the pouch of Douglas is a non-specific sign of ectopic pregnancy. In 10–20 per cent of ectopic pregnancies, a pseudogestational sac is seen as a small, centrally located endometrial fluid collection surrounded by a single echogenic rim of endometrial tissue undergoing decidual reaction.

Laparoscopy should be considered in women with hCG above the discriminatory level and absence of an intrauterine gestational sac on ultrasound.

## Management

The classical approach to the treatment of ectopic pregnancy has always been surgical (salpingectomy or salpingotomy), either by laparotomy or laparoscopy.

With the wider use of ultrasound, an early diagnosis is now possible in many cases before the onset of symptoms. Non-surgical (medical) therapeutic approaches have been introduced, such as puncture and aspiration of the ectopic sac, local injections of prostaglandins, potassium chloride, hyperosmolar glucose or methotrexate. The advantages of treatment that does not involve surgery or the use of potentially toxic drugs are obvious. With earlier diagnosis it has also become apparent that spontaneous regression of tubal pregnancies is more common than previously thought. This has led to non-interventional expectant management, which is based on the assumption that a significant proportion of all tubal pregnancies will resolve without any treatment. Unfortunately, not all patients will be suitable for this type of treatment or for a simple follow-up, and strict criteria must be observed in the selection of patients. Ultrasound examinations combined with serial hCG assessments are prerequisites for successful expectant management or in the follow-up of the patient treated medically.

## Gestational trophoblastic disorders

## Definitions

Gestational trophoblastic disorder is a term commonly applied to a spectrum of inter-related diseases originating from the placental trophoblast. The main categories of GTD are complete hydatidiform mole,

partial hydatidiform mole and choriocarcinoma. Complete or classical hydatidiform mole is described as a generalized swelling of the villous tissue, diffuse trophoblastic hyperplasia and no embryonic or fetal tissue. Partial hydatidiform mole is characterized by focal swelling of the villous tissue, focal trophoblastic hyperplasia and embryonic or fetal tissue. The abnormal villi are scattered within macroscopically normal placental tissue that tends to retain its shape.

## Epidemiology and risk factors

### Incidence rate
Estimates of the incidence of the various forms of GTD vary, mainly because few countries have registries and complete and partial moles have often been treated as a single entity in epidemiological studies. The estimated incidence of complete mole is 1 per 1000–2000 pregnancies (see Table 8.1), whereas the incidence of partial mole is around 1 per 700 pregnancies. The vast majority of complete and partial moles abort spontaneously during the first trimester, and the incidence of molar pregnancies has been estimated to be 2 per cent of all miscarriages. The incidence of choriocarcinoma varies from 1 in 10 000 to 1 in 50 000 pregnancies, or, expressed as a percentage of hydatidiform mole, 3–10 per cent.

### Risk factors
High maternal age and a previous history of molar pregnancy have consistently been shown to influence the risk of hydatidiform mole and choriocarcinoma, whereas the evidence that the rate of molar pregnancies varies according to the dietary habits of some ethnic groups remains controversial. The ABO blood groups of the parents appear to be a factor in choriocarcinoma development, i.e. women with blood group A have been shown to have a greater risk than blood group O women.

## Clinical features

### General and gynaecological examination
Patients with a complete mole present with vaginal bleeding, uterine enlargement greater than expected for gestational age and an abnormally high level of serum hCG. Medical complications include pregnancy-induced hypertension, hyperthyroidism, hyperemesis,

anaemia and the development of ovarian theca lutein cysts. The ovarian hyperstimulation and enlargement of both ovaries may subsequently lead to ovarian torsion or rupture of theca lutein cysts.

The primary symptoms of choriocarcinoma are gynaecological, i.e. vaginal bleeding, in only 50–60 per cent of the cases. Many women will present with dyspnoea, neurological symptoms and abdominal pain a few weeks or months and sometimes up to 10–15 years after their last pregnancy.

### P Understanding the pathophysiology

**Complete hydatidiform moles**
These have a diploid chromosomal constitution totally derived from the paternal genome and usually resulting from the fertilization of an oocyte by a diploid spermatozoon. The maternal chromosomes may be either inactivated or absent, remaining only inside the mitochondria.

**Partial moles**
Partial moles are usually triploid and of diandric origin, having two sets of chromosomes from paternal origin and one from maternal origin. Most have a 69XXX or 69XXY genotype derived from a haploid ovum, with either reduplication of the paternal haploid set from a single sperm or, less frequently, from dispermic fertilization. Triploidy of digynic origin, due to a double maternal contribution, is not associated with placental hydatidiform changes.

**Choriocarcinoma**
Choriocarcinoma is a highly malignant tumour that arises from the trophoblastic epithelium and metastasizes readily to the lungs, liver and brain. Around 50 per cent of choriocarcinomas follow a molar pregnancy, 30 per cent occur after a miscarriage and 20 per cent after an apparently normal pregnancy. Choriocarcinomas can occur after an extrauterine pregnancy and will present with signs and symptoms similar to those classically outlined for ectopic pregnancy. There have been a few well-documented examples of choriocarcinoma arising from villous tissue in an otherwise normally developed placenta, suggesting that most or possibly all choriocarcinomas that follow an apparently normal pregnancy are in reality metastases from a small intraplacental choriocarcinoma.

### *Arteriography*

Arteriography was first used in the in-utero diagnosis of molar pregnancy. Because of cost, maternal discomfort and morbidity, it was rapidly replaced by ultrasound imaging in the 1960s. In women with persistent GTD or with chemotherapy-resistant disease, angiography has proved to be of great value in the diagnostic work-up of myometrial invasion and surgical management.

### *Ultrasound examination*
Molar changes can now be detected from the second month of pregnancy by ultrasound, which typically reveals a uterine cavity filled with multiple sonolucent areas of varying size and shape ('snow-storm appearance') without associated embryonic or fetal structure (Fig. 8.7).

### *Laboratory examinations*
The measurement of plasma hCG is pivotal in the diagnosis and follow-up of GTD.

### *Other investigations*
These must include a histological examination of the sample confirming the trophoblastic hyperplasia and a chest X-ray to exclude the presence of lung metastasis.

## Management

Following uterine evacuation, 18–29 per cent of patients with a complete mole and 1–11 per cent of

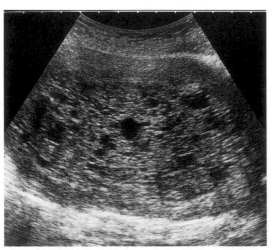

**Figure 8.7** Ultrasound view of a complete hydatidiform mole at the end of the first trimester.

patients with a partial mole will develop a persistent trophoblastic tumour. Pulmonary complications due to trophoblastic embolization are frequently observed following the evacuation of a molar pregnancy, and the prognosis for these patients depends on the severity of the symptoms. Thus early diagnosis reduces the risk of severe complications and in particular respiratory failure.

Serial measurement of hCG levels is the gold standard for diagnosis and monitoring the therapeutic response of GTD. After evacuation of a molar pregnancy, the hCG level should be monitored weekly until undetectable, followed by monthly monitoring for 6–24 months.

## New developments

Ultrasound imaging has improved the diagnostic capability of early pregnancy disorders. The diagnosis of suspected miscarriages and life-threatening ectopic pregnancies is now more accurate and less invasive than it has ever been in the past. Ultrasound and, in particular, transvaginal sonography combined with fast and accurate

hCG testing are the best routine tools that obstetricians and gynaecologists can offer women with an abnormal early pregnancy.

## Key Points

- The miscarriage of an early pregnancy is the commonest medical complication.
- Human chorionic gonadotrophin is a placental-specific protein that can be detected in maternal plasma and urine 7 and 14 days after ovulation, respectively.
- Transvaginal ultrasound should demonstrate a gestational sac from 4.4–4.6 weeks after the last menstrual period.
- Mortality from ectopic pregnancy remains high, as its incidence has increased over the last 15 years (1–2 per cent of pregnancies).
- Screening algorithms incorporating plasma hCG and transvaginal sonography should allow the diagnosis of most ectopic pregnancies before tubal rupture.
- Complete and partial hydatidiform moles can be complicated by persistent trophoblastic disease and the patient should be offered follow-up.

## CASE HISTORY

Miss SP is a single, 24-year-old Caucasian who weighs 64 kg. She presents with a 2-day history of right iliac fossa pain and some vaginal bleeding. Her last period was 6 weeks prior to the onset of pain and her periods have been regular. She has not been using regular contraception but has a regular partner. She admits to some breast tenderness and feeling nauseous first thing in the morning. She has no significant past medical history and has never previously been pregnant. She is otherwise fit and well.

On examination, she looks well and is afebrile. She has some guarding and rebound tenderness in the right iliac fossa. Vaginal examination confirms tenderness in the right iliac fossa and there is no unusual vaginal discharge.

Her pregnancy test is positive.

## Discussion

### What is the differential diagnosis?
There are several causes for bleeding in early pregnancy. She could have a threatened or incomplete miscarriage. It is unlikely that this is a complete miscarriage, as she has only

had a light bleed. It is also possible she might have had a missed miscarriage. However, the most likely diagnosis is ectopic pregnancy and this must be excluded before assuming another cause. It is also possible that she may have an early pregnancy that is intact, with other pathology such as an ovarian cyst that may have ruptured, torted or haemorrhaged. She may even have accompanying appendicitis.

### How would you make a diagnosis?
As the patient seems systemically well but the diagnosis of ectopic pregnancy has not been excluded, blood should be taken for blood count, grouping and saving and intravenous access must be maintained. An ultrasound scan will confirm whether or not the gestation is intrauterine and viable. Vaginal ultrasound would probably be of most benefit at this stage. If there is no intrauterine pregnancy and no obvious ectopic pregnancy, a laparoscopy is still indicated to exclude an ectopic pregnancy. The optimum management may include laparoscopic removal of the ectopic pregnancy through a salpingotomy or even salpingectomy.

## Additional reading

Jurkovic D. Ultrasound and early pregnancy. In: Jauniaux E (ed.) Carforth: Parthenon Publishing, 1996.

O'Brien PMS, Grudzinskas JG (eds). *Problems of early pregnancy – advances in diagnosis and management.* London: RCOG, 1997.

Royal College of Radiologists/Royal College of Obstetricians and Gynaecologists. *Guidance on ultrasound procedures in early pregnancy.* London: RCR/RCOG, 1995.

# Benign disease of the uterus and cervix

## OVERVIEW

Benign disease of the cervix and body of the uterus is extremely common. Cervical ectropion and fibroids are often present without symptoms, but are also common problems encountered in almost every gynaecological outpatient clinic. Adenomyosis and endometriosis, other important benign conditions, are considered in Chapter 10.

Benign disease of the uterus may conveniently be classified in terms of the tissue of origin: the uterine cervix, the endometrium or the myometrium.

## Epithelium: the uterine cervix

The transformation zone is a special feature of the ecto-cervix, and corresponds to that portion of the uterine cervix visible during speculum examination. Within this zone the stratified squamous epithelium of the vagina meets the columnar epithelium of the cervical canal. The anatomical site of the squamocolumnar junction fluctuates under hormonal influence, and the high cell turnover of this tissue is important in the pathogenesis of cervical carcinoma, discussed in Chapter 12. The columnar epithelium is normally visible with the speculum during the ovulatory phase of the menstrual cycle, during pregnancy and in women taking the combined oral contraceptive pill, in whom oestrogen levels are elevated. In contrast, only squamous epithelium is visible in a postmenopausal woman not taking hormone replacement therapy.

### Cervical ectropion

The presence of a large area of columnar epithelium on the ectocervix can be associated with excessive mucus secretion, leading to a complaint of vaginal discharge. The appearance of the cervix is termed cervical ectropion or, very inappropriately, a 'cervical erosion'. The latter term is best avoided, as it conveys quite the wrong impression of what is really a normal phenomenon. Ectropion can be associated with excessive but non-purulent vaginal discharge, as the surface area of columnar epithelium containing mucus-secreting glands is increased. If the discharge associated with cervical ectropion becomes troublesome to the patient, discontinuing the oral contraceptive pill or, alternatively, ablative treatment under local anaesthesia using a thermal probe can reduce it. This treatment involves a metal probe that heats the tissue to around 100 °C, destroying the epithelium to a depth of 3–4 mm. The technique is sometimes confusingly termed 'cold coagulation' to distinguish it from more destructive diathermy or laser treatment of the cervix. A less glandular epithelium regenerates after the procedure.

Cervical ectropion may also give rise to postcoital bleeding, as fine blood vessels present within the columnar epithelium are easily traumatized. This symptom may be very distressing as well as embarrassing, but a direct question should always be asked when taking the gynaecological history because of its association with cervical carcinoma. Reassurance about the cause and treatment as described above can be given after obtaining a normal cervical cytology result.

## Nabothian follicles

Within the transformation zone of the ectocervix the exposed columnar epithelium undergoes squamous metaplasia. Glands contained within columnar epithelium may become roofed over with squamous cells, resulting in the formation of small (2–3 mm) mucus-filled cysts visible on the ectocervix. These are termed Nabothian follicles, and are of no pathological significance. Larger (up to 10 mm) Nabothian follicles are occasionally identified coincidentally during transvaginal ultrasound scanning, but do not require treatment.

## Endometrium

The uterine endometrium comprises glands and stroma with a complex architecture, including blood vessels and nerves. As discussed in detail in Chapter 4, during the follicular phase of the menstrual cycle, proliferation of tissue from the basal layer occurs, followed by secretory changes under the influence of progesterone after ovulation and finally shedding as progesterone levels fall, with corpus luteum regression. Disturbances of prostaglandin biosynthesis within the endometrium may give rise to menstrual disorders (see Chapter 5), but the increased use of endoscopy and ultrasound has given more specific appreciation of visible abnormalities of the endometrium.

## Endometrial polyps

Historically, a diagnosis of 'dysfunctional uterine bleeding' was made in women with menstrual disturbance in whom curettage provided a histologically normal sample of endometrium. In current practice, hysteroscopy or ultrasound enables the identification of endometrial polyps that may be the cause of abnormal bleeding, especially intermenstrual bleeding. These polyps typically occur in women aged over 40 years. Intermenstrual bleeding in younger women is more likely to be a consequence of combined or progestogen-only contraceptive pill use or the wearing of an intrauterine contraceptive device (IUCD), and is less likely to require investigation. In perimenopausal or postmenopausal women with abnormal bleeding, the first priority is to exclude endometrial malignancy, but in many patients the cause will turn out to be a benign polyp that can be removed at hysteroscopy. Reflecting typical clinical experience, polyps were detected by outpatient hysteroscopy in 11 per cent of 2581 women referred for the investigation of menstrual symptoms.

After the menopause the endometrium is normally atrophic, but hormone replacement therapy does provide endometrial stimulation, leading to polyp formation. Women presenting special diagnostic problems are those taking tamoxifen for the treatment of breast cancer. This agent is a partial oestrogen agonist with inhibitory effects on breast tissue. However, the endometrium is stimulated, sometimes leading to polyp formation or even endometrial hyperplasia and malignancy. Ultrasound assessment is difficult because the drug affects the sonographic properties of the inner myometrium, giving the misleading impression of a greatly thickened endometrium.

## Asherman's syndrome

When the endometrium has been damaged, in particular when it has been removed down to or beyond the basal layer, normal regeneration does not occur, and instead there is fibrosis and adhesion formation, termed Asherman's syndrome. This phenomenon is exploited therapeutically in endometrial resection, a surgical treatment for menorrhagia in which the endometrium is resected using a diathermy loop or is ablated with a laser, in each case beyond the basal layer into the myometrium so that regeneration cannot occur. The result is reduced, or absent, menstrual shedding.

Asherman's syndrome occurs as an adverse consequence of excessive curettage, especially at the time of evacuation of retained placental tissue after miscarriage or secondary postpartum haemorrhage. In a hysteroscopic follow-up study after surgical evacuation following retained placenta, the prevalence of adhesions within the endometrial cavity was 20 per cent, and these were strongly associated with menstrual symptoms. Treatment options for Asherman's syndrome include maintaining separation of the uterine walls by insertion of a large inert IUCD such as a Lippes loop (now obsolete other than for this purpose) or hysteroscopic lysis of intrauterine adhesions.

Other causes of Asherman's syndrome relevant in particular parts of the world are tuberculosis and schistosomiasis.

## Complications of cervical stenosis

When premalignant disease of the cervix was treated by knife cone biopsy, rather than the currently preferred technique of diathermy loop excision (see Chapter 12), subsequent cervical stenosis was common. This is now less commonly seen, but it may give rise to haematometra as menstrual blood accumulates in the endometrial cavity. Suggestive features in the history are amenorrhoea associated with severe cyclical dysmenorrhoea-like pain, with a previous history of cervical surgery. In postmenopausal women, cervical stenosis may give rise to pyometra, in which accumulated secretions become a focus of infection. Underlying malignancy may also lead to pyometra. Treatment is by careful surgical dilatation of the cervix and endometrial biopsy under antibiotic cover. Finally, a cervix not completely stenosed but scarred from previous surgery may fail to dilate during labour (cervical dystocia), necessitating Caesarean section.

## Myometrium: uterine fibroids

### Pathology

A fibroid is a benign tumour of uterine smooth muscle, termed a leiomyoma. The gross appearance is of a firm, whorled tumour located adjacent to and bulging into the endometrial cavity (submucous fibroid), centrally within the myometrium (intramural fibroid), at the outer border of the myometrium (subserosal fibroid) or attached to the uterus by a narrow pedicle containing blood vessels (pedunculated fibroid) (Fig. 9.1). Fibroids can arise separately from the uterus, especially in the broad ligament, presumably from embryonal remnants. The typical whorled appearance may be altered following degeneration, three forms of which are recognized: red, hyaline and cystic.

Red degeneration follows an acute disruption of the blood supply to the fibroid during active growth, classically during pregnancy. This may present with the sudden onset of pain and tenderness localized to an area of the uterus, associated with a mild pyrexia and leukocytosis. The symptoms and signs typically resolve over a few days and surgical intervention is rarely required.

Hyaline degeneration occurs when the fibroid more gradually outgrows its blood supply, and may progress to central necrosis, leaving cystic spaces at the centre, termed cystic degeneration. As the final stage in the natural history, calcification of a fibroid may be detected incidentally on an abdominal X-ray in a postmenopausal woman. Rarely, malignant or sarcomatous degeneration has been said to occur, but

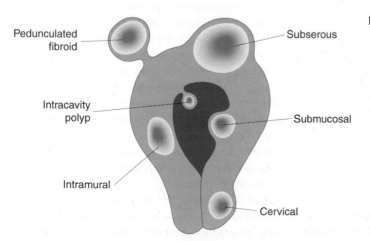

**Figure 9.1** Typical location of uterine fibroids.

Pedunculated fibroid

Subserous

Intracavity polyp

Submucosal

Intramural

Cervical

## P  Understanding the pathophysiology

### Aetiology

A range of hypotheses accounting for the pathogenesis of fibroids has been explored. The key features of uterine leiomyomata are their occurrence during the reproductive years, where ovarian hormone levels are high, their diverse manifestation as either single or multiple tumours, and the existence of racial and familial predisposition. The possibility of abnormal oestrogen receptor expression has been explored and discounted: both main progesterone receptor subtypes are expressed similarly in myoma and normal myometrium. Thus myoma tissue is still influenced by ovarian hormones. Experimentally, progesterone has been shown to stimulate the production of both an apoptosis-inhibiting protein and epidermal growth factor (EGF) in cultured myoma tissue. Oestradiol has the effect of stimulating expression of the EGF receptor.

Reduced expression of growth inhibitory factors such as monocyte chemotactic protein-1 (MCP-1) may play a part in the loss of inhibition required for fibroid growth. Treatment by ovarian suppression (see below) is associated with an increase in matrix metalloproteinase (MMP) expression and a decrease in metalloproteinase inhibitory (TIMP) activity, which suggests that ovarian hormones have a role in maintaining the architecture of a myoma once formed.

Cytogenetic studies have identified specific features of uterine myoma tissue compared to normal myometrium and to leiomyosarcoma. It appears that cells within an individual myoma are monoclonal in origin, but cells from different myomas within the same uterus are of independent origin. It is likely that the clonal expansion of tumour cells precedes the development of cytogenetic aberrations, but the latter may determine the clinical course, depending on the extent to which control over growth is lost. Some evidence for this is provided by cytogenetic analysis, which showed a greater proportion of karyotypic abnormality in larger, compared to smaller, fibroids. The most common cytogenetic aberrations detected have been on chromosomes 12, 6, 3 and 7, a ring chromosome 1, and translocation involving chromosomes 12 and 14. Relevant areas of chromosomes 12, 6 and 7 are thought to contain putative growth-regulating or tumour-suppressor genes. It is not yet clear to what extent the cytogenetic features can be correlated with the clinical picture.

The possibility of malignant transformation of a fibroid to a leiomyosarcoma has traditionally been cited as a reason to recommend surgery for fibroids, with a stated risk of up to 0.5 per cent. However, current opinion is that where a sarcoma develops in the presence of fibroids, the association is coincidental and malignant transformation of a fibroid is unlikely. The cytogenetic evidence gives some basis for reassurance on this point, as the typical findings in leiomyosarcoma tissue are of more extensive genetic instability with frequent deletions, especially involving chromosomes 1 and 10.

malignancy probably arises through a separate pathway of chromosomal deletions (see the box above) and the real possibility of malignant change in a fibroid is vanishingly small.

## Clinical features

Fibroids are common, being detectable clinically in about 20 per cent of women over 30 years of age. Autopsy studies with systematic histology of the uterus show a prevalence of up to 50 per cent. Risk factors for clinically significant fibroids are nulliparity, obesity, a positive family history and African racial origin. The great majority do not cause symptoms but may be identified coincidentally, for example at the time of taking a cervical smear or performing laparoscopic sterilization. Common presenting complaints are menstrual disturbance and pressure symptoms, especially urinary frequency. Pain is unusual except in the special circumstance of acute degeneration discussed above. Menorrhagia may occur coincidentally in a woman with fibroids; it is likely that only submucous fibroids distorting the endometrial cavity and increasing the surface area are truly causal.

Subfertility may result from mechanical distortion or occlusion of the Fallopian tubes, and an endometrial cavity grossly distorted by submucous fibroids may prevent implantation of a fertilized ovum. Once a pregnancy is established, however, the risk of miscarriage is not increased. In late pregnancy, fibroids located in the cervix or lower uterine segment may be the cause of an abnormal lie. After delivery, postpartum haemorrhage may occur due to inefficient uterine contraction.

Abdominal examination might indicate the presence of a firm mass arising from the pelvis, and on bimanual examination the mass is felt to be part of the uterus, usually with some mobility.

## Differential diagnosis

Other causes of an abdominopelvic mass in a woman in the reproductive years need to be considered. The uterus enlarged with fibroids is typically firm in contrast to a uterus enlarged with a pregnancy. An ovarian tumour, whether benign or malignant, primary or secondary, may enlarge to occupy the pelvis and be clinically difficult to differentiate from a uterine fibroid. Leiomyosarcomas typically present with a history of a rapidly enlarging abdominopelvic mass. There may be less mobility of the uterus than expected with a fibroid and general signs of cachexia.

## Investigations

Often the clinical features alone will be sufficient to establish the diagnosis. A haemoglobin concentration will help to indicate anaemia if there is clinically significant menorrhagia. Ultrasonography is useful to distinguish a uterine from an ovarian mass. Imaging of the renal tract may be helpful in the presence of a large fibroid to exclude hydronephrosis due to pressure from the mass on the ureters. Clinical suspicion of sarcoma will be an indication for needle biopsy or, more likely, urgent laparotomy.

## Treatment

Conservative management is appropriate where asymptomatic fibroids are detected incidentally. It may be useful to establish the growth rate of the fibroids by repeat clinical examination or ultrasound after a 6–12-month interval. Where treatment is required, the only practical currently available medical treatment is ovarian suppression using a gonadotrophin-releasing hormone (GnRH) agonist. Unfortunately, while very effective in shrinking fibroids, when ovarian function returns, the fibroids regrow to their previous dimensions. Mifepristone (an antiprogestogen) has been shown to be effective in shrinking fibroids at a low dose, but is not available for use in this indication. The optimal dose, duration of treatment and long-term effects have yet to be established.

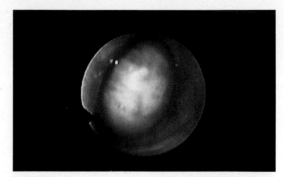

**Figure 9.2** Hysteroscopic appearance of a fibroid polyp within the endometrial cavity. (Kindly supplied by Mr ED Alexopoulos.)

The choice of surgical treatment is determined by the presenting complaint and the patient's aspirations for menstrual function and fertility. Menorrhagia associated with a submucous fibroid or fibroid polyp (Fig. 9.2) may be treated by hysteroscopic resection. Where a bulky fibroid uterus causes pressure symptoms, the options are myomectomy with uterine conservation, or hysterectomy. Myomectomy will be the preferred option where preservation of fertility is required, but care must be taken in the management of a subsequent pregnancy, as the uterus may be predisposed to rupture. It is traditionally held that uterine rupture during pregnancy is more likely when the endometrial cavity has been entered during myomectomy, but, not surprisingly, there are few data to confirm or refute this. In any event, the decision to undertake myomectomy in a woman who desires future fertility needs to be carefully considered and the benefits and risks fully discussed with the patient. An important point for the preoperative discussion is that there is a small but significant risk of uncontrolled bleeding during myomectomy, which could lead to the need for hysterectomy.

Hysterectomy and myomectomy can be facilitated by GnRH agonist pretreatment over a 2-month period to reduce the bulk and vascularity of the fibroids. Useful benefits of this approach are to enable a Pfannensteil (low transverse) rather than a midline abdominal incision, or to facilitate vaginal rather than abdominal hysterectomy, both of which are conducive to more rapid recovery and fewer postoperative complications. A technical problem with myomectomy after GnRH agonist pre-treatment is that the tissue planes around the fibroid are less easily defined, but on the positive side, blood loss and the likely need for transfusion are reduced.

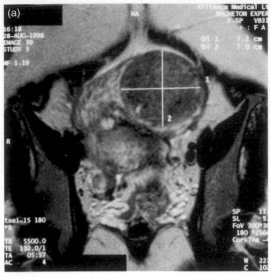
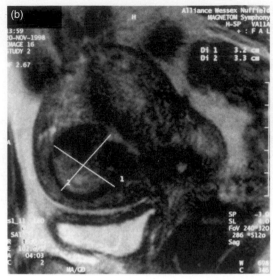

**Figure 9.3** Magnetic resonance imaging appearances of uterine fibroids (a) before and (b) after uterine artery embolization. (Kindly supplied by Dr N Hacking.)

## Management

Pelvic examination often reveals an enlarged and tender uterus. If the woman has no symptoms and the uterus is not enlarged, no treatment is indicated. If the woman is symptomatic, hysterectomy is usually the preferred treatment, since adenomyosis does not respond well to hormonal treatment.

### New developments

Endoscopic surgical treatments for fibroids have proved disappointing: myolysis using a diathermy needle to destroy the tissue is followed by intense adhesion formation. Given the requirement for a substantial blood supply to support growth, interruption of the arterial supply to the tumour is a theoretically attractive concept. In practice, this is feasible by the radiological technique of percutaneous selective catheterization of the uterine arteries. Microparticles are released into the vessels, causing occlusion of both uterine arteries. Sufficient collateral circulation is present from the ovarian arteries to sustain normal uterine metabolic requirements, and women experience a substantial reduction in fibroid bulk, together with improvement in menstrual symptoms over the following 6 months. Currently available follow-up data suggest that the symptomatic improvement is sustained. Figures 9.3a and b show contrast-enhanced magnetic resonance imaging (MRI) of a fibroid uterus before and after embolization of the uterine arteries.

### Key Points

- Cervical ectropion is a very common finding and may be associated with chlamydial infection.
- The aetiology of fibroids is unknown, but growth is oestrogen dependent.
- Fibroids are common, being detectable clinically in about 20 per cent of women over 30 years of age.
- Risk factors for fibroids are nulliparity, obesity, a positive family history and African racial origin.
- Factors contributing to menorrhagia may include a mechanical obstruction to venous drainage and also increased total surface area of the endometrium and disorders of prostaglandin synthesis and metabolism.
- The mechanism whereby fibroids affect fertility is unclear.
- Hysteroscopic techniques for the removal of submucous fibroids are becoming popular to avoid major surgery.
- Hormone replacement therapy is not contraindicated in postmenopausal women with fibroids.

## CASE HISTORY

Mrs AP, a 37-year-old African woman who works as a cleaner in a local hospital, presents with a history of increasingly heavy, regular, painful periods. She also complains of increased urinary frequency, especially on standing. There is no irregular bleeding and the smear history is normal. She has two children but still wishes to retain her fertility as she is planning a third. She is married, a non-smoker and otherwise fit and well. On examination, the abdomen is distended and there is a pelvic mass consistent with that of a 20-week size pregnancy. Vaginal examination confirms this and ultrasound scan shows two large fibroids that are intramyometrial but also subserous.

### Discussion

*How would you manage this patient?*
The important factor here is that Mrs AP has fibroids large enough to cause compression symptoms and menorrhagia. If fibroids do not cause symptoms, they can be observed. The other important feature is that she wishes to retain her fertility and therefore hysterectomy may be contraindicated.

Myomectomy can be attempted and obviously there is a risk of bleeding and the patient must be warned that she may lose the uterus if this is performed by laparotomy.

A more modern option is embolization (i.e. obstructing the uterine artery by an injection of a variety of substances to cause necrosis of the fibroid).

## Additional reading

Alexopoulos ED, Fay TN, Simonis CD. A review of 2581 out-patient diagnostic hysteroscopies in the management of abnormal uterine bleeding. *Gynaecol Endoscopy* 1999; **8**: 105–10.

Lethaby A, Vollenhoven B, Sowter M. Pre-operative gonadotropin-releasing hormone analogue before hysterectomy or myomectomy for uterine fibroids (Cochrane Review). In: *The Cochrane Library*, Issue 2. Oxford: Update Software, 1999.

Rein MS, Powell WL, Walters FC et al. Cytogenetic abnormalities in uterine myomas are associated with myoma size. *Mol Hum Reprod* 1998; **4**: 83–6.

# Endometriosis and adenomyosis

## OVERVIEW

Endometriosis remains a challenging condition for clinicians and patients alike. Difficulties exist in relationship to explanation of its aetiology, pathophysiology and progression and to its recognition, both from symptoms and at endoscopy. Similar problems exist in determining who and when to treat and for how long once the diagnosis has been made.

## Introduction

Endometriosis is most simply defined as the presence of endometrial surface epithelium and/or the presence of endometrial glands and stroma outside the lining of the uterine cavity. One of the first definitive descriptions of endometriosis as a specific clinical condition was by Sampson in 1921.

Endometriosis is one of the commonest benign gynaecological conditions. It has been estimated that between 10 and 15 per cent of women presenting with gynaecological symptoms have the condition. This estimate of prevalence is based on identifying lesions at laparoscopy undertaken for pain or investigation of subfertility. Rather confusingly, the condition is also sometimes seen in asymptomatic women, for example at the time of laparoscopic sterilization.

Clinical diagnosis is usually made following the laparoscopic observation of haemorrhagic or fibrotic lesions in the pelvic peritoneal or the serosal surface of various pelvic organs. Lesions can be very small, for example 2–3 mm, or can be extensive, in some cases completely obliterating the normal anatomy of the pelvis. These ectopic endometrial tissues respond in varying degrees to the clinical changes in ovarian hormones. Unlike normal endometrium, they do not have an ordered blood supply, but there is an in-growth of new capillaries. Cyclical bleeding can occur within, and from, the endometriotic deposits and this contributes to a local inflammatory reaction. With healing and subsequent fibrosis, overlying peritoneal damage will lead to adhesions between associated organs. Ovarian implants lead to the formation of chocolate cysts or endometriomas. There is therefore a spectrum of appearances that reflect the stage in the evolution of the condition at which the patient is seen.

## Pathogenesis

It is not known why some women acquire this disease. Its persistence and spread are dependent on the cyclical secretion of steroid hormones from the ovaries,

## P  Understanding the pathophysiology

The precise aetiology of endometriosis remains unknown. Several theories exist to explain the process through which endometriosis develops and there is clinical evidence to support each of these concepts. However, no single theory can explain the location of endometriotic deposits in all the sites reported.

### Menstrual regurgitation and implantation

It has been suggested that endometriosis results from the retrograde menstrual regurgitation of viable endometrial glands and tissue within the menstrual fluid and subsequent implantation on the peritoneal surface. In animals, experimental endometriosis can be induced by placement of menstrual fluid or endometrial tissue in the peritoneal cavity. Endometriosis is also commonly found in women with associated abnormalities of the genital tract, causing obstruction to the vaginal outflow of menstrual fluid, lending credence to this theory.

### Coelomic epithelium transformation

There is a common origin for the cells lining the Müllerian duct, the peritoneal cells and the cells of the ovary. It has been proposed that these cells undergo de-differentiation back to their primitive origin and then transform into endometrial cells. This transformation into endometrial cells may be due to hormonal stimuli of ovarian origin by as yet unidentified chemical substances liberated from uterine endometrium or those produced from inflammatory irritation.

### Genetic and immunological factors

It has been suggested that genetic and immunological factors may alter the susceptibility of a woman and allow her to develop endometriosis. There appears to be an increased incidence in first-degree relatives of patients with the disorder and racial differences, with increased incidence amongst oriental women and a low prevalence in women of Afro-Caribbean origin.

### Vascular and lymphatic spread

Vascular and lymphatic embolization to distant sites has been demonstrated and explains the rare findings of endometriosis in sites outside the peritoneal cavity. This will explain foci in sites outside the peritoneal cavity, such as joints, skin, kidney and lung.

There is almost certainly an interaction between one or more of these theoretical processes to allow the development and subsequent growth of ectopic endometrial tissue to the fully developed endometriotic lesion.

since it is found almost exclusively in women in the reproductive age group with functioning ovaries. It can also be maintained in women who have undergone oophorectomy but are then given exogenous hormone replacement treatment. It has been suggested that the frequency of this disease has increased in recent years, and factors such as environmental pollution with dioxins have been implicated on the basis of primate studies. However, another view is that the apparent increase may reflect the greater use of diagnostic laparoscopy to investigate pain symptoms and the acceptance of the more subtle appearances of endometriosis as viewed endoscopically. There seems to be no association between the extent of the disease process seen at laparoscopy and the patient's age or symptomatology.

## Histological subtypes

It is possible to link a number of histological subtypes of endometriotic deposits, specific appearances at laparoscopy and a variety of morphological components to the presence of steroid receptors and hormonal responsiveness in terms of proliferative and secretory change in relationship to ovarian steroid hormone stimulation. These are summarized in Table 10.1.

### Free implants

These have a polypoidal cauliflower-like structure and grow along the surface or cover a cystic structure. They are characterized by the presence of a surface epithelium supported by endometrial stroma. Endometrial glands may be present in an identifiable form or may be absent. Cyclical changes with both secretory differentiation and menstrual bleeding have been observed in such lesions (Fig. 10.1). These lesions are highly responsive to alterations in oestrogen secretion; hence they are very sensitive to hormonal suppressive therapies.

### Enclosed implants

At this next stage of development the implant has become covered with a surface layer of peritoneum and thus located within tissue or within part of a free-growing lesion. These lesions will present as wedge-shaped extensions of stroma (ramification), often deep in local tissue planes connecting lesions with one another. In a minority of lesions there are clear-cut

**Table 10.1**  Endometrial deposits – correlation between histological, morphological and functional activity

| Histological subtype | Components | Hormonal response | Laparoscopic appearance |
| --- | --- | --- | --- |
| Free | Surface epithelium, glands and stroma | Proliferative, secretory and menstrual changes | Haemorrhagic vesicle/bleb |
| Enclosed | Glands and stroma | Proliferative, variable Secretory change No menstruation | Papule and (later) nodule |
| Healed | Glands only | No response | White nodule or flattened fibrotic scar |

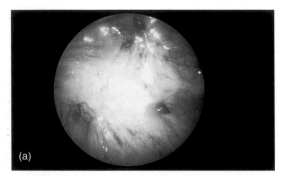 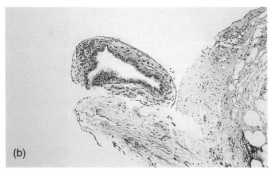

**Figure 10.1**  (a) Red lesion on peritoneum. (b) High-power section of peritoneum with red lesions. Gland lined with endometrial-like epithelium and surrounded by stroma. Secretory activity not seen (biopsy taken on day 15 of cycle). (Source: *An Atlas of Endometriosis*. Shaw, Robert W. Copyright 1993, Parthenon Publishing Group.)

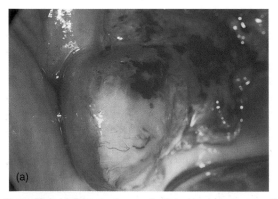 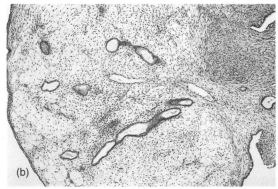

**Figure 10.2**  (a) Extensive haemorrhagic lesions indicative of active, symptomatic disease. (b) Biopsy from active lesions on day 24 of cycle. Histology shows oedematous connective tissue, haemosiderin-laden macrophages and complex glandular structures with secretory activity. (Source: *An Atlas of Endometriosis*. Shaw, Robert W. Copyright 1993, Parthenon Publishing Group.)

changes in response to the menstrual cycle, with evidence of proliferative and secretory change and menstrual bleeding. However, capillary and venous dilatation is seen during the luteal phase of the ovarian cycle. The lesions react in a similar way to basal endometrium and such lesions are only likely to be partly responsive to a hormone treatment approach (Fig. 10.2).

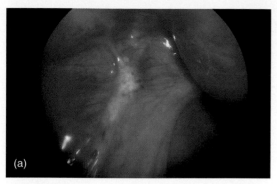
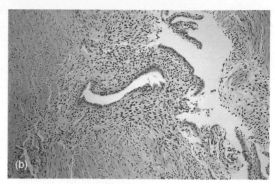

**Figure 10.3** (a) Puckered blue-black lesion with surrounding white fibrous plaque – classical 'powder-burn' lesion but may represent a less active form of disease. (b) High-power biopsy of lesion showing fibrous tissue and endometriotic glands, which are inactive with no active bleeding (biopsy taken on day 21 of cycle). (Source: *An Atlas of Endometriosis.* Shaw, Robert W. Copyright 1993, Parthenon Publishing Group.)

## Healed lesions

These have the feature of cystically dilated glands containing a thin glandular epithelium supported by small numbers of stromal cells surrounded by connective tissue. This absence of functional stromal tissue and the enclosure of the implant by increasing the amounts of scar tissue make the lesions insensitive to hormonal stimuli.

## Ovarian endometriosis

Endometriosis involving the ovary may present either as a superficial form with haemorrhagic lesions or in a more severe form as an enclosed haemorrhagic cyst.

The superficial lesions have the varying appearances seen with involvement of the peritoneum. They commonly present as superficial haemorrhagic lesions and red vesicles or blue-black 'powder-burn' lesions (Fig. 10.3). Such haemorrhagic lesions are commonly associated with adhesion formation. Adhesions are of particular relevance when they involve the posterior aspect of the ovaries, since they then rapidly lead to fixation within the ovarian fossa (Fig. 10.4).

The word endometrioma is used to describe endometriotic (or chocolate) cysts of the ovary. The name arises from the characteristic dark brown chocolate-coloured content of the cyst. Histological evaluation of an endometrioma shows there is a wide variation in the presence of endometriotic tissue. The cyst wall can be lined by free endometrial tissue, histologically and functionally similar to that of endometrial lining. However, in many instances of the long-standing presence of an endometrioma, the cyst wall becomes covered only by thickened fibrotic reactive tissue, with no specific features of glandular or stromal tissue.

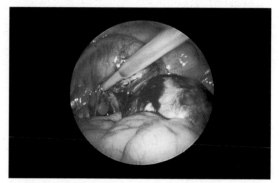

**Figure 10.4** Endometrioma on left ovary with adhesions to descending colon. (Source: *An Atlas of Endometriosis.* Shaw, Robert W. Copyright 1993, Parthenon Publishing Group.)

Endometriomas are thought to be formed from lesions that commence on the outer surface of the ovary. As they grow larger, there is inversion of the ovarian cortex and, with increasing inflammatory reaction at the site of inversion, this becomes occluded. The inverted ovarian cortex slowly becomes distended and filled with the 'chocolate' fluid from repeated 'menstrual bleeds'. Leakage from the cyst wall leads commonly to adhesion formation around the endometriomas, particularly on the posterior surface of the ovary within the ovarian fossa or to the posterior aspect of the broad ligament.

## Symptoms

Patients with endometriosis have extremely variable symptoms. Some symptoms may vary depending on the site of the ectopic endometrial lesion, but there is

**Table 10.2** Symptoms of endometriosis in relationship to site of lesion

| Site | Symptoms |
| --- | --- |
| Female reproductive tract | Dsymenorrhoea<br>Lower abdominal and pelvic pain<br>Dyspareunia<br>Rupture/torsion endometrioma<br>Low back pain<br>Infertility |
| Urinary tract | Cyclical haematuria/dysuria<br>Ureteric obstruction |
| Gastrointestinal tract | Dyschezia<br>Cyclical rectal bleeding<br>Obstruction |
| Surgical scars/umbilicus | Cyclical pain and bleeding |
| Lung | Cyclical haemoptysis<br>Haemopneumothorax |

a lack of correlation between the apparent extent of the disease, as judged laparoscopically, and the intensity of symptoms. Indeed, the disease may be a coincidental finding during open surgery or during investigation of a patient complaining of infertility. It may be possible to relate the variety of symptoms in patients with endometriosis to the siting of the deposits (summarized in Table 10.2), but often there is little direct correlation to more specific siting of lesions.

It can be seen that many of these symptoms are shared by a number of other common gynaecological conditions, or disorders of urogenital or gastrointestinal system origin. This cross-over of symptoms means that many patients with endometriosis have a delay from the time of onset of symptoms to the time of diagnosis of the disorder. They may well have been treated for other conditions prior to its definitive diagnosis. No one symptom is totally predictive of endometriosis, but one symptom is highly suggestive, that of spasmodic dysmenorrhoea, particularly if severe enough to warrant time off work and if unresponsive to normal analgesics. If this symptom is also associated with pain on postmenstrual days, pelvic pain throughout the cycle or deep pain at intercourse (deep dyspareunia), this should further heighten the suspicion of endometriosis. The occurrence of abnormal cyclical bleeding at the time of menstruation, from the rectum, bladder or umbilicus, is strongly suggestive of the presence of the disease. Heavy periods are probably the cause rather than an effect of endometriosis, as exposure to menstrual flow is the main risk factor for developing the condition.

## Physical examination

Endometriosis is suggested by the clinical findings on vaginal examination of thickening or nodularity of the uterosacral ligaments, tenderness in the pouch of Douglas, an ovarian mass or masses and a fixed retroverted uterus. However, pelvic tenderness alone is non-specific, and differential diagnoses for restricted mobility of the uterus include chronic pelvic inflammatory disease (rare in the UK) and uterine, ovarian or cervical malignancy. In these conditions, other suggestive features are usually present. Specific diagnosis requires visualization of the peritoneal cavity and biopsy of lesions in uncertain cases, either at laparoscopy or laparotomy.

## Non-invasive tests

### CA 125 levels
CA 125 is a glycoprotein expressed by some epithelial cells of coelomic origin. Serum levels are raised in a significant proportion of patients with ovarian epithelial carcinoma. It is noted that patients with severe endometriosis may also have elevated CA 125 levels but these are not to comparable to those in patients with ovarian cancer. In those with elevated CA 125, levels often fall during treatment, and rises in CA 125 correlate well with recurrence of disease.

However, in the majority of individuals, measurement of CA 125 alone cannot be diagnostic of the presence of endometriosis.

### Ultrasound
Ultrasound is of limited value in the diagnosis of endometriosis, other than for the assessment of ovarian cysts that might turn out to be endometriomata. A characteristic feature of an endometrioma is a

homogeneous hypoechoic collection of low-level echoes within an ovarian cyst.

## Magnetic resonance imaging

Magnetic resonance imaging (MRI) potentially offers significant gains in the imaging of endometriosis compared with ultrasound when there are ovarian cysts or invasion of surrounding organs such as the bowel, bladder or rectovaginal septum. The image quality can be useful for planning technically difficult surgery. However, in the majority of patients, MRI is of little benefit, as peritoneal deposits are only a few millimetres in diameter and are not well seen.

## Laparoscopy

Laparoscopy remains the 'gold standard' means of diagnosing this condition. As shown in Figures 10.1 and 10.2, the laparoscopic features of endometriotic deposits are quite variable, and inexperienced laparoscopists may miss lesions unless they are very extensive, fail to recognize atypical lesions, and in many because of a failure to do an adequate visualization of the whole of the pelvis, particularly the ovarian fossa. Laparoscopy allows direct visualization of endometriotic lesions and the possibility of biopsy of suspicious areas and also staging of the disease in terms of the extent of adhesions and the number and size of lesions. It also allows for concurrent therapy at the time of laparoscopy in the form of diathermy or laser treatment in selected cases.

## Endometriosis and subfertility

It is estimated that between 30 and 40 per cent of patients with endometriosis complain of difficulty in conceiving. In many patients there is a multifactorial pathogenesis to this subfertility. It has yet to be shown how the presence of a few small endometriotic deposits might render a patient subfertile. In the more severe stages of endometriosis there is commonly anatomical distortion, with peri-adnexal adhesions and destruction of ovarian tissue when endometriomas develop – hence a more readily explainable relationship is apparent. A number of possible and variable mechanisms have been postulated to connect mild endometriosis with subfertility. These vary from endocrine disorders including anovulation, altered prolactin secretion and luteinized unruptured follicle syndrome, to disorders of sperm or oocyte function (Table 10.3).

**Table 10.3** Infertility and endometriosis – possible mechanisms

| | |
|---|---|
| Ovarian function | Luteolysis caused by prostaglandins |
| | Oocyte maturation defects |
| | Endocrinopathies |
| | Luteinized unruptured follicle syndrome |
| | Altered prolactin release |
| | Anovulation |
| Tubal function | Impaired fimbrial oocyte pick-up |
| | Altered tubal mobility |
| Coital function | Deep dyspareunia – reduced coital frequency |
| Sperm function | Antibodies causing inactivation |
| | Macrophage phagocytosis |
| Early pregnancy failure | Prostaglandin induced |
| | Immune reaction |
| | Luteal phase deficiency |

Currently there is no simple explanation of how mild endometriosis may prevent conception occurring. For this reason many investigators would question the benefit of any form of medical or surgical treatment in such cases. Clearly, if, apart from her subfertility the patient also has symptoms associated with endometriosis, appropriate therapy is indicated. However, it is accepted that endometriosis is a disease that tends to persist and often progress with time. There is an argument that offering therapy at an early stage may prevent further progression of the disease, the end result of which may well be mechanical disruption to tubal–ovarian function. For these reasons, endometriosis involving the posterior aspect of the ovary and the ovarian fossa is often treated at an early stage, whereas endometriosis occurring only on the uterosacral ligaments may well be left untreated. From the balance of evidence, conclusions have been drawn that, apart from mechanical damage, endometriosis does not cause subfertility. This view has been substantiated by the failure of medical therapies in placebo-controlled trials to improve conception rates. However, this widely held viewpoint may well be brought into question following publication of the findings from a Canadian multicentre study in which surgical (laparoscopic) ablation of deposits was compared with no intervention. Surgical destruction did improve cumulative pregnancy rates in this study, but further confirmatory trials are awaited. With regard to hormonal therapy, the evidence is very clear that this treatment does not improve subsequent fertility.

## Treatment

Patients with endometriosis are often difficult to treat, not only from a physical point of view, but also often because of associated psychological issues. For some patients the label of endometriosis in itself may create its own problems, since it is known to be a recurrent disorder throughout the whole of reproductive life. Whilst there is no standard formula for treatment, nor indeed a cure, it is important to tailor treatment for the individual according to her age, symptoms, extent of the disease and her desire for future childbearing. Problems also arise when minimal endometriosis is detected in a patient presenting with pain and there is real uncertainty as to whether the condition is coincidental or causal. In this situation a full explanation of the associated diagnostic uncertainty is required.

## Drug therapy

### Analgesics
Non-steroidal anti-inflammatory drugs (NSAIDs) are potent analgesics and are very helpful in reducing the severity of dysmenorrhoea and pelvic pain. However, they have no specific impact on the disease and its progression and hence their use is for symptom control. There may be additional benefit in combining these agents with paracetamol or codeine, so as to avoid the main adverse effect of NSAIDs, which is gastrointestinal upset.

### Combined oral contraceptive agents
Oral contraceptive agents are known to reduce the severity of dysmenorrhoea and menstrual blood loss in many patients. They may be of some benefit, but are often of little help when given in the standard manner with regular monthly withdrawal bleeds. Two or three packs of pills taken without a break may be beneficial in avoiding the exacerbation of symptoms associated with menstruation. Explanation that missing a withdrawal bleed is not harmful is often needed.

### Danazol/gestrinone
Danazol and gestrinone are hormonal, ovarian suppressive, medical treatments comparable in their effect of reducing the severity of symptoms for endometriosis. Danazol is given in a dose of between 400 and 800 mg daily and gestrinone in a dose of 2.5 mg twice weekly. In most instances the drugs are well tolerated, but many women do experience androgenic side effects, e.g. weight gain, greasy skin and acne. The drugs are normally given in courses of between 3 and 6 months. In longer-term administration of the drugs there may be alterations in lipid profiles or liver function, which need to be monitored. Prescribing of danazol has recently been restricted owing to a possible association with ovarian cancer.

### Progestogens
Synthetic progestogens such as medroxyprogesterone acetate and dydrogesterone have been given on a continuous basis to produce pseudo-decidualization of the endometrium and comparable changes in endometriotic lesions. The dose of agents required to be effective is quite high, and side effects, including breakthrough bleeding, weight gain, fluid retention and weight changes, are not uncommon.

### Gonadotrophin-releasing hormone agonists
Gonadotrophin-releasing hormone agonists (GnRH-A) are as effective as danazol in relieving the severity and symptoms of endometriosis and differ only in their side effects. These drugs induce a state of hypogonadotrophic hypogonadism or pseudo-menopause with low circulating levels of oestrogen. Side effects include symptoms seen at the menopause, in particular hot flushes and night sweats. Despite these side effects, the drugs are well tolerated and they have become established agents in the treatment of endometriosis. They are available as multiple, daily-administered intranasal sprays or as slow-release depot formulations, each lasting for 1 month or more. Apart from the symptomatic side effects described above, the low circulating oestrogen levels can affect bone metabolism in ways comparable to those seen at the natural menopause. Therefore, with continuing long-term use there can be reduction in bone mineral density, seen

most acutely in the trabecular bone of the lumbar spine. Bone loss of some 5 per cent can occur over a 6-month course of treatment, but for the majority of patients this is readily replaced as ovarian function returns on ceasing the drug therapy. The administration of low-dose hormone replacement therapy (HRT) along with the GnRH-A analogues, the so-called 'add back' therapy, may offer a way of preventing the adverse effects of oestrogen deficiency, although information about the long-term results of this approach to treatment is so far lacking.

## Surgical treatment

### Conservative surgery

Laparoscopic surgery with techniques such as intra-abdominal lasers has become the standard for the surgical management of endometriosis. It is now much simpler and safer to eradicate visible endometriotic lesions with diathermy, $CO_2$ or KTP lasers. Likewise, endometriotic cysts can be drained and opened and the inner cyst wall or lining destroyed and vaporized with the laser. In many instances, because of the severe adhesive disease found with endometriomas, open surgery may still be necessary. Conservative approaches have reduced the need for open surgery with its long recovery times, and this allows patients to delay treatment until such time as definitive surgery may become necessary.

### Definitive surgery

Where there are severe symptoms or progressive disease or in women whose families are complete, definitive surgery for the relief of dysmenorrhoea and pain is often necessary. This takes the form of hysterectomy and bilateral salpingo-oophorectomy. The removal of the ovaries and subsequent ovarian hormone production is beneficial in achieving long-term symptom relief. Paradoxically, such patients can receive HRT subsequent to surgery. To minimize the risk of recurrence, the commencement of HRT is often deferred for a period of time following surgery, particularly when active disease was found to be present at the time of laparotomy, and this delay is typically a period of 6 months or more.

Definitive surgery is also required for large adherent endometriotic cysts and for the small proportion of patients who have deep-seated endometriosis involving the bowel or bladder. Endometriosis thus remains a disorder of which we still have little understanding and, at present, little hope of a permanent cure other than definitive surgery in the form of pelvic clearance. New treatment options, both medical and laparoscopic surgery, have expanded the potential for delay in surgery, but for most sufferers the disease remains one of repeat recurrences throughout their reproductive life.

## Adenomyosis

Adenomyosis is often incorrectly termed internal endometriosis because of the histological features of the disorder in which endometrial glands are found deep within the myometrium. Adenomyosis is increasingly being viewed as a separate pathological entity affecting a different population of patients with an as yet unknown and different aetiology.

Patients with adenomyosis are usually multiparous and diagnosed in their late thirties or early forties. They present with increasingly severe secondary spasmodic dysmenorrhoea and increased menstrual blood loss (menorrhagia). Examination of patients may be useful with the findings most often of a bulky and sometimes tender uterus, particularly if examined perimenstrually. Ultrasound examination of the uterus may be helpful on occasions when adenomyosis is particularly marked or localized to one area. Then ultrasound may show alterations of echogenicity within the myometrium from the localized, haemorrhage-filled, distended endometrial glands. In some instances where there is a very localized area of adenomyosis, this may give an irregular nodular development within the uterus, very similar to that of uterine fibroids. MRI provides excellent images of the myometrium, endometrium and areas of adenomyosis and is now the investigation of choice.

Given the practical difficulty in making the diagnosis of adenomyosis preoperatively, conservative surgery and medical treatments are so far poorly developed. In general, any treatment that induces amenorrhoea will be helpful as it will relieve pain and excessive bleeding. Effective agents such as danazol, gestrinone and GnRH-A used in the treatment of endometriosis may also be beneficial for this condition. On ceasing treatment, however, the symptoms rapidly return in the majority of patients, and hysterectomy remains the only definitive treatment. Where well-localized islands of adenomyosis can be identified within the myometrium, there is the potential for laparoscopic laser surgery, and some reports of benefit have appeared in the literature.

## ⚲ Key Points

- Endometriosis is one of the commonest gynaecological conditions and at present affects between 10 and 25 per cent of women with symptoms of gynaecological origin.
- Growth of endometriosis is oestrogen dependent. Endometriosis is associated with tubal and ovarian damage and the formation of adhesions and can compromise fertility.
- The commonest presenting symptoms other than infertility are painful periods and dyspareunia.
- The typical peritoneal lesion is described as a 'powder burn'. The medical treatment of endometriosis involves suppressing oestrogen and progesterone levels to prevent cyclical changes and includes treatment with progestogens, gestrinone or GnRH agonists.
- The surgical treatment of endometriosis is either minimally invasive, using laparoscopic techniques, or radical, with total abdominal hysterectomy and bilateral salpingo-oophorectomy.
- Adenomyosis is a common condition, presenting with painful periods, and is common in women in their late thirties or early forties.

## Additional reading

Jacobson TZ, Barlow DH, Koninckx PR, Olive D, Farquhar C. Laparoscopic surgery for subfertility associated with endometriosis (Cochrane Methodology Review). In: *The Cochrane Library*, Issue 4. Chichester, UK: John Wiley & Sons, 2003.

Sampson JA. Perforating haemorrhagic (chocolate) cysts of the ovary. *Arch Surg* 1921; **3**: 245–323.

Sampson JA. Peritoneal endometriosis due to menstrual dissemination of endometrial tissue into the peritoneal cavity. *Am J Obstet Gynecol* 1927; **14**: 422–69.

# Benign tumours of the ovary

## OVERVIEW

Benign ovarian cysts are common, frequently asymptomatic and often resolve spontaneously. They are the fourth commonest gynaecological cause of hospital admission. By the age of 65 years, 4 per cent of all women will have been admitted to hospital for this reason.

Ninety per cent of all ovarian tumours are benign, although this varies with age. Of the tumours that require surgery, 13 per cent in premenopausal women are malignant and 45 per cent in postmenopausal women are malignant. The main objectives of management are to exclude malignancy and to avoid cyst accidents, without causing undue morbidity or impairing future fertility in younger women.

Ovarian tumours may be physiological or pathological, and may arise from any tissue in the ovary. Most benign ovarian tumours are cystic. The finding of solid elements makes malignancy more likely. However, fibromas, thecomas, dermoids and Brenner tumours usually have solid elements.

## Pathology

### Physiological cysts

Physiological cysts are simply large versions of the cysts which form in the ovary during the normal ovarian cycle. Most are asymptomatic incidental findings at pelvic examination or ultrasound scan. Although they may occur in any premenopausal woman, they are most common in young women. They are an occasional complication of ovulation induction, when they are commonly multiple. They may also occur in premature female infants and in women with trophoblastic disease.

### Follicular cyst

Lined by granulosa cells, this is the commonest benign ovarian tumour and is most often found incidentally. It results from the non-rupture of a dominant follicle, or the failure of atresia in a non-dominant follicle. A follicular cyst can persist for several menstrual cycles and may achieve a diameter of up to 10 cm. Smaller cysts are more likely to resolve, but may require intervention if symptoms develop or if they do not resolve after 8–16 weeks. Occasionally, they may continue to produce oestrogen, causing menstrual disturbances and endometrial hyperplasia.

### Luteal cyst

Less common than follicular cysts, these are more likely to present with intraperitoneal bleeding. This is more common on the right side, possibly as a result of increased intraluminal pressure secondary to ovarian vein anatomy. They may also rupture. This usually happens on days 20–26 of the cycle. Corpora lutea are not called luteal cysts unless they are more than 3 cm in diameter.

## Benign germ cell tumours

Germ cell tumours are among the commonest ovarian tumours seen in women less than 30 years of age. Overall, only 2–3 per cent are malignant, but in the under-twenties this proportion may rise to a third. Malignant tumours are usually solid, although benign forms also commonly have a solid element. Thus the traditional classification into solid or cystic germ cell tumours, signifying malignant or benign respectively, may be misleading. As the name suggests, they arise from totipotential germ cells, and may therefore contain elements of all three germ layers (embryonic differentiation). Differentiation into extra-embryonic tissues results in ovarian choriocarcinoma or endodermal sinus tumour. When neither embryonic nor extra-embryonic differentiation occurs, a dysgerminoma results.

### Dermoid cyst (mature cystic teratoma)

The benign dermoid cyst is the only benign germ cell tumour that is common. It results from differentiation into embryonic tissues. It accounts for around 40 per cent of all ovarian neoplasms and is most common in young women. The median age of presentation is 30 years (Comerci et al., 1994). It is bilateral in about 11 per cent of cases. However, if the contralateral ovary is macroscopically normal, the chance of a concealed second dermoid is very low (1–2 per cent), particularly if preoperative ultrasound is normal.

A dermoid is usually a unilocular cyst less than 15 cm in diameter, in which ectodermal structures are predominant. Thus it is often lined with epithelium like the epidermis and contains skin appendages, teeth, sebaceous material, hair and nervous tissue. Endodermal derivatives include thyroid, bronchus and intestine, and the mesoderm may be represented by bone, cartilage and smooth muscle.

Occasionally only a single tissue may be present, in which case the term monodermal teratoma is used. The classic examples are carcinoid and struma ovarii, which contains hormonally active thyroid tissue. Primary carcinoid tumours of the ovary rarely metastasize, but 30 per cent may give rise to typical carcinoid symptoms (Saunders et al., 1960). Thyroid tissue is found in 5–20 per cent of cystic teratomas. The term 'struma ovarii' should be reserved for tumours composed predominantly of thyroid tissue and as such comprise only 1.4 per cent of cystic teratomas. Only 5–6 per cent of struma ovarii produce sufficient thyroid hormone to cause hyperthyroidism. Some 5–10 per cent of struma ovarii develop into carcinoma.

The majority (60 per cent) of dermoid cysts are asymptomatic. However, 3.5–10 per cent may undergo torsion. Less commonly (1–4 per cent), they may rupture spontaneously, either suddenly, causing an acute abdomen and a chemical peritonitis, or slowly, causing chronic granulomatous peritonitis. As the latter may also arise following intraoperative spillage, great care should be taken to avoid this event, and thorough peritoneal lavage must be performed if it does occur. During pregnancy, rupture is more common due to external pressure from the expanding gravid uterus or to trauma during delivery.

About 2 per cent are said to contain a malignant component, usually a squamous carcinoma in women over 40 years old. Poor prognosis is indicated by non-squamous histology and capsular rupture. Amongst women aged under 20 years, up to 80 per cent of ovarian malignancies are due to germ cell tumours (see Chapter 13).

### Mature solid teratoma

These rare tumours contain mature tissues just like the dermoid cyst, but there are few cystic areas. They must be differentiated from immature teratomas, which are malignant (see Chapter 13).

## Benign epithelial tumours

The majority of ovarian neoplasia, both benign and malignant, arise from the ovarian surface epithelium.

They are therefore essentially mesothelial in nature, deriving from the coelomic epithelium overlying the embryonic gonadal ridge, from which develop Müllerian and Wolffian structures. Therefore, this may result in development along endocervical (mucinous cystadenomata), endometrial (endometrioid) or tubal (serous) pathways or uroepithelial (Brenner) lines respectively. Although benign epithelial tumours tend to occur at a slightly younger age than their malignant counterparts, they are most common in women over 40 years.

## Serous cystadenoma

This is the most common benign epithelial tumour and is bilateral in about 10 per cent. It is usually a unilocular cyst with papilliferous processes on the inner surface and occasionally on the outer surface. The epithelium on the inner surface is cuboidal or columnar and may be ciliated. Psammoma bodies are concentric calcified bodies which occur occasionally in these cysts, but more frequently in their malignant counterparts. The cyst fluid is thin and serous. They are seldom as large as mucinous tumours.

## Mucinous cystadenoma

These constitute 15–25 per cent of all ovarian tumours and are the second most common epithelial tumour. They are typically large, unilateral, multilocular cysts with a smooth inner surface. A specimen at Hammersmith Hospital, London, weighed over 14 kg! The lining epithelium consists of columnar mucus-secreting cells. The cyst fluid is generally thick and glutinous.

A rare complication is pseudomyxoma peritonei, which is more often present before the cyst is removed than following intraoperative rupture. Pseudomyxoma peritonei is commonly associated with mucinous tumours of the appendix. Synchronous tumours of the ovary and appendix are common. These are usually well-differentiated carcinomas or borderline tumours (Wertheim et al., 1994). They result in seedling growths which continue to secrete mucin, causing matting together and consequent obstruction of bowel loops. The 5-year survival rate is approximately 50 per cent, but by 10 years as few as 18 per cent are alive.

## Endometrioid cystadenoma

Benign endometrioid cysts are difficult to differentiate from ovarian endometriosis.

## Brenner tumours

These account for only 1–2 per cent of all ovarian tumours, and are bilateral in 10–15 per cent of cases. They probably arise from Wolffian metaplasia of the surface epithelium. The tumour consists of islands of transitional epithelium (Walthard nests) in a dense fibrotic stroma, giving a largely solid appearance. The vast majority are benign, but borderline or malignant specimens have been reported. Almost three-quarters occur in women over the age of 40 and about half are incidental findings, being recognized only by the pathologist. Although some can be large, the majority are less than 2 cm in diameter. Some secrete oestrogens, and abnormal vaginal bleeding is a common presentation.

## Clear cell (mesonephroid) tumours

These arise from serosal cells showing little differentiation, and are only rarely benign. The typical histological appearance is of clear or 'hobnail' cells arranged in mixed patterns.

# Benign sex cord stromal tumours

Sex cord stromal tumours represent only 4 per cent of benign ovarian tumours. They occur at any age, from prepubertal children to elderly, postmenopausal women. Many secrete hormones and present with the results of inappropriate hormone effects.

## Granulosa cell tumours

These are all malignant tumours but are mentioned here because they are generally confined to the ovary when they present and so have a good prognosis. However, they do grow very slowly and recurrences are often seen 10–20 years later. They are largely solid in most cases. Call–Exner bodies are pathognomonic but are seen in less than half of granulosa cell tumours. Some produce oestrogens and most appear to secrete inhibin.

## Theca cell tumours

Almost all are benign, solid and unilateral, typically presenting in the sixth decade. Many produce oestrogens in sufficient quantity to have systemic effects such as precocious puberty, postmenopausal bleeding, endometrial hyperplasia and endometrial cancer. They rarely cause ascites or a pleural effusion.

## Fibroma

These unusual tumours are most frequent around 50 years of age. Most are derived from stromal cells and are similar to thecomas. They are hard, mobile and lobulated with a glistening white surface. Less than 10 per cent are bilateral. While ascites occurs with many of the larger fibromas, Meig's syndrome – ascites and pleural effusion in association with a fibroma of the ovary – is seen in only 1 per cent of cases.

## Sertoli–Leydig cell tumours

These are usually of low-grade malignancy. Most are found around 30 years of age. They are rare, comprising less than 0.2 per cent of ovarian tumours. They are often difficult to distinguish from other ovarian tumours because of the variety of cells and architecture seen. Many produce androgens, and signs of virilization are seen in three-quarters of patients. Some secrete oestrogens. They are usually small and unilateral.

## Age distribution of ovarian tumours

In younger women, the most common benign ovarian neoplasm is the germ cell tumour; amongst older women, it is the epithelial cell tumour (Fig. 11.1). The percentage of ovarian neoplasms that are benign also changes with the age of the woman (Fig. 11.2).

## Presentation

The presentation of benign ovarian tumours is as follows.
- Asymptomatic
- Pain
- Abdominal swelling
- Pressure effects
- Menstrual disturbances
- Hormonal effects
- Abnormal cervical smear

## Asymptomatic

Many benign ovarian tumours are found incidentally in the course of investigating another unrelated problem or during a routine examination while performing a cervical smear or at an antenatal clinic. As pelvic ultrasound, and particularly transvaginal scanning, is now used more frequently, physiological cysts are detected more often. Where ultrasound was used in trials of screening for ovarian cancer, the majority of tumours detected were benign. About 50 per cent of simple cysts less than 6 cm in diameter will resolve spontaneously if observed over a period of 6 months. A further 25 per cent regress in the following 2 years. Use of an oral contraceptive pill does not encourage the resolution of physiological cysts.

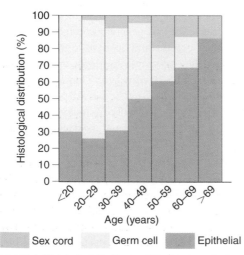

**Figure 11.1** Histological distribution (%) of benign ovarian neoplasia treated surgically by age.

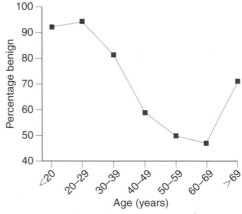

**Figure 11.2** The proportion of surgically treated ovarian tumours that are benign falls with increasing age until the eighth decade. (Modified from Koonings et al., 1989.)

## Pain

Acute pain from an ovarian tumour may result from torsion, rupture, haemorrhage or infection. Torsion usually gives rise to a sharp, constant pain caused by ischaemia of the cyst. Areas may become infarcted. Haemorrhage into the cyst may cause pain as the capsule is stretched. Intraperitoneal bleeding mimicking ectopic pregnancy may result from rupture of the tumour. This happens most frequently with a luteal cyst. Chronic lower abdominal pain sometimes results from the pressure of a benign ovarian tumour, but is more common if endometriosis or infection is present.

## Abdominal swelling

Patients seldom note abdominal swelling until the tumour is very large. A benign mucinous cyst may occasionally fill the entire abdominal cavity. The bloating of which women complain so often is rarely due to an ovarian tumour.

## Miscellaneous

Gastrointestinal or urinary symptoms may result from pressure effects. In extreme cases, oedema of the legs, varicose veins and haemorrhoids may result. Sometimes uterine prolapse is the presenting complaint in a woman with an ovarian cyst.

Occasionally patients complain of menstrual disturbances, but this may be coincidence rather than due to the tumour. Rarely, sex cord stromal tumours present with oestrogen effects such as precocious puberty, menorrhagia and glandular hyperplasia, breast enlargement or postmenopausal bleeding. Secretion of androgens may cause hirsutism and acne initially, progressing to frank virilism with deepening of the voice or clitoral hypertrophy. Very rarely indeed, thyrotoxicosis may result from ectopic secretion of thyroid hormone.

Rarely, a patient with an abnormal cervical smear will be found to have an ovarian tumour, the removal of which is followed by resolution of the cytological abnormality. Surprisingly, these are often benign tumours.

## Differential diagnosis

The differential diagnosis of benign ovarian tumours is broad, reflecting the wide range of presenting symptoms.

### S Differential diagnosis of benign ovarian tumours

**Pain**
Ectopic pregnancy
Spontaneous abortion
Pelvic inflammatory disease
Appendicitis
Meckel's diverticulum
Diverticulitis

**Abdominal swelling**
Pregnant uterus
Fibroid uterus
Full bladder
Distended bowel
Ovarian malignancy
Colorectal carcinoma

**Pressure effects**
Urinary tract infection
Constipation

**Hormonal effects**
All other causes of menstrual irregularities, precocious puberty and postmenopausal bleeding.

A full bladder should be considered in the differential diagnosis of any pelvic mass. In premenopausal women, a gravid uterus must always be considered. Fibroids can be impossible to distinguish from ovarian tumours. Rarely, a fimbrial cyst may grow sufficiently to cause anxiety.

Ectopic pregnancy may present as a pelvic mass and lower abdominal pain, especially if there has been chronic intraperitoneal bleeding. Often a ruptured, bleeding corpus luteum will be mistaken for an ectopic gestation. It may be difficult to differentiate between appendicitis and an ovarian cyst. Cooperation between gynaecologist and surgeon is essential to avoid unnecessary surgery on simple ovarian cysts in young women and the effects this may have upon subsequent fertility. Pelvic inflammatory disease may give rise to a mass of adherent bowel, a hydrosalpinx or pyosalpinx.

If the tumour is ovarian, malignancy must be excluded. In the vast majority of cases this can only be done by a laparotomy. Even then, careful histological examination may be necessary to exclude invasion. Frozen section will only rarely be of value. A pelvic mass may also be caused by a rectal tumour or diverticulitis. Hodgkin's disease may present as a pelvic mass of enlarged pelvic lymph nodes.

## Investigation

The investigations required will depend upon the circumstances of the presentation. Patients presenting with acute symptoms will usually require emergency surgery, whereas asymptomatic patients or women with chronic problems may benefit from more detailed preliminary assessment.

### Gynaecological history

Details of the presenting symptoms and a full gynaecological history should be obtained with particular reference to the date of the last menstrual period, the regularity of the menstrual cycle, any previous pregnancies, contraception, medication and family history (particularly of ovarian, breast or bowel cancer).

### General history and examination

Indigestion or dysphagia might indicate a primary gastric cancer metastasizing to the pelvis. Similarly, a history of altered bowel habit or rectal bleeding would suggest diverticulitis or rectal carcinoma. However, ovarian carcinoma may also present with these features.

If the patient has presented as an acute emergency, look for evidence of hypovolaemia. Hypotension is a relatively late sign of blood loss, as the blood pressure will be maintained for some time by peripheral arteriolar and central venous vasoconstriction. When decompensation occurs, it often does so very rapidly. It is vital to recognize the early signs – tachycardia and cold peripheries.

The breasts should be palpated and the neck, axillae and groins examined for lymphadenopathy.

A malignant ovarian tumour may cause a pleural effusion. This is much less commonly found with a benign tumour. Some patients may have ankle oedema. Very occasionally, foot drop may be noted as a result of compression of pelvic nerve roots. This would not occur with a benign tumour, but suggests a malignancy with lymphatic involvement.

### Abdominal examination

The abdomen should be inspected for signs of distension by fluid or by the tumour itself. Dilated veins may be seen on the lower abdominal wall. Gentle palpation will reveal areas of tenderness, and peritonism may be elicited by asking the patient to cough or suck in and blow out her abdominal wall. Male hair distribution may suggest a rare androgen-producing tumour.

The best way of detecting a mass that arises from the pelvis is to palpate gently with the radial border of the left hand, starting in the upper abdomen and working caudally. This is the reverse of the process taught to every medical student for feeling the liver edge. Using only the right hand is the commonest reason for failing to detect pelvi-abdominal masses.

Shifting dullness is probably the easiest way of demonstrating ascites, but it remains a very insensitive technique. It is always worth listening for bowel sounds in any patient with an acute abdomen. Their complete absence in the presence of peritonism is an ominous sign.

### Bimanual examination

This is an essential component of the assessment because, even in expert hands, ultrasound examination is not infallible. By palpating the mass between both the vaginal and abdominal hands, its mobility, texture and consistency, the presence of nodules in the pouch of Douglas and the degree of tenderness can all be determined (Fig. 11.3). While it is impossible to make a firm diagnosis with bimanual examination, a hard, irregular, fixed mass is likely to be invasive.

### Ultrasound

Transabdominal and transvaginal ultrasound can demonstrate the presence of an ovarian mass with reasonable sensitivity and fair specificity and, although

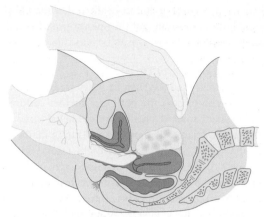

**Figure 11.3** Bimanual examination involves palpating the pelvic organs between both hands.

it cannot distinguish reliably between benign and malignant tumours, solid ovarian masses are more likely to be malignant than their cystic counterparts. The use of colour-flow Doppler may increase the reliability of ultrasound. Neither computerized tomographic scanning nor magnetic resonance imaging has significant advantages over ultrasound in this situation, and both are more expensive.

## Ultrasound-guided diagnostic ovarian cyst aspiration

This investigation has been introduced gradually into gynaecological practice from the subspecialty of assisted reproduction, where ultrasound-guided egg collection is now commonplace. This has happened without the benefit of appropriate trials to indicate its potential efficacy.

Unfortunately, this technique has up to a 71 per cent false-negative rate and a 2 per cent false-positive rate for the cytological diagnosis of malignancy (Diernaes et al., 1987). There is a risk of disseminating malignant cells along the needle track or into the peritoneal cavity, but the size of that risk is not established. The cyst often fills again with fluid.

Overall, ultrasound-guided aspiration of ovarian cysts cannot be recommended as a diagnostic tool.

## Radiological investigations

A chest X-ray is essential to detect metastatic disease in the lungs or a pleural effusion that may be too small to detect clinically. Occasionally an abdominal X-ray may show calcification, suggesting the possibility of a benign teratoma. An intravenous urogram is often performed but is seldom useful. A barium enema is indicated only if the mass is irregular or fixed, or if there are bowel symptoms. A computerized tomography scan is seldom indicated.

## Blood test and serum markers

It is always sensible to measure the haemoglobin, and an elevated white cell count would suggest infection. Platelet count and clotting screen may be useful in the rare case of a large intra-abdominal bleed. Blood may be cross-matched if necessary.

Serum markers have yet to establish a role in the routine management of most ovarian tumours. However, a raised serum CA 125 is strongly suggestive of ovarian carcinoma, especially in postmenopausal women. Women with extensive endometriosis may also have elevated levels, but the concentration is usually not as high as is seen with malignant disease. The beta-human chorionic gonadotrophin (β-hCG) concentration might be measured to exclude an ectopic pregnancy, but trophoblastic tumours and some germ cell tumours secrete this marker. Oestradiol levels may be elevated in some women with physiological follicular cysts and sex cord stromal tumours. Androgen concentrations may be increased by Sertoli–Leydig tumours. Raised alpha-fetoprotein levels suggest a yolk sac tumour.

## Management

The management will depend upon the severity of the symptoms, the age of the patient and therefore the risk of malignancy, and her desire for further children.

## The asymptomatic patient

### The older woman
Women over 50 years of age are far more likely to have a malignancy and have little to gain from the conservative management of a pelvic mass more than 5 cm in diameter (Rulin & Preston, 1987). Physiological cysts are, by definition, unlikely. However, the capacity of the postmenopausal ovary to generate benign cysts is greater than previously thought, occurring in

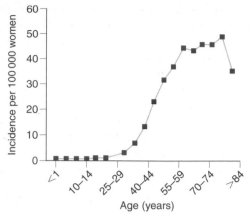

**Figure 11.4** The incidence of ovarian cancer in England and Wales (Office of Population Censuses and Surveys, 1985). Note how uncommon ovarian cancer is before the age of 35 years.

up to 17 per cent of asymptomatic women (Levine et al., 1992). More than 50 per cent of small, simple cysts will resolve spontaneously, but almost 30 per cent will remain static (Levine et al., 1992). Even in this age group, only 29–50 per cent of all ovarian cysts will be malignant (Fig. 11.4).

Therefore, efforts have been made to define criteria that would enable unnecessary surgery to be avoided in this older age group. Evaluation of the cyst with tumour markers, ultrasound and colour-flow Doppler studies, and careful follow-up suggest that simple, unilateral cysts less than 6 cm in diameter with CA 125 less than 35 mU/mL and normal vascular resistance patterns are likely to be benign and may safely be managed conservatively (Goldstein, 1993; Bailey et al., 1998). In these cases, if there is no change in the cyst at the second ultrasound at 3 months, follow-up with 6-monthly ultrasound and CA 125 estimation is safe. Most will resolve in 3 years, but some do persist for up to 7 years.

The role of laparoscopic surgery in the assessment and treatment of apparently benign cysts in this age group is controversial (Fowler & Carter, 1995; Parker, 1995). Whilst the small cysts described above may be managed without surgery, there may be a small minor role for the laparoscopic assessment and treatment of larger (perhaps up to 10 cm) but otherwise apparently benign cysts. Nonetheless, this should only be in the hands of those who are both laparoscopically experienced and prepared to perform definitive surgery for an unexpected ovarian carcinoma under the same anaesthetic. Complete and intact removal of the cyst should be achieved. For the more general gynaecologist,

laparoscopy may be useful to confirm that the ultrasound lesion is ovarian, but the open approach is still recommended if the ovary is to be removed.

### Premenopausal women

Young women aged less than 35 years are both more likely to wish to have the option of further children and less likely to have a malignant epithelial tumour. However, ovarian cysts more than 10 cm in diameter are unlikely to be physiological or to resolve spontaneously. A normal follicular cyst up to 3 cm in diameter requires no further investigation. A clear unilocular cyst of 3–10 cm identified by ultrasound should be re-examined 12 weeks later for evidence of diminution in size. If the cyst persists, such women may be followed with 6-monthly ultrasound and CA 125 estimations as described above. The use of a combined oral contraceptive is unlikely to accelerate the resolution of a functional cyst (Steinkampf & Hammond, 1990), and hormonal treatment of endometriosis does not usually benefit an endometrioma. If the cyst does enlarge, laparoscopy or laparotomy may be indicated.

---

**Criteria for observation of an asymptomatic ovarian tumour**

- Unilateral tumour
- Unilocular cyst without solid elements
- Premenopausal women – tumour 3–10 cm in diameter
- Postmenopausal women – tumour 2–6 cm in diameter
- Normal CA 125
- No free fluid or masses suggesting omental cake or matted bowel loops

---

## The patient with symptoms

If the patient presents with severe, acute pain or signs of intraperitoneal bleeding, an emergency laparoscopy or laparotomy will be required. More chronic symptoms of pain or pressure may justify pelvic ultrasound if no mass can be felt, but ultrasound is unlikely to contribute to the investigation of a woman in whom both ovaries can be clearly felt to be of a normal size.

### The pregnant patient

An ovarian cyst in a pregnant woman may undergo torsion or may bleed. There is said to be an increased incidence of these complications in pregnancy, although the evidence for this is poor. Very occasionally, a cyst can prevent the presenting fetal part from engaging. A dermoid cyst may rupture or leak slowly, causing peritonitis. However, an ovarian cyst is usually discovered incidentally at the antenatal clinic or on ultrasound, and occasionally at Caesarean section.

The pregnant woman with an ovarian cyst is a special case because of the dangers to the fetus of surgery. These have probably been exaggerated in the past, and no urgent operation should be postponed solely because of a pregnancy. Thus, if the patient presents with acute pain due to torsion or haemorrhage into an ovarian tumour or if appendicitis is a possibility, the correct course is to undertake a laparotomy regardless of the stage of the pregnancy. The likelihood of labour ensuing is small. However, the operation should be covered by tocolytic drugs and performed in a centre with intensive neonatal care when possible.

If an asymptomatic cyst is discovered, it is prudent to wait until after 14 weeks' gestation before removing it. This avoids the risk of removing a corpus luteal cyst upon which the pregnancy might still be dependent. In the second and third trimester, the management of an asymptomatic ovarian cyst may be either conservative or surgical. The risks to the mother and fetus of an elective procedure need to be balanced against the chances of a cyst accident, an unexpected malignancy or spontaneous resolution. Cysts less than 10 cm in diameter that have a simple appearance on ultrasound are unlikely to be malignant or to result in a cyst accident, and may therefore be followed ultrasonographically: many will resolve spontaneously (Thornton & Wells, 1987). If the cyst is unresolved 6 weeks postpartum, surgery may be undertaken then. The role for cyst aspiration in pregnancy, either diagnostically or therapeutically, is small.

Ovarian cancer is uncommon in pregnancy, occurring in less than 3 per cent of cysts. However, a cyst with features suggestive of malignancy on ultrasound, or one that is growing, should be removed surgically. The tumour marker CA 125 is not useful in the pregnant woman, since elevated levels occur frequently as an apparently physiological change. Management may need to include a Caesarean hysterectomy, bilateral salpingo-oophorectomy and omentectomy.

### The female fetus

Fetal ovarian androgen synthesis commences at 12 weeks', and oestradiol and progesterone at 20 weeks', gestation. Thus small follicular cysts up to 7 mm in diameter may occur in up to a third of newborn girls. However, larger cysts are rare and, usually, isolated findings. Most are follicular cysts, although luteal cysts, cystic teratomata and granulosa cell tumours also occur. They may undergo torsion or haemorrhage, and occasionally necrosis of the pedicle may result in the 'disappearance' of the ovary. Rarely, small-bowel compression may cause polyhydramnios, but diaphragmatic splinting and consequent pulmonary hypoplasia does not seem to occur. Most resolve spontaneously, either antenatally or, more commonly, postnatally. Consideration may need to be given to the antenatal aspiration of a very large cyst if it is felt that it may obstruct labour or be ruptured during vaginal delivery, although this is reported rarely. Therefore, delivery by Caesarean section is not indicated. Cysts that have not resolved by 6 months of age should be explored surgically.

### The prepubertal girl

Ovarian cysts are uncommon and often benign. Teratomata and follicular cysts are the most common. Theca and granulosa cell tumours may secrete hormones. Presentation may be with abdominal pain or distension, or precocious puberty, either isosexual or heterosexual. Management depends upon the relief of symptoms, exclusion of malignancy and conservation of maximum ovarian tissue without jeopardizing fertility.

## Treatment

Treatment is mostly surgical, although there may be a few women in whom cyst aspiration is indicated.

## Therapeutic ultrasound-guided cyst aspiration

The theoretical advantages of this technique are that surgery is avoided and cyst accidents are reduced. However, it assumes that the cyst fluid is unable to re-accumulate, and that both physiological (likely to resolve spontaneously) and malignant cysts can be reliably excluded beforehand. Cytological assessment of the aspirated fluid is performed routinely but cannot be relied upon to exclude malignancy (see above).

The role of this technique therefore remains controversial. The best candidate is a young woman with a unilateral, unilocular, anechoic, thin-walled cyst less than 10 cm in diameter. The recurrence rate is 27 per cent if the fluid is clear and 68 per cent if it is bloodstained (De Crespigny et al., 1989). A tumour in a young woman that appears to be largely solid on ultrasound is likely to be a germ cell tumour and requires removal. An acutely painful ovary may be due to torsion, and surgery is essential.

There may be a small place for cyst aspiration in women in whom surgery is considered to be high risk, either because of coexisting medical problems or because dense pelvic adhesions envelop the ovaries.

## Examination under anaesthesia

Prior to any laparoscopy or laparotomy for a suspected ovarian tumour, it is prudent to perform a bimanual examination under anaesthesia to confirm the presence of the mass.

## Laparoscopic procedures

Laparoscopy may be of value if there is uncertainty about the nature of the pelvic mass. Thus it may be possible to avoid a laparotomy when there is no pathology. However, it can be difficult to exclude ovarian disease in the presence of marked pelvic inflammatory disease.

The second indication for laparoscopy is if the patient has a cyst suitable for laparoscopic surgery (Nezhat et al., 1989). This decision should be made after a full history and careful bimanual examination, ultrasound assessment and a thorough laparoscopic appraisal of the whole abdominal cavity, particularly the contralateral ovary. The patient should be aware of the possibility, and consented for, a laparotomy in case malignancy is found or unexpected laparoscopic complications are encountered.

### Indications for laparoscopy

- Uncertainty about the nature of the mass
- Tumour suitable for laparoscopic surgery
  - age less than 35 years
  - ultrasound shows no solid component
  - simple ovarian cyst
  - endometrioma

The advantages are those of laparoscopic surgery in general: less postoperative pain, shorter hospital stay and quicker return to normal activities. It may also result in less adhesion formation than an open procedure, although the evidence is not convincing. However, the consequences of spillage of cyst contents, incomplete excision of the cyst wall and an unexpected histological diagnosis of malignancy are considerable disadvantages. Up to 83 per cent of malignant ovarian tumours found by chance at a laparoscopic operation for a 'cyst' are treated inadequately (Maiman et al., 1991). Dermoid cysts are better removed by laparotomy because of the serious consequences of leakage of the cyst contents.

Laparoscopic surgery is best reserved for young women, under 35 years of age, in whom the likelihood of malignant disease is small and in whom conservation of ovarian tissue is more important. These operations require considerable expertise in laparoscopic manipulation and should not be attempted without appropriate training.

## Laparotomy

A clinical diagnosis may not be possible without a laparotomy and even then histological examination is essential for a confident conclusion. Frozen section is seldom of value in this situation, as a thorough examination of the tumour is required to exclude invasive disease.

If there is any possibility of invasive disease, a longitudinal skin incision should be used to allow adequate exposure in the upper abdomen. If wider exposure is required after making a transverse incision, the ends of the wound can be extended cranially to fashion a flap from the upper edge of the wound. A sample of ascitic fluid or peritoneal washings should be sent for cytological examination at the beginning of the operation. It is essential to explore the whole abdomen thoroughly and to inspect *both* ovaries.

In a young woman less than 35 years of age, an ovarian tumour is very unlikely to be malignant. Even if the mass is a primary ovarian malignancy, it is likely to be a germ cell tumour that is responsive to chemotherapy. Thus, ovarian cystectomy or unilateral oophorectomy is a sensible and safe treatment for unilateral ovarian masses in this age group (Bianchi et al., 1989). It is sometimes said that the contralateral ovary should be bisected and a sample sent for histology in case the tumour is malignant. In practice, most gynaecologists are unwilling to biopsy an apparently healthy ovary lest this results in infertility from peri-ovarian adhesions. Even when the lesion is bilateral, every effort should be made to conserve ovarian tissue. This policy is made possible by the effectiveness of modern chemotherapy for germ cell tumours.

Since epithelial cancer is so much more likely in a woman over the age of 44 years with a unilateral ovarian mass, she is probably best advised to have a total abdominal hysterectomy, bilateral salpingo-oophorectomy and infracolic omentectomy. However, there is evidence to suggest that unilateral oophorectomy in selected cases of epithelial carcinoma confined to one ovary may give equally good results as the traditional radical approach (Mangioni et al., 1989). It would seem reasonable to individualize the treatment of women aged 35–44 years where there are greater benefits to the patient from a conservative approach and where the risks may well be less. If conservative surgery is planned, preliminary hysteroscopy and curettage of the uterus are essential to exclude a concomitant endometrial tumour; a thorough laparotomy is especially important and an appropriate plan of action must be decided in advance with the patient should more widespread disease be found.

## Key Points

- Asymptomatic, simple ovarian cysts often resolve spontaneously.
- Ovarian cysts are very rarely malignant before the age of 35, especially when less than 10 cm in diameter.
- Solid ovarian tumours are often malignant – in young women these are usually germ cell or sex cord stromal tumours.
- There is only a limited place for aspiration of cysts.
- Conservative management is appropriate for most young women:
  - observation of cystic lesions <10 cm,
  - unilateral oophorectomy even for solid lesions.

- Women over 45 years of age with a unilocular ovarian cyst greater than 6 cm or with any other type of ovarian tumour should usually be advised to have a total abdominal hysterectomy and bilateral salpingo-oophorectomy.
- A bimanual examination under anaesthesia should be performed prior to any surgery for ovarian tumours to confirm that a mass is still palpable.

## References

Bailey CL, Ueland FR, Land GL et al. The malignant potential of small cystic ovarian tumours in women over 50 years of age. *Gynecol Oncol* 1998; **69**: 3–7.

Bianchi UA, Favalli G, Sartori E et al. Limited surgery in non-epithelial ovarian cancer. In: Conte PF, Ragni N, Rosso R, Vermorken JB (eds), *Multimodal treatment of ovarian cancer*. New York: Raven Press, 1989, 119–26.

Comerci JT, Licciardi F, Bergh PA, Gregori C, Breen JL. Mature cystic teratoma: a clinicopathological evaluation of 517 cases and review of the literature. *Obstet Gynecol* 1994; **84**: 22–8.

De Crespigny LC, Robinson HP, Davoren RA, Fortune D. The 'simple' ovarian cyst: aspirate or operate? *Br J Obstet Gynaecol* 1989; **96**: 1035–9.

Diernaes E, Rasmussen J, Soersen T, Hasche E. Ovarian cysts: management by puncture? *Lancet* 1987; **i**: 1084.

Fowler JM, Carter JR. Laparoscopic management of the adnexal mass in postmenopausal women. *J Gynecol Tech* 1995; **1**: 7–10.

Goldstein SR. Conservative management of small postmenopausal cystic masses. *Clin Obstet Gynecol* 1993; **36**(2): 395–401.

Koonings PP, Campbell K, Mishell DR, Grimes DA. Relative frequency of primary ovarian neoplasms: a 10 year review. *Obstet Gynecol* 1989; **74**: 921–6.

Levine D, Gosink B, Wolf SI, Feldesman MR, Pretorius DH. Simple adnexal cysts: the natural history in postmenopausal women. *Radiology* 1992; **184**: 653–9.

Maiman M, Seltzer V, Boyce J. Laparoscopic excision of ovarian neoplasms subsequently found to be malignant. *Obstet Gynecol* 1991; **77**: 563–5.

Mangioni C, Chiari S, Colombo N et al. Limited surgery in epithelial ovarian cancer. In: Conte PF, Ragni N, Rosso R,

Vermorken JB (eds), *Multimodal treatment of ovarian cancer*. New York: Raven Press, 1989, 127–32.

Nezhat C, Winer WK, Nezhat F. Laparoscopic removal of dermoid cysts. *Obstet Gynecol* 1989; **73**: 278–81.

Office of Population Censuses and Surveys. *Cancer statistics registration 1981*. London: HMSO, 1985.

Parker WH. Laparoscopic management of the adnexal mass in postmenopausal women.*J Gynecol Tech* 1995; **1**: 3–6.

Rulin MC, Preston AL. Adnexal masses in postmenopausal women. *Obstet Gynecol* 1987; **70**: 579–81.

Saunders AM, Hertzman VO. Malignant carcinoid teratoma of the ovary. *Can Med Assoc J* 1960; **83**: 602–5.

Steinkampf MP, Hammond KR. Hormonal treatment of functional ovarian cysts: a randomised, prospective study. *Fertil Steril* 1990; **54**: 775–7.

Thornton JG, Wells M. Ovarian cysts in pregnancy: does ultrasound make traditional management inappropriate? *Obstet Gynecol* 1987; **69**: 717–20.

Wertheim I, Fleischhacker D, McLachlin CM, Rice LW, Berkowitz RS, Goff BA. Pseudomyxoma peritonei: a review of 23 cases. *Obstet Gynecol* 1994; **84**: 17–21.

## Additional reading

Bourne TH, Campbell S, Reynolds KM. Screening for early familial ovarian cancer with transvaginal ultrasonography and colour flow imaging. *BMJ* 1993; **306**: 1025–9.

Campbell S, Bhan V, Royston P, Whitehead MI, Collins WP. Transabdominal ultrasound screening for early ovarian cancer. *BMJ* 1989; **299**: 1363–7.

# Chapter 12

# Malignant disease of the uterus and cervix

## OVERVIEW

Although cervical screening has reduced the incidence of cervical cancer, overall the rate is rising in younger women. Surgery remains the mainstay of treatment for early-stage disease, whilst radiotherapy is used for more advanced stages. Post-menopausal bleeding is the commonest presenting symptom of endometrial cancer. Although formerly endometrial cancer was thought to carry a good prognosis, it is now recognized that the 5-year survival is similar to that of cervical carcinoma.

## Malignant disease of the cervix

### Introduction

There are two main types of cervical cancer – squamous cell carcinoma and adenocarcinoma. The squamous cancer is preceded by a premalignant phase that usually lasts for about 10 years. The same may be true of adenocarcinoma but much less is known about these lesions. Cervical cytological is designed to detect squamous abnormalities of the cervix but does detect some glandular abnormalities. With regular, frequent screening, most are detected at the premalignant phase and can be treated readily. As a result of screening there has been a fall in the incidence of cervical cancer that has affected squamous cancers far more than adenocarcinoma of the cervix.

### Epidemiology

Cervical cancer is the second commonest cancer in women worldwide and is nearly as common as breast cancer. In the developing world, cervical cancer is very much more common than breast cancer. The reverse is true in the developed world. The age-related incidence changed dramatically in England in the last century, with the disease becoming far more common in younger women in the 1980s. Each year there are approximately 1500 deaths in England and Wales from carcinoma of the cervix. The rate has fallen steeply in recent years because of cervical cytology screening.

### Aetiology

The cause of cervical cancer is unknown. There is increasing evidence that infection by certain strains of human papillomavirus (HPV) is one factor. It is probable that 80–90 per cent of sexually active women acquire HPV infection of the genital tract at some stage in their lives, in much the same way that most people become infected with the Epstein–Barr virus that causes glandular fever. With HPV infection so common in relation to cervical cancer, it is obvious that one or more other factors must play a part for cancer to develop. HPV types 16 and 18 are the most commonly associated with cervical cancer, but many other types are also found. The range of types and proportions of each type vary markedly in different parts of the world. The association between HPV infection and cervical cancer has led to the development of vaccines both to prevent and to treat this disorder and its precursors. While it is now technically possible to construct a large range of different vaccines, many years of fieldwork will be necessary to evaluate their efficacy, acceptability and effect upon the prevalence of other HPV subtypes.

## Pathophysiology

### Transformation zone

The ectocervix is covered by squamous epithelium, a stratified epithelium very similar to skin, but lacking keratin, the protein that makes skin waterproof. The canal of the cervix, however, is lined by columnar epithelium, only one cell thick, and the point where these two epithelia meet is called the squamocolumnar junction (SCJ).

The position of the SCJ varies throughout the reproductive life (Fig. 12.1). During infancy it lies just at the external os, but as the cervix increases in volume during puberty and also pregnancy, the SCJ is said to roll out onto the ectocervix. The delicate columnar epithelium exposed to the acid environment of the vagina undergoes a process of metaplasia whereby it becomes squamous epithelium.

The transformation zone is that part of the cervix that extends from the widest part of skin that was originally columnar epithelium into the current SCJ. This area is often characterized by Nabothian follicles, which are retention cysts from previous endocervical glands that have been covered by the advancing squamous epithelium.

The area of columnar epithelium seen on the ectocervix appears red because the single-cell thickness of columnar epithelium allows the vascular stroma to be seen. This red area has been incorrectly called cervical erosion. To further compound this error, for many years women with this normal red appearance on their cervix were treated for cervical erosion by cautery under general anaesthetic.

### Dysplasia

The process of metaplasia can be disrupted by external influences and can lead to disordered squamous epithelium called dysplastic epithelium. HPV is now implicated in this process, although HPV infection alone does not appear to be sufficient to cause dysplasia. Smoking and immune suppression appear to be additional factors which may act as co-agents.

Dysplastic epithelium lacks the normal maturation of cells as they move from the basal layer to the superficial layer. The nuclei tend to be larger, more variable in size and shape and more actively dividing than in healthy squamous epithelium.

Dysplasias are now usually referred to as cervical intraepithelial neoplasia (CIN). They are graded as mild, moderate or severe, depending on the degree of cytological atypia and also the thickness of the epithelium involved. CIN I affects only the deepest third of the epithelium from the basal layer upwards, with maturation seen more superficial to that. CIN II affects two-thirds of the thickness of the epithelium, while CIN III shows no maturation throughout the full thickness. A simpler classification (the Bethesda system) of these abnormalities has been proposed where HPV infection alone and CIN I are grouped together as 'low-grade squamous intraepithelial lesions (LSIL)' and CIN II and III as 'high-grade SIL (HSIL)'.

### Natural history of CIN

It has been known for many years that CIN will progress to cervical carcinoma in some instances. The rate of invasion of CIN III lesions is said to be 36 per cent over 20 years, but all these women had been treated. In a small series of women diagnosed by punch biopsy and not treated, 90 per cent developed invasive cancer. Initially it was believed that CIN III tended to develop from CIN I and II, and only CIN III lesions would progress to invasive cancer. Most authors now believe that CIN III lesions probably arise as such. Apparent progression from CIN I to CIN III is explained on the basis of a smaller area of CIN III only becoming apparent with time as the lesions enlarge.

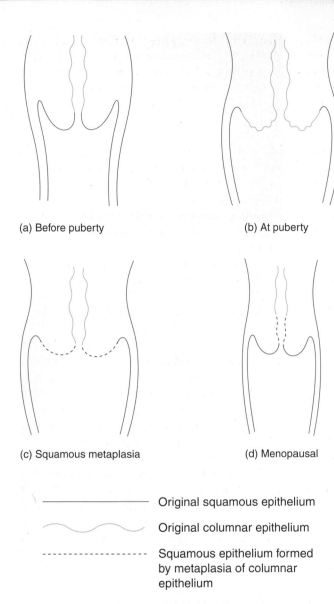

(a) Before puberty

(b) At puberty

(c) Squamous metaplasia

(d) Menopausal

**Figure 12.1** The position of the squamocolumnar junction varies throughout reproductive life.

———————————— Original squamous epithelium

∼∼∼∼∼∼∼∼∼∼∼∼ Original columnar epithelium

- - - - - - - - - - - - - - - Squamous epithelium formed by metaplasia of columnar epithelium

The risk of invasion of CIN I and II abnormalities has not been clearly defined. While the risk for CIN I appears to be much less than for CIN III, the difficulty is in defining whether the abnormality in the cervix is truly a pure CIN lesion or whether there are small areas of more significant abnormalities. Certainly cervical malignancies are seen in association with CIN I abnormalities.

## Cytology – cervical smears

Exfoliative cervical cytology is a technique developed by Papanicolaou to collect the cells that had been shed from the skin of the cervix, spread them on a glass slide and stain them using a specially developed technique. Originally cells were washed from the vagina and collected in the posterior fornix. However, a more efficient technique of exfoliative cytology involves scraping the cervix to collect cells directly.

The normal cells shed from healthy squamous epithelium have extremely small nuclei that are flattened and pyknotic. On the other hand, cells from dysplastic epithelium where little maturation has occurred have large nuclei, a large degree of cytological atypia and increased nuclear:cytoplasmic ratio. Smears may show borderline nuclear changes or mild, moderate or severe dyskaryosis. Women with moderate or severe dyskaryosis are referred for colposcopy. Most experts also recommend referral of women with mild dyskaryosis, but some say the smear should be repeated and the woman referred only if subsequent smears are not normal. Three normal smears are required before a woman can be returned to routine screening after a smear showing mild dyskaryosis.

A very small number of smears are reported to show abnormal glandular cells or borderline nuclear changes in glandular cells. Such women are always referred to colposcopy urgently because of the high risk of invasive cancer of the cervix or endometrium.

The sensitivity of cervical cytology is about 50 per cent, but because CIN takes about 10 years on average to become invasive, missed lesions are detected on second and third subsequent samples. The specificity of cervical cytology is about 92 per cent, with the result that about 8 per cent of the normal population having smears will be reported to have a dyskaryotic result.

## Colposcopy

The colposcope is a binocular operating microscope with magnification of between 5 and 20 times. It has been used to examine the cervix in detail to identify CIN and pre-clinical invasive cancer.

The cervix is first examined for abnormal vessel patterns known to be associated with premalignant and malignant lesions of the cervix. To assist in the identification of abnormal vessels, the cervix may be washed with normal saline and may be viewed through a green filter, which highlights the blood vessels as black lines. Application of 3–5 per cent acetic acid to the area highlights CIN as white, compared with the pink of the squamous epithelium (Fig. 12.2). The acetic acid coagulates protein of cytoplasm and nuclei and since abnormal epithelium is of a high nuclear density, this prevents light from passing through the epithelium, which thus appears white. Acetowhite epithelium and an abnormal subepithelial capillary pattern may be revealed as mosaicism or punctation. Mosaic vessels are arranged parallel to the surface, giving a crazy paving appearance, whereas punctation is formed by dilated vessels viewed end on. Abnormal branching vessels are suggestive of microinvasive carcinoma (Fig. 12.3).

Schiller's test identifies normal squamous epithelium. Normal, mature squamous epithelium contains abundant glycogen that stains dark brown with iodine, and the test involves the application of Lugol's iodine

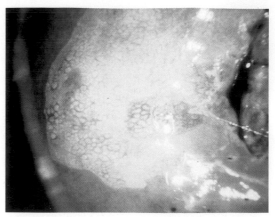

**Figure 12.2** This figure shows acetowhite epithelium. (Courtesy of Mr KS Metcalf.)

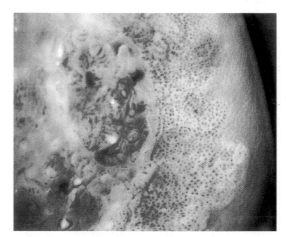

**Figure 12.3** Abnormal vascular patterns. (Courtesy of Mr KS Metcalf.)

solution to the ectocervix. The normal squamous epithelium will stain dark brown, whereas columnar epithelium, abnormal squamous epithelium and immature normal squamous epithelium will not.

Usually a colposcopic-directed biopsy will be taken from the most abnormal areas of the epithelium to confirm the diagnosis. Colposcopy is considered complete if healthy columnar epithelium is identified within the endocervical canal. If the transformation zone extends up the canal out of view, colposcopy is unsatisfactory because there may be more abnormal lesions in the canal out of sight.

## Treatment of CIN

Cervical intraepithelial neoplasia has the potential to be an invasive malignancy but does not have malignant

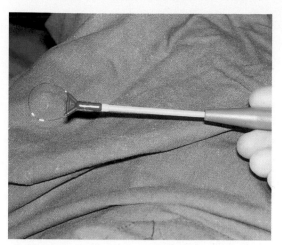

**Figure 12.4** A LLETZ loop. (Courtesy of Mr KS Metcalf.)

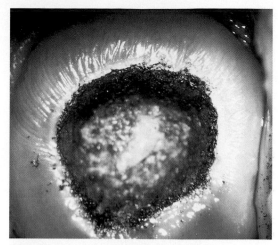

**Figure 12.5** The cervix after LLETZ. (Courtesy of Mr KS Metcalf.)

properties. Because of this, treatment involves completely removing the abnormal epithelium. This can be done either by an excisional technique or by destroying the abnormal epithelium. It should be remembered that CIN within cervical glands can extend as far as 5 mm into the stroma of the cervix. Treatment, therefore, must be directed to a depth of at least 5 mm. In practice, the best results are obtained when the cervix is treated to 10 mm.

Ablative techniques, such as cold coagulation, cryotherapy and laser vaporization, may be used to destroy the abnormal epithelium. The advantages of ablative therapy are that it is quick, cheap and an easy technique to learn. The principal disadvantage is that no histology is available for review. In all large series of ablative therapy, a small number of invasive cancers were overlooked at the time of original diagnosis and were treated in error with ablation. Approximately 1 per cent of patients treated for CIN III will have an unsuspected invasive carcinoma. Using ablative therapy, this will not be discovered until the patient is symptomatic or returns for follow-up.

Excisional techniques include the now popular large loop excision of transformation zone (LLETZ) using a diathermy generator (Fig. 12.4). Other excisional techniques use a carbon dioxide laser, a diathermy wire (NETZ) or a scalpel with the old-fashioned knife cone biopsy (Fig. 12.5). LLETZ has become extremely popular because it is quick and easy to perform. However, its major disadvantage is that it is not easy to tailor the excision to the exact area of the abnormality. In consequence, a high rate of incomplete excision is seen in up to 40 or even 50 per cent of cases. Laser cone biopsy and NETZ, on the other hand, allow very accurate excision with good visibility but are more difficult techniques to learn and require slightly longer to perform than LLETZ. Knife cone biopsy requires a general anaesthetic and has a higher incidence of both primary and secondary haemorrhage. Excellent histology can be obtained with a laser or NETZ with much lower morbidity.

The follow-up of patients treated for CIN is controversial. In some areas of the UK, one or two follow-up colposcopies are offered, but in others follow-up is entirely by cytology. The published data suggest that women who have undergone treatment for CIN III have a 9 per cent recurrence rate over 10 years and a fourfold increased incidence of invasive carcinoma compared with the background population, which remains elevated for 20 years. It seems unlikely that these figures are achieved by treatment given in less expert hands. Certainly they suggest that women should be offered smears every year for the first 10 years after treatment.

## Invasive carcinoma of the cervix

### Clinical presentation

Many early lesions and microinvasive carcinomas are asymptomatic and are detected by cervical screening. Those with larger lesions present with postcoital bleeding, intermenstrual bleeding or postmenopausal bleeding. Some patients will complain of a profuse, offensive vaginal discharge, which may be blood-stained. Other symptoms, such as pain, are uncommon until a very late stage.

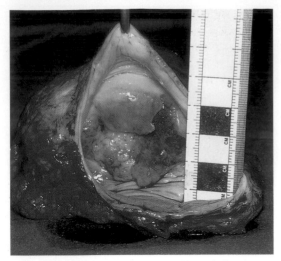

**Figure 12.6** A hysterectomy specimen with cervical cancer. (Courtesy of Mr KS Metcalf.)

In all patients with abnormal vaginal bleeding, the possibility of either a cervical or uterine carcinoma should be considered and only be discounted after both have been formally excluded. Sometimes cervical cancer presents with bleeding during pregnancy.

Cancer of the cervix may not be clinically obvious to a general practitioner until it has become very large. It may look like a friable polyp or an ulcerated area. It often bleeds on contact. However, it is usually easier to feel a cervical cancer than to see it because the cervix becomes stony hard. The surface may be friable. As the carcinoma grows into the surrounding tissue, the cervix becomes less and less mobile. Figure 12.6 shows a hysterectomy specimen with cervical carcinoma. A combined vaginal and rectal examination will allow a more thorough clinical assessment of the paracervical tissues. Occasionally pyometra occurs, causing uterine enlargement.

## Pathophysiology

Most cervical carcinomas are of the squamous cell type, resembling the epithelium of the ectocervix. The other principal type is adenocarcinoma with cells resembling the epithelium lining the endocervical canal. Because cervical screening is less effective in preventing adenocarcinoma of the cervix, this type has become more common in recent years and now accounts for 15–20 per cent of cases. Both of these carcinomas arise close to the SCJ, where the process of metaplasia is shifting the path of differentiation from glandular epithelium of the canal lining to squamous epithelium of the ectocervix. Presumably both the adenocarcinoma and the squamous carcinoma arise from the same precursor cells and, interestingly, the biological behaviour of both common types of carcinoma is very similar (see Fig. 12.1).

Carcinoma of the cervix may spread by direct infiltration and via the lymphatic vessels. The tumour may spread downwards into the vaginal wall, forward into the bladder, laterally into the parametrium and paracolpos, or posteriorly into the rectum. Lymphatic spread occurs outwards in the parametrium to the external and internal iliac nodes, including those in the obturator fossa, and to the common iliac and para-aortic nodes. Blood spread occurs late in the process.

## Staging

The FIGO classification is based on an examination under anaesthetic with an intravenous urogram and cystoscopy (Table 12.1). Special imaging techniques and the results of subsequent surgical findings are not included. The staging is designed to be applicable whether the patient is treated in the developing world, where high technology imaging is not available, or by radiotherapy, where later surgical findings cannot be included.

## Treatment

### Pre-clinical lesions – Stage Ia

Patients who have preclinical invasive disease that invades to a depth of less than 3 mm and a width of 7 mm can be treated safely by complete local excision. This is usually in the form of a colposcopically directed cone biopsy type of procedure performed with a knife, laser, LLETZ or NETZ.

Patients with disease invading to a depth of between 3 and 5 mm have a risk of nodal disease of approximately 5 per cent and probably have a higher risk of local recurrence. Accordingly, unless the patient is very keen to be treated conservatively, these patients should be offered radical treatment.

### Clinical invasive cervical carcinoma – Stage Ib–IV

Treatment for clinical invasive carcinoma is by surgery, radiotherapy or a combination of the two. Chemotherapy has gained an important place in conjunction with radiotherapy such that chemoradiation has replaced radiotherapy in all women sufficiently fit to undergo this more toxic treatment.

If the disease is apparently confined to the cervix, either surgery or chemoradiotherapy may be offered.

**Table 12.1** The 1998 FIGO staging classification for cervical cancer

| Stage | Description |
|-------|-------------|
| 0 | Pre-invasive carcinoma (carcinoma in situ, CIN) |
| I | Carcinoma confined to the cervix (corpus extension should be disregarded) |
| Ia | Invasive cancer identified only microscopically All gross lesions, even with superficial invasion, are Stage Ib cancers Depth of measured stromal invasion should not be greater than 5 mm and no wider than 7 mm[a] |
| Ia1 | Measured invasion no greater than 3 mm in depth and no wider than 7 mm |
| Ia2 | Measured depth of invasion greater than 3 mm and no greater than 5 mm and no wider than 7 mm |
| Ib | Clinical lesions confined to the cervix or pre-clinical lesions greater than Ia |
| Ib1 | Clinical lesions no greater than 4 cm in size |
| Ib2 | Clinical lesions greater than 4 cm in size |
| II | Carcinoma extending beyond the cervix and involving the vagina (but not the lower third) and/or infiltrating the parametrium (but not reaching the pelvic side wall) |
| IIa | Carcinoma has involved the vagina |
| IIb | Carcinoma has infiltrated the parametrium |
| III | Carcinoma involving the lower third of the vagina and/or extending to the pelvic side wall (there is no free space between the tumour and the pelvic side wall) |
| IIIa | Carcinoma involving the lower third of the vagina |
| IIIb | Carcinoma extending to the pelvic wall and/or hydronephrosis or non-functioning kidney due to ureteric obstruction caused by tumour |
| IVa | Carcinoma involving the mucosa of the bladder or rectum and/or extending beyond the true pelvis |
| IVb | Spread to distant organs |

[a] The depth of invasion should not be more than 5 mm from the base of the epithelium, either surface or glandular, from which it originates. Vascular space involvement, either venous or lymphatic, should not alter the staging.

Both forms of treatment are probably equally effective, although for premenopausal women in particular, surgery is thought to offer lower morbidity. Once the disease has spread outside the cervix, chemoradiotherapy is usually the mainstay of treatment.

### Surgery

The standard surgical procedure for carcinoma of the cervix is a Wertheim hysterectomy, which involves removal of the uterus and the paracervical tissues surrounding the cervix and the upper vagina. In addition, the pelvic lymph nodes are carefully dissected as a therapeutic manoeuvre to remove as many of the nodes as possible. The pelvic lymph nodes include the external iliac, internal iliac, common iliac, obturator and presacral nodes.

The dissection of the pelvic nodes is both diagnostic and therapeutic. If a large number of nodes are involved, it is usual to offer the patient adjuvant radiotherapy. However, if only one or two lymph nodes are involved, the pelvic dissection may well be therapeutic. The ovaries may be conserved, particularly if the patient has a squamous tumour.

Although the vagina is shortened by 2–3 cm, the remaining vagina is pliable and physical sexual function is preserved. The principal complications seen following this procedure are related to difficulty with complete bladder emptying because of division of the parasympathetic nerve supply to the bladder that runs within the uterosacral ligament.

Careful attention to bladder emptying to prevent urinary retention is important in the immediate postoperative period. On rare occasions, patients suffer from lymphoedema of the legs and mons pubis. This is more common after postoperative radiotherapy.

### Radiotherapy

Radical radiotherapy for cervical carcinoma involves the use of a linear accelerator to treat the whole pelvis with external beam therapy to shrink the central carcinoma and also to treat the possible sites of regional metastasis. Internal sources are then placed in the upper vagina and within the canal of the cervix to provide a very high dose to the central tumour. The external beam therapy is usually given in approximately 25 fractions over a 5-week period, followed by two internal treatments in the following week. Most patients tolerate this treatment well, although some damage to the bladder and bowel is inevitable.

Diarrhoea during treatment is usual, although this often settles after treatment is finished. A radiation menopause is induced in premenopausal women and inevitably there is some loss of elasticity within the vagina with narrowing. This can be reduced by the use of vaginal dilators and early resumption of intercourse.

Radiotherapy is also used in an adjuvant setting following surgery if more than one or two lymph nodes are positive, if excision margins are close or if the tumour was bulky and had a high chance of recurrence. In advanced cancer of the cervix, radiotherapy may be used in a palliative setting to reduce vaginal bleeding and discharge and to assist in local control of the disease. Chemotherapy may also be used in an adjuvant setting. Response rates are typically 60 per cent, and chemotherapy may be used in the neoadjuvant setting prior to surgery rather than following surgery.

### Carcinoma of the cervix and pregnancy

Difficult problems may arise if a woman with cervical carcinoma is also pregnant. In early pregnancy, external irradiation may be given; abortion of a dead fetus will follow and then local irradiation with caesium can be given. Later in pregnancy, the uterus must be emptied by hysterotomy or Caesarean section before radiotherapy can be given. Many surgeons prefer to treat these cases by Wertheim hysterectomy at the time of Caesarean section.

### Pelvic exenteration

Pelvic exenteration may be considered in a few selected cases of recurrent disease after radiotherapy, where the disease has spread into the bladder or rectum but where there is no evidence of distant metastases. The morbidity of this surgery can be considerable.

Anterior exenteration consists of removal of the uterus, vagina and bladder, with implantation of the ureters into an artificial bladder made from an ileal loop. If the rectum also has to be removed in a total exenteration, a terminal colostomy is formed.

### Carcinoma of the cervical stump after hysterectomy

The stump of cervix left after subtotal hysterectomy is just as prone to the development of carcinoma as when the uterus is intact, and the results of treatment are much worse. Intracavitary radiotherapy is prejudiced because an intrauterine tube cannot be used, and

vaginal irradiation may not deliver a dose sufficient to destroy the growth without risk of damage to the bladder or rectum. Surgical treatment is prejudiced by the previous operation.

### Palliative treatment

Palliative treatment is required for the distressing symptoms that may arise in the advanced stages of the disease. Patients with growths that are too advanced for curative treatment and those with recurrent disease must be kept free from pain and as comfortable as possible. Expert nursing is necessary, especially when incontinence compels frequent changing of pads and sheets. The help of the palliative care team is invaluable.

### Prognosis

The prognosis of invasive cervical carcinoma varies, depending mainly on the volume and stage of disease. An illustrative general statement might be that the expectation of 5-year survival is:
– Stage I: 80%
– Stage II: 74%
– Stage III: 47%
– Stage IV: 25%.

In Stages Ib and IIa there is little difference between the results of surgery and radiotherapy. Of those who die, 61 per cent do so within 2 years, 79 per cent do so within 3 years and only 1–2 per cent die after 5 years.

## Malignant disease of the body of the uterus

## Introduction

The most common malignant disease affecting the uterus is endometrial carcinoma, which arises from the lining of the uterus. However, sarcomas also arise from the stroma of the endometrium or from the myometrium, and these are discussed later in the chapter.

## Epidemiology

While endometrial cancer can occur in women in their twenties, the vast majority of cases occur in women over 45 years of age. The incidence rises steeply from

**Table 12.2**   Risk factors for endometrial cancer

- Obesity
- Impaired carbohydrate tolerance
- Nulliparity
- Late menopause
- Unopposed oestrogen therapy
- Functioning ovarian tumours
- Previous pelvic irradiation
- Family history of carcinoma of breast, ovary or colon

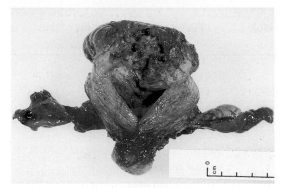

**Figure 12.7**  A uterus with adenocarcinoma of the endometrium. (Courtesy of Mr KS Metcalf.)

about age 45 years to about 55 years and remains at the same high rate thereafter. It is curious that the incidence of a tumour thought to be oestrogen associated should rise so rapidly at a time when endogenous levels of oestrogens are falling.

## Aetiology

The cause of endometrial carcinoma is unknown, although a number of factors that increase the risk of endometrial cancer are listed in Table 12.2. Many of the factors are related to an increase in oestrogen levels. In the postmenopausal period, the majority of circulating oestrogen is derived from aromatization of peripheral androgens. This conversion takes place principally in adipose tissue. In addition, postmenopausal women with diabetes have increased oestrogen levels.

Women who use oral contraception or progestogens have up to a 50 per cent reduction in the incidence of endometrial cancer and the protection lasts for many years after stopping these drugs. Cigarette smoking has also been associated with the reduced risk of endometrial cancer.

Increasing evidence suggests that it is simplistic to view excess oestrogen as the prime factor in the development of endometrial cancer. The interaction between oestrogen, insulin and insulin-like growth factor-1 may be more important.

## Pathology

The commonest subtype of endometrial carcinoma is called endometrioid because it resembles the normal proliferative endometrium, although the architecture is much more complicated. Squamous metaplasia can occur within adenocarcinomas and this can result in an adenoacanthoma or an adenosquamous carcinoma. Papillary serous and clear cell carcinomas are particularly aggressive forms of endometrial carcinoma, and primary squamous cell carcinoma of the endometrium is extremely rare.

## Clinical presentation

Most women with endometrial carcinoma will present with postmenopausal bleeding. However, a postmenopausal discharge, particularly a bloodstained discharge, may well be associated with carcinoma. In the premenopausal period, many women with endometrial carcinoma will present with intermenstrual bleeding, but one-third will present with heavy periods only.

Figure 12.7 shows a uterus with adenocarcinoma of the endometrium.

## Diagnosis

Traditionally, postmenopausal bleeding was investigated by a dilatation and curettage. More recently, however, diagnosis has shifted to the outpatient setting, with the ultrasound determination of endometrial thickness and outpatient sampling of the endometrium using instruments such as a Pipelle sampler in cases where the ultrasound suggests that the endometrium is more than 5 mm thick. If the sampler has been fully introduced into the uterus and no malignant tissue is identified, the test can be

**Table 12.3** FIGO staging of carcinoma of the corpus uteri

| Stage | Description |
| --- | --- |
| I | The carcinoma is confined to the corpus |
| II | The carcinoma has involved the corpus and the cervix but has not extended outside the uterus |
| III | The carcinoma has extended outside the uterus but not outside the true pelvis |
| IV | The carcinoma has extended outside the true pelvis or has obviously involved the mucosa of the bladder or rectum Bullous oedema as such does not permit a case to be allotted to Stage IV |

regarded as negative. Outpatient hysteroscopy may be undertaken, although it is rarely necessary. Ultrasound also allows the ovaries to be imaged, as a number of patients with postmenopausal bleeding will have ovarian pathology. It is important to advise women to return if the bleeding recurs.

## Staging

The FIGO classification and staging of endometrial carcinoma are shown in Table 12.3.

## Treatment

### Surgery

The treatment of choice in patients with endometrial carcinoma is total abdominal hysterectomy and bilateral salpingo-oophorectomy. Most women with Stage II disease are not diagnosed until after the hysterectomy has been performed. In such women, the prognosis is much the same as for Stage I. Radical hysterectomy and bilateral pelvic lymphadenectomy with para-aortic node sampling is only performed if the cervical spread is clearly recognized before surgery. Even then, it is often wiser to treat the patient with radiotherapy like a cervical cancer.

Lymphadenectomy has not achieved an established place in the treatment of endometrial cancer in the UK. If spread to the lymph nodes has occurred, the para-aortic nodes will be involved in more than 50 per cent of such cases because of direct spread along the lymphatics that accompany the ovarian vessels. While a therapeutic lymphadenectomy can be achieved in the pelvis, complete removal of all para-aortic lymph nodes is very much more difficult. Indeed, in the USA, where lymphadenectomy is recommended, most surgeons perform no more than node sampling – a procedure without therapeutic value and of limited prognostic value. The age, the obesity and the high rate of co-morbidity in these women detract further from the widespread adoption of lymphadenectomy in women with endometrial cancer.

### Radiotherapy

The role of postoperative radiotherapy has also come under review in recent years. Formerly, deep myometrial invasion was regarded as an indication for this adjuvant treatment. However, a study in Holland confirmed the results of a much older Norwegian study that showed no evidence of benefit. It seems more sensible to withhold radiotherapy initially, offering it only to the small number of women who develop recurrent disease. In this group of women, salvage radiotherapy offers a 50 per cent cure rate.

Treatment needs to be individualized for the patient with more advanced disease, but surgery is not usually the first line of treatment. Pelvic radiotherapy is performed and then occasionally residual disease may be removed surgically. Some centres report good results with radiation to para-aortic nodal disease but that is not the general experience.

### Progestogens

The only value of progestogens is in the palliation of recurrent disease. Good results are obtained rarely and only with well-differentiated tumours containing oestrogen receptors.

## Prognosis

Carcinoma of the endometrium has traditionally been the poor relation of gynaecological malignancies, with the majority of cases being treated outside major cancer centres. Such an approach stems from the belief that the cancer carries a good prognosis. However, the 5-year survival figures approximate to those of cancer of the cervix (Table 12.4).

**Table 12.4** Five-year survival for women with endometrial cancer

| Stage | 5-year survival (%) |
| --- | --- |
| Stage I | 83 |
| Stage II | 71 |
| Stage III | 39 |
| Stage IV | 27 |

Prognosis of the disease is related to stage, which now includes grade of disease, myometrial invasion and lymph node involvement. Other factors such as age and body morphology are also important: the higher the age, the more likely the patient is to succumb to the disease.

## Sarcoma and mixed mesodermal tumours of the uterus

## Mixed mesodermal tumours

This includes tumours that contain heterologous mesenchymal elements. In adults they often present as a large fleshy mass protruding from the uterine wall into the uterine cavity. Histological examination shows that it contains some elements resembling sarcoma and others resembling carcinoma, together with bizarre components such as cartilage and striped muscle. Metastasis via the bloodstream is common, as is local recurrence after removal. The patient complains of bleeding from the uterus, and sometimes of pain. Tumours of this type occasionally follow uterine irradiation. The prognosis is poor.

Sarcoma botryoides (embryonal rhabdomyosarcoma) is a variety of the same type of tumour that is seen in infants and young children. There is a blood-stained, watery discharge and the vagina is found to contain grape-like masses of soft growth, usually arising from the cervix. Among the myxomatous cells of the tumour, primitive striped muscle cells (rhabdomyoblasts) can be demonstrated. Local recurrence often follows removal, and distant metastases occur.

## Leiomyosarcoma

Leiomyosarcoma arise in the uterine muscle. Very rarely, such a tumour may arise by transformation of a previously benign fibromyoma; this occurs in less than 0.2 per cent of fibroids. Sarcoma also occasionally arises in the stroma of the endometrium – endometrial stromal sarcoma.

Tumours of this group grow more rapidly and are softer than fibromyomata. They may increase in size after the menopause, when fibromyomata remain unchanged or shrink. On naked-eye inspection, the tumour may be seen to have invaded the uterine wall or the capsule of the fibromyoma, and the cut surface often shows small haemorrhages and areas of degenerative softening. Microscopically, they consist of spindle-shaped or rounded cells, many of them pleomorphic, with little stroma and primitive blood vessels. Histological diagnosis of malignancy depends on the number of mitoses per high-power field (HPF). Patients with more than ten mitoses per HPF are regarded as having malignant disease. Distant metastasis via the bloodstream and direct spread to adjacent structures often occur.

These tumours occur in adults, who usually complain of uterine bleeding. Rapid growth of the tumour, with increasing pain, may give rise to suspicion of its nature, but in many cases the diagnosis is made only after the tumour has been removed. In rare cases, a sarcoma may be slow growing, and its nature discovered only when it recurs after operation.

## Treatment

If the diagnosis is suspected in adults before operation, total hysterectomy and bilateral salpingo-oophorectomy is performed, followed by external radiotherapy. In many cases the diagnosis is made only after hysterectomy has been performed for supposed fibromyomata; a decision about whether to proceed to additional radiotherapy must then be taken, depending on the extent and nature of the disease. The prognosis is poor, except for leiomyosarcoma arising in a fibromyoma.

In children, as with many other forms of malignant disease, the prognosis with conventional treatment has been very poor. The modern use of a combination of external irradiation and chemotherapy has altered the outlook and allowed a less radical surgical approach to be taken. Exenteration is now rarely indicated in the treatment of these tumours.

## Key Points

- The cause of cervical cancer is unknown, but HPV infection appears to play some role. Most women become infected with HPV at some stage in their lives but very few develop cervical cancer.
- The advent of regular cervical screening and colposcopy has reduced the incidence and mortality of invasive cervical cancer dramatically.
- Squamous cell carcinoma is the most common type and has a similar prognosis to adenocarcinoma.
- Metastatic spread is mainly lymphatic.
- Treatment is dependent on surgical staging. Surgery is most often performed in young women with Stage I disease.
- Radiotherapy is used for older and less fit patients regardless of the size of the tumour.

- Chemoradiotherapy is used for those with large-volume or advanced stage tumours who are fit enough to cope with the increased toxicity.
- The 5-year survival for carcinoma of the uterus is similar to cervical cancer stage for stage.
- While oestrogen may play a part in the aetiology, insulin and insulin growth factors are also important.
- Postmenopausal bleeding is the most common presenting symptom.
- Total abdominal hysterectomy and bilateral salpingo-oophorectomy is the treatment of choice for Stage I and most Stage II disease.

# Carcinoma of the ovary and Fallopian tube

## OVERVIEW

Carcinoma of the ovary is most common in the wealthy nations of the world. There are just under 6000 cases each year in the UK. While the incidence of ovarian cancer is similar to that of endometrium and of cervix, more women die from ovarian cancer than from carcinoma of the cervix and body of the uterus combined.

Most ovarian tumours are of epithelial origin. These are rare before the age of 35 years, but the incidence increases with age to a peak in the 50–70-year-old age group (Fig. 13.1). Most epithelial tumours are not discovered until they have spread widely. Some of these 'ovarian' tumours probably arise from the Fallopian tube, tumours of which are usually recognized only when at a relatively early stage. Surgery and chemotherapy, mainly with carboplatin or cisplatin and paclitaxel, form the mainstay of treatment for epithelial tumours. The results are poor: less than 25 per cent of women with ovarian cancer are alive at 5 years.

Only 3 per cent of ovarian cancers are seen in women younger than 35 years and most of these are non-epithelial cancers such as germ cell tumours. In contrast to epithelial tumours, germ cell tumours can be treated very successfully with conservative surgery and modern multi-drug chemotherapy. Fertility can often be conserved.

## CANCER OF THE OVARY

### Aetiology

#### 'Incessant ovulation' theory

Epithelial tumours are most frequently associated with nulliparity, an early menarche, a late age at menopause and a high estimated number of years of ovulation. Oral contraceptive use reduces the risk fourfold (The Cancer and Steroid Hormone Study, 1987). However, even without oral contraceptives, increasing age at first birth reduces the risk of ovarian cancer. This and other anomalies cast doubt upon the 'incessant ovulation' theory.

### Subfertility treatment

Subfertility, especially when it is unexplained, is associated with both ovarian and endometrial cancer. However, case-controlled studies have suggested that

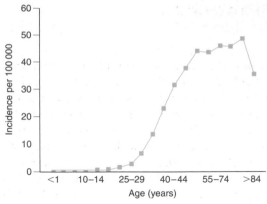

**Figure 13.1** The incidence of ovarian cancer in England and Wales (Office of Population Censuses and Surveys, 1985).

there might possibly be a link between ovarian cancer and prolonged attempts at induction of ovulation (Venn et al., 1995).

## Genetic factors

### Familial ovarian cancer

- Familial ovarian cancer is rare – 5–10%
- Suggestive history
- At least two first-degree relatives with ovarian, breast or colorectal carcinoma
- Cases usually diagnosed before 50 years of age
- Defective genes include *BRCA1* and *BRCA2*
- The risk of ovarian cancer (40%) in these families is less than the risk of breast cancer (80%)
- Genetic testing cannot guarantee to detect all defective genes

## Familial ovarian cancer

There is a family history in between 5 and 10 per cent of women with epithelial ovarian cancers – usually serous adenocarcinomas (Kasprzak et al., 1999). A woman with one affected close relative has a lifetime risk of 2.5 per cent, twice the risk in the general population. With two affected close relatives, the lifetime risk increases to 30–40 per cent (Ponder, 1994). A particular feature of familial cancers is the relatively early age at which they occur.

Most of these families also have cases of breast or colorectal cancer in the family. The defective gene in the breast/ovary families is most commonly the tumour-suppressor gene *BRCA1* (81 per cent). *BRCA2* is defective in about 14 per cent. Families with colorectal cancer have defects in the DNA repair genes, but this is seldom found in association with familial ovarian cancer (Kasprzak et al., 1999). A woman who has inherited a defective *BRCA1* gene in a well-documented family has a 60 per cent risk of breast cancer by 50 years of age and an 80 per cent lifetime risk. However, the risk of ovarian cancer is much lower, being nearer 40 per cent.

## Management of women with a family history of ovarian cancer

Genetic testing for *BRCA1* is now possible but is impracticable and unreliable because mutations are found far less often than expected, even in women with a strong family history. There are very considerable problems in interpreting the results in women with only one or two affected relatives. There may be a spectrum of mutations with very different levels of risk. Even a negative test result may not provide the expected reassurance.

Once identified with the help of a clinical geneticist, women with a high risk of ovarian and breast cancer are difficult to advise. The main risk is breast cancer, but prophylactic, bilateral mastectomy is a very drastic step for any woman to take. None of the available screening tests for ovarian cancer is very effective, and false-positive results can result in unnecessary surgery. Annual ovarian ultrasonography with colour-flow Doppler studies and serum CA 125 estimation every 6–12 months are recommended, but it is uncertain how much protection this offers. Prophylactic bilateral oophorectomy, usually combined with hysterectomy, is recommended for clearly defined high-risk women after completion of their family at about 45 years of age (Kasprzak et al., 1999). This does not remove the risk entirely, as carcinoma of the peritoneum has occurred after this procedure.

## Classification of ovarian tumours

Ovarian tumours can be solid or cystic. They may be benign or malignant and in addition there are those that, while having some of the features of malignancy, lack any evidence of stromal invasion. These are called borderline tumours.

Primary ovarian tumours are divided into epithelial type (implying an origin from surface epithelium), sex cord gonadal type (also known as sex cord stromal type, or sex cord mesenchymal type, and originating from sex cord mesenchymal elements), and germ cell type.

## Simplified histological classification of ovarian tumours

I **Common epithelial tumours (benign, borderline or malignant)**
  A. Serous tumour
  B. Mucinous tumour
  C. Endometrioid tumour
  D. Clear cell (mesonephroid) tumour
  E. Brenner tumour
  F. Undifferentiated carcinomas
II **Sex cord stromal tumours**
  A. Granulosa stroma cell tumour
  B. Androblastoma: Sertoli–Leydig cell tumour
  C. Gynandroblastoma
III **Germ cell tumours**
  A. Dysgerminoma
  B. Endodermal sinus tumour (yolk sac tumour)
  C. Embryonal cell tumour
  D. Choriocarcinoma
  E. Teratoma
  F. Mixed tumours
IV **Metastatic tumours**

## Pathology of epithelial tumours

Well-differentiated epithelial carcinomas tend to be more often associated with early-stage disease, but the degree of differentiation does correlate with survival, except in the most advanced stages. Diploid tumours tend to be associated with earlier stage disease and a better prognosis. Cell type is not of itself prognostically significant. Comparing patients stage for stage and grade for grade, there is no difference in survival between different epithelial types. However, mucinous and endometrioid lesions are likely to be associated with an earlier stage and lower grade than serous cystadenocarcinomas.

## Serous carcinoma

Most serous carcinomas have both solid and cystic elements but some may be mainly cystic. They often affect both ovaries. Well-differentiated tumours have a papillary pattern with stromal invasion. Psammoma bodies (calcospherules) are often present. At the other end of the spectrum is the anaplastic tumour composed of sheets of undifferentiated neoplastic cells in masses within a fibrous stroma. Occasional glandular structures may be present which enable a diagnosis of adenocarcinoma to be made. All gradations between these two are seen, sometimes in the same tumour.

## Mucinous carcinoma

Malignant mucinous tumours account for 10 per cent of the malignant tumours of the ovary. They are usually multilocular, thin-walled cysts with a smooth external surface containing mucinous fluid. Mucinous tumours are amongst the largest tumours of the ovary and may reach enormous dimensions. A cyst diameter of 25 cm is quite common.

## Endometrioid carcinoma

These are ovarian tumours that resemble endometrial carcinomas. There is little to characterize an ovarian tumour as being of endometrioid type by naked-eye examination. Most are cystic, often unilocular, and contain turbid brown fluid. Five to 10 per cent are seen in continuity with recognizable endometriosis. Ovarian adenoacanthoma, with benign-appearing squamous elements, accounts for almost 50 per cent of some series of endometrioid tumours.

It is important to note that 15 per cent of endometrioid carcinomas of the ovary are associated with endometrial carcinoma in the body of the uterus. In most cases these are two separate primary tumours.

## Clear cell carcinoma (mesonephroid)

These are the least common of the malignant epithelial tumours of the ovary, accounting for 5–10 per cent of ovarian carcinomas. The appearance from which the tumours derive their name is the clear cell pattern but, in addition, some areas show a tubulo-cystic pattern with the characteristic 'hob-nail' appearance of the lining epithelium.

Because there is a very strong association between clear cell tumours of the ovary and ovarian endometriosis, and because clear cell and endometrioid tumours frequently coexist, it has been suggested that the clear cell tumour may be a variant of endometrioid tumour.

## Borderline epithelial tumours

Ten per cent of all epithelial tumours of the ovary are of borderline malignancy. These show varying degrees of nuclear atypia and an increase in mitotic activity, multi-layering of neoplastic cells and formation of cellular buds, but no invasion of the stroma. Most borderline tumours remain confined to the ovaries and this may account for their much better prognosis. Peritoneal lesions are present in some cases and, although a few are true metastases, many do not progress and some even regress after removal of the primary tumour. The histological diagnosis of borderline malignancy can be difficult, particularly in mucinous tumours. Most borderline tumours are serous or mucinous in type.

## Natural history

Some two-thirds of patients with ovarian cancer present with disease that has spread beyond the pelvis. This is probably due to the insidious nature of the signs and symptoms of carcinoma of the ovary, but may sometimes be due to a rapidly growing tumour. Due to the non-specific nature of most of these symptoms, a diagnosis of ovarian cancer is seldom considered until the disease is in an advanced stage.

## Metastatic spread

The pelvic peritoneum and other pelvic organs become involved by direct spread (Table 13.1). The peritoneal fluid, flowing to lymphatic channels on the undersurface of the diaphragm, carries malignant cells to the omentum, to the peritoneal surfaces of the small and large bowel and the liver, and to the parietal

**Table 13.1** Pelvic and para-aortic node metastases

| | Nodes involved (%) | |
| --- | --- | --- |
| | Pelvic nodes | Para-aortic nodes |
| Stage I–II | 30 | 19 |
| Stage III–IV | 67 | 65 |

peritoneal surface throughout the abdominal cavity and on the surface of the diaphragm. Metastases on the undersurface of the diaphragm may be found in up to 44 per cent of what otherwise seems to be stage I–II disease.

Lymphatic spread commonly involves the pelvic and the para-aortic nodes. Spread may also occur to nodes in the neck or inguinal region. Haematogenous spread usually occurs late in the course of the disease. The main areas involved are the liver and the lung, although metastases to bone and brain are sometimes seen.

## Clinical staging

Peritoneal deposits on the surface of the liver do not make the tumour Stage IV; the parenchyma must be involved (Table 13.2). Similarly, the presence of a pleural effusion is insufficient to put the tumour in Stage IV unless malignant cells are found on cytological examination of the pleural fluid.

## Diagnosis

Abdominal pain or discomfort are the commonest presenting complaints and distension or feeling a lump the next most frequent. Patients may complain of indigestion, urinary frequency, weight loss or, rarely, abnormal menses or postmenopausal bleeding. A hard abdominal mass arising from the pelvis is highly suggestive, especially in the presence of ascites. A fixed, hard, irregular pelvic mass is usually felt best by combined vaginal and rectal examination (Fig. 13.2, page 148). The neck and groin should also be examined for enlarged nodes.

**Table 13.2** FIGO staging *for* primary ovarian carcinoma

| Stage | | FIGO definition |
|---|---|---|
| I | | Growth limited to ovaries |
| | Ia | Growth limited to one ovary<br>No ascites<br>No tumour on external surface<br>Capsule intact |
| | Ib | Growth limited to both ovaries<br>No ascites<br>No tumour on external surfaces<br>Capsule intact |
| | Ic | Tumour either Stage Ia or Ib but tumour on surface of one or both ovaries *or*<br>with capsule ruptured *or*<br>with ascites present containing malignant cells *or*<br>with positive peritoneal washings |
| II | | Growth involving one or both ovaries with pelvic extension |
| | IIa | Extension and/or metastases to the uterus or tubes |
| | IIb | Extension to other pelvic tissues |
| | IIIc | Tumour either Stage IIa or IIb but tumour on surface of one or both ovaries *or*<br>with capsule ruptured *or*<br>with ascites present containing malignant cells *or*<br>with positive peritoneal washings |
| III | | Growth involving one or both ovaries with peritoneal implants outside the<br>  pelvis or positive retroperitoneal or inguinal nodes<br>Superficial liver metastases equals Stage III |
| | IIIa | Tumour grossly limited to the true pelvis with negative nodes but with<br>  histologically confirmed microscopic seeding of abdominal peritoneal surfaces |
| | IIIb | Tumour with histologically confirmed implants on abdominal peritoneal surfaces,<br>  none exceeding 2 cm in diameter<br>Nodes are negative |
| | IIIc | Abdominal implants >2 cm in diameter or positive retroperitoneal<br>  or inguinal nodes |
| IV | | Growth involving one or both ovaries with distant metastases<br>If pleural effusion is present, there must be positive cytology to allot a case to Stage IV<br>Parenchymal liver metastasis equals Stage IV |

Haematological investigations include a full blood count, urea, electrolytes and liver function tests. A chest X-ray is essential. It is sometimes advisable to carry out a barium enema or colonoscopy to differentiate between an ovarian and a colonic tumour and to assess bowel involvement from the ovarian tumour itself. An intravenous pyelogram (IVP) is occasionally useful. Ultrasonography may help to confirm the presence of a pelvic mass and detect ascites before it is clinically apparent. In conjunction with CA 125 estimation, it may be used to calculate a 'risk of malignancy score'. In most women, the diagnosis is far from certain before the laparotomy, and the operation is undertaken on the basis that there is a large mass that needs to be removed regardless of its nature.

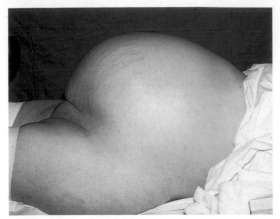

**Figure 13.2** Abdominal distension with underlying ovarian mass and ascites. (Courtesy of Mr K Metcalf.)

## Markers for epithelial tumours

CA 125 is the only marker in common clinical use. It can also be raised in benign conditions such as endometriosis. CA 125 is useful for monitoring women receiving chemotherapy to assess response. A persistent rise in CA 125 may precede clinical evidence of recurrent disease by several months in some cases. However, the values can be normal in the presence of small tumour deposits.

## Screening

Because carcinoma of the ovary tends to be asymptomatic in the early stages and most patients present with advanced disease, much effort has been made to define a tumour marker which could be used for screening purposes. So far, none has become available that is truly specific and that is suitable for the early detection of epithelial carcinoma (Oram and Jeyarajah, 1994). Ultrasound is not suitable as a primary screening tool because of expense and a high false-positive rate. The most promising approach is a combination of CA 125 with ultrasound for those women with persistently raised values.

In our present state of knowledge and with the available technology, screening the general population is neither useful nor safe. Patients should be enrolled in trials to assess new screening techniques, but should not be led to believe that these have proven value.

## Surgery

### Surgery for epithelial ovarian cancer

**Primary surgery – to determine diagnosis and remove tumour**
- Total abdominal hysterectomy
- Bilateral salpingo-oophorectomy
- Infracolic omentectomy

**Conservative primary surgery**
- Young, nulliparous woman with Stage Ia disease
- No evidence of synchronous endometrial cancer
- Unilateral salpingo-oophorectomy

**Interval debulking surgery**
- Women with bulky disease after primary surgery
- Must respond after two to four courses of chemotherapy
- Chemotherapy resumed after surgery

**Second-look surgery**
- At the end of chemotherapy
- No place in current management

**Borderline tumours**
- Ovarian cystectomy or oophorectomy adequate in young women
- Hysterectomy and bilateral salpingo-oophorectomy in older women

Surgery is the mainstay of both the diagnosis and the treatment of ovarian cancer. A vertical incision is required for an adequate exploration of the upper abdomen. A sample of ascitic fluid or peritoneal washings with normal saline should be taken for cytology. The pelvis and upper abdomen are explored carefully to identify metastatic disease.

The therapeutic objective of surgery for ovarian cancer is the removal of all tumour. While this is achieved in the majority of Stage I cases and in some Stage II, it is usually impossible in more advanced disease. Because of the diffuse spread of tumour throughout the peritoneal cavity and the retroperitoneal nodes, microscopic deposits will persist in almost all cases, even when all macroscopic tumour appears to have been excised. Thus, while surgery alone may be curative in many Stage I cases, additional therapy is essential for most of the remainder.

The resection of all visible tumour usually requires a total hysterectomy, bilateral salpingo-oophorectomy and infracolic omentectomy. However, in a young nulliparous woman with a unilateral tumour and no ascites, unilateral salpingo-oophorectomy may be justifiable after careful exploration to exclude metastatic disease and curettage of the uterine cavity to exclude a synchronous endometrial tumour. If the tumour is subsequently found to be poorly differentiated or if the washings are positive, a second operation to clear the pelvis will be necessary.

Borderline disease usually presents as a Stage Ia tumour confined to one ovary. It is often not recognized as malignant. If an ovarian cystectomy has been performed in a young woman and it seems likely that the disease has been removed completely, there is probably little to be gained from further surgery but the risk of recurrence (36 per cent) is higher than after oophorectomy (15 per cent) or pelvic clearance (2.5 per cent). In cases of doubt, a second laparotomy should be performed to explore the abdomen thoroughly and to remove the rest of the affected ovary. Older women who have no wish to have children have little to gain from conservative surgery, and it is probably still prudent to recommend bilateral oophorectomy and hysterectomy.

When bulky disease remains after initial surgery, a second laparotomy may be performed on those women who respond after two to four courses of chemotherapy. The chemotherapy is then resumed as soon as possible after the second operation. This is called 'interval debulking'. A large European study of this approach suggests that the median survival in this poor-prognosis group may be increased by 6 months and that the survival at 3 years may be improved from 10 per cent to 20 per cent (Van der Berg et al., 1995). This has led to the use of initial chemotherapy in women in whom the disease is unlikely to be resectable. Confirmation of malignancy is made by cytology or guided biopsy, and surgery follows if the tumour responds. It remains to be seen if this is an effective strategy.

Second-look surgery is defined as a planned laparotomy at the end of chemotherapy. The objectives are, first, to determine the response to previous therapy in order to document accurately its efficacy and to plan subsequent management, and second, to excise any residual disease. While there is no doubt that second-look surgery gives the most accurate indication of the disease status, the evidence suggests that neither the surgical resection of residual tumour nor the opportunity to change the treatment has any effect on the patient's survival. Second-look procedures therefore have no place outside clinical trials at the present time.

## Selecting patients for postoperative treatment

Women with Stage Ia or Ib disease and well or moderately differentiated tumours may not require further treatment. The benefit of adjuvant therapy for women with Stage Ic disease remains uncertain, but many oncologists advise chemotherapy. All other patients with invasive ovarian carcinoma require adjuvant therapy. There is no evidence that adjuvant therapy affects the outcome in women with borderline tumours.

## Radiotherapy

Radiotherapy is now almost never used in the routine management of ovarian carcinoma. A potential exception is radio-immunotherapy in which radioactive yttrium is linked to a monoclonal antibody which recognizes an antigen found on most ovarian cancers. This is given intraperitoneally. It remains an experimental treatment.

## Chemotherapy

### Chemotherapy for epithelial ovarian cancer

- Stage II–IV – possibly Stage Ic
- Carboplatin or cisplatin and paclitaxel

Chemotherapy is given both to prolong clinical remission and survival, and for palliation in advanced and recurrent disease. Chemotherapy is commenced as soon as possible after surgery and is usually given for five or six cycles at 3–4-weekly intervals.

The platinum drugs, cisplatin and its analogue carboplatin, are heavy metal compounds which cause cross-linkage of DNA strands in a similar fashion to alkylating agents. These are considered to be the most effective drugs in general use in the management of ovarian carcinoma, and are the most widely used cytotoxic drugs either alone or in combination.

Cisplatin is a very toxic drug. Until the advent of the 5-hydroxytryptamine (5HT) antagonists (ganesetron and ondansetron), severe nausea and vomiting, sometimes lasting several days, were a serious problem. Permanent renal damage will occur unless cisplatin is given with adequate hydration with intravenous fluids. Peripheral neuropathy and hearing loss are reported with increasing cumulative doses. Electrolyte disturbances, such as hypomagnesaemia, are seen occasionally. Unlike most chemotherapeutic agents, marrow toxicity is not usually a problem, with the exception of anaemia.

Carboplatin is as effective as cisplatin in the treatment of ovarian cancer and is the most commonly used first-line drug, either alone or in combination with paclitaxel. It causes less nausea and vomiting than cisplatin and has no significant renal toxicity. Neurotoxicity is rare and hearing loss is subclinical. The lack of renal toxicity means that there is no need to give carboplatin with intravenous hydration. The dose is calculated in relation to the glomerular filtration rate, using the area under the curve (AUC) formula.

Paclitaxel (Taxol) is given in combination with cisplatin or carboplatin as first-line treatment, but may be used alone when the disease recurs. It is usually given as a 4-hour infusion after a premedication regimen of dexamethasone 20 mg, diphenhydramine 50 mg and ranitidine or cimetidine to prevent hypersensitivity reactions. Paclitaxel is derived from the bark of the Pacific yew tree (*Taxus brevifolia*) and has a mechanism of action that is unique among cytotoxic drugs.

Sensory neuropathy and neutropenia are more common with higher doses, and infusions for 24 hours result in a higher incidence of grade 4 neutropenia. Other forms of toxicity such as myalgia and arthralgia are dose dependent but never severe. Nausea and vomiting are very mild, but loss of body hair is usually total irrespective of dose and schedule. Bradycardia and hypotension usually do not cause symptoms.

## Results – epithelial tumours

### Results of treatment of epithelial tumours

- Borderline tumours
  - excellent long-term prognosis in most cases
  - most of those who die have pseudomyxoma peritonei
- Invasive tumours – 5-year survival rates
  - 90% for Stage Ia and Ib well or moderately differentiated tumours
  - 10% for Stage III
  - 23% overall

## Borderline epithelial tumours

Women with borderline ovarian epithelial tumours confined to the ovaries have a good long-term prognosis, with very few women dying from their disease. Even with extra-ovarian spread, the 15-year survival for serous borderline epithelial tumours is around 90 per cent. For Stage III mucinous tumours, the 15-year survival rate is only 44 per cent. Most of those who die have pseudomyxoma peritonei. With the exception of those with pseudomyxoma peritonei, the overall prognosis is good.

## Invasive epithelial ovarian cancer

Survival for epithelial ovarian cancer is dependent mainly on stage, size of residual tumour at the end of initial surgery and grade of tumour. The 5-year survival ranges from 60 to 70 per cent for women with Stage I disease to 10 per cent for Stage III–IV. Since the majority of patients present with advanced disease, the overall 5-year survival in the UK is only 23 per cent.

While women with Stage I tumours with grade 1 or 2 histology have a 5-year survival rate of over 90 per cent, those with poorly differentiated tumours do much worse. In more advanced tumours, the amount of residual tumour at the end of initial surgery is significant in terms of prognosis.

The survival figures for cancer of the ovary have changed little over the last 20 years and remain poor for women with advanced disease despite more radical surgery and improvements in chemotherapy. Most studies do show some improvement in median survival in patients with minimal residual disease following surgery and who respond to post-surgical treatment. However, this benefit has not been sufficiently long lasting to affect 5-year survival rates. There is no doubt that even if long-term survival has not been improved, modern cytotoxic therapy has improved the quality of life for many patients with advanced ovarian cancer in spite of the side effects.

## Non-epithelial tumours

Non-epithelial tumours constitute approximately 10 per cent of all ovarian cancers. Because of their rarity and their sensitivity to intensive chemotherapy, it is especially appropriate to refer these patients for specialist care.

## Sex cord stromal tumours

### Non-epithelial tumours

- Sex-cord stromal tumour
- Granulosa cell tumour
- Theca cell tumour
- Sertoli–Leydig tumour
- Germ cell tumour
- Dysgerminoma
- Yolk sac (endodermal sinus) tumour
- Teratoma

### *Granulosa and theca cell tumours*

The most common sex cord stromal tumours are the granulosa and theca cell tumours. They often produce steroid hormones, in particular oestrogens, which can cause postmenopausal bleeding in older women and sexual precocity in pre-pubertal girls. Granulosa cell tumours usually secrete inhibin. This can be used to monitor the effects of treatment.

Theca cell tumours are usually benign. Granulosa cell tumours occur at all ages, but are found predominantly in postmenopausal women. The staging system for these tumours is the same as for epithelial tumours. Most present as Stage I. Bilateral tumours are present in only 5 per cent of cases.

#### Pathology

Granulosa cell tumours are normally solid, but cystic spaces may develop when they become large. Some are predominantly cystic. Like most tumours of the sex cord stromal tumour group, the cut surface is often yellow because of neutral lipid related to sex steroid hormone production. Areas of haemorrhage are also common.

#### Treatment

The surgical treatment is the same as for epithelial tumours. Unilateral oophorectomy is indicated only in young women with Stage Ia disease. The effect of adjunctive therapy is difficult to assess, as granulosa cell tumours can recur up to 20 years after the initial diagnosis. Radiotherapy has been largely replaced by chemotherapy in advanced or recurrent cases. In cases of late recurrence, further surgery should be considered before any other therapy is given. The 5-year survival is around 80 per cent overall, but recurrence is associated with a high mortality.

### *Sertoli–Leydig cell tumours*

Half of these rare neoplasia produce male hormones which can cause virilization. Rarely, oestrogens are secreted. The prognosis for the majority who have localized disease is good, and treatment is the same as for granulosa cell tumours.

## Germ cell tumours

### *Dysgerminomas*

Dysgerminomas account for 2–5 per cent of all primary malignant ovarian tumours. Nearly all occur in young women less than 30 years old. They spread mainly by lymphatics. All cases need a chest X-ray and a computerized tomography (CT) scan. Serum alpha-fetoprotein (AFP) and beta-human chorionic gonadotrophin (β-hCG) must be assayed to exclude the ominous presence of elements of choriocarcinoma, endodermal sinus tumour or teratoma. Occasionally some cases of pure dysgerminoma have raised levels of β-hCG. Pure dysgerminomas have a good prognosis as they are normally Stage I tumours (75 per cent), most being Stage Ia.

#### Pathology

Dysgerminomas are solid tumours which have a smooth or nodular, bosselated external surface. They are soft or rubbery in consistency, depending upon the proportion of fibrous tissue contained in them. They may reach a considerable size: the mean diameter is 15 cm. Approximately 10 per cent are bilateral; they are alone among malignant germ cell tumours in having a significant incidence of bilaterality. Elements of immature teratoma, yolk sac tumour or choriocarcinoma are found in about 10 per cent of dysgerminomas. Very thorough sampling of all dysgerminomas must be undertaken by the histopathologist to exclude the presence of these more malignant germ cell elements, as this indicates a worse prognosis.

## Other germ cell tumours

### Yolk sac (endodermal sinus) tumours

Yolk sac (endodermal sinus) tumour is the second most common malignant germ cell tumour of the ovary, making up 10–15 per cent overall and reaching a higher proportion in children. It may present as an acute abdomen due to rupture of the tumour following necrosis and haemorrhage. The tumour is usually well encapsulated and solid. Areas of necrosis and haemorrhage are often seen, as are small cystic spaces. Its consistency varies from soft to firm and rubbery and its cut surface is slippery and mucoid. It often secretes AFP, which can be used to monitor treatment.

### Teratoma

Mature teratomas are benign, the most common being the cystic teratoma or dermoid cyst found at all ages but particularly in the third and fourth decades. Not all solid teratomas are immature type.

Immature teratomas are composed of a wide variety of tissues and comprise about 1 per cent of all ovarian teratomas. They are unilateral in almost all cases and appear as solid masses that have smooth and bosselated surfaces. The cut surface shows mainly solid tissue, although small cystic spaces are visible. Blood levels of $\beta$-hCG and AFP should be estimated, even when the tumour appears to be a straightforward immature teratoma.

### Treatment

A malignant germ cell tumour should be suspected prior to surgery if a young woman has what appears to be a predominantly solid tumour on ultrasound examination. Such patients should be referred to a gynaecological oncologist.

### Treatment of non-epithelial tumours

- Sex cord stromal tumours
- Mainly treated by surgery – hysterectomy and bilateral salpingo-oophorectomy
- Unilateral salpingo-oophorectomy only in young women with Stage Ia disease
- Chemotherapy (when required) same regimens as used for epithelial tumours
- Germ cell tumours
- Mainly conservative surgery because the patients are usually young
- Combination chemotherapy is highly effective when required

Early disease is treated by surgery. In young women with Stage Ia disease, unilateral oophorectomy may suffice, but in older patients hysterectomy and bilateral salpingo-oophorectomy is recommended. Women are suitable for conservative surgery if they have a unilateral encapsulated tumour, no ascites, no evidence of abnormal lymph nodes at surgery and a negative CT scan of the para-aortic nodes.

Stage I malignant teratomas and dysgerminomas may be followed up closely without further treatment. For the remainder, chemotherapy has replaced radiotherapy, particularly in the young age groups in which this tumour is most common, as fertility is likely to be preserved. Short courses of cisplatin chemotherapy given in combination with bleomycin and etoposide (BEP) are curative in the 90 per cent of patients without adverse features. More intensive regimens are used for patients with adverse features.

## CANCER OF THE FALLOPIAN TUBE

Primary carcinoma of the Fallopian tube is extremely rare, comprising only 0.3 per cent of gynaecological malignancies. However, only early Fallopian tube carcinomas can be distinguished with certainty from ovarian disease. A study of screening for ovarian cancer detected three cases of early Fallopian tube carcinoma and 19 ovarian tumours, a relative prevalence 25 times greater than expected. This suggests that Fallopian tube carcinoma may be more common than is realized.

Primary carcinoma is usually unilateral. The mean age at diagnosis is 56 years. Many of the patients are nulliparous (45 per cent), and infertility is reported in up to 71 per cent of these women. Tumour spread is identical to that of ovarian cancer, and metastases to pelvic and para-aortic nodes are common. Most tumours involving the Fallopian tube are metastatic from ovarian cancer, but secondary spread from the breast and gastrointestinal tract also occurs.

## Pathology

Carcinoma of the Fallopian tube usually distends the lumen with tumour. The tumour may protrude through the fimbrial end and the tube may be retort shaped, resembling a hydrosalpinx. It is usually very similar to the serous adenocarcinoma of the ovary

histologically. There may be evidence of in-situ disease in the tubal epithelium.

## Staging

The FIGO clinical staging is similar to that used for ovarian cancer (Table 13.3). Probably because of the difficulty in distinguishing between advanced ovarian and advanced Fallopian tube carcinoma, 74 per cent of Fallopian tube carcinomas are diagnosed at Stage I–IIa; the remaining 26 per cent are Stage IIb–IV.

**Table 13.3**   FIGO staging for Fallopian tube carcinoma

| Stage | | FIGO definition |
|---|---|---|
| 0 | | Carcinoma in situ – limited to the tubal mucosa |
| I | | Growth limited to the Fallopian tubes |
| | Ia | One tube involved with extension into the submucosa or muscularis |
| | | Not penetrating the serosal surface |
| | | No ascites |
| | Ib | Both tubes involved but otherwise as for Ia |
| | Ic | One or both tubes with extension through or onto the tubal serosa *or* |
| | | ascites with malignant cells *or* |
| | | positive peritoneal washings |
| II | | Growth involving one or both Fallopian tubes with pelvic extension |
| | IIa | Extension or metastases to the uterus or ovaries |
| | IIb | Extension to other pelvic organs |
| | IIIc | Stage IIa or IIb plus ascites with malignant cells *or* |
| | | positive peritoneal washings |
| III | | Tumour involves one or both Fallopian tubes with peritoneal implants outside the pelvis or positive retroperitoneal or inguinal nodes |
| | | Superficial liver metastases equals Stage III |
| | | Tumour appears limited to the true pelvis but with histologically proven malignant extension to the small bowel or omentum |
| | IIIa | Tumour is grossly limited to the true pelvis with negative lymph nodes but with histologically confirmed microscopic seeding of abdominal peritoneal surfaces |
| | IIIb | Tumour involving one or both Fallopian tubes with histologically confirmed implants of abdominal peritoneal surfaces, none exceeding 2 cm in diameter |
| | | Lymph nodes are negative |
| | IIIc | Abdominal implants >2 cm in diameter or positive retroperitoneal or inguinal nodes |
| IV | | Growth involving one or both Fallopian tubes with distant metastases |
| | | If pleural effusion is present, there must be positive cytology |
| | | Parenchymal liver metastases equals Stage IV |

## Clinical presentation and management

Most cases of cancer of the Fallopian tube are diagnosed at laparotomy. The diagnosis is seldom considered preoperatively. The usual presenting symptom is postmenopausal bleeding and the diagnosis should be considered particularly if the patient also complains of a watery discharge and lower abdominal pain. Unexplained postmenopausal bleeding or abnormal cervical cytology without obvious cause demands a careful bimanual examination and pelvic ultrasound. Laparoscopy may be required in doubtful cases.

The management of cancer of the Fallopian tube is the same as for cancer of the ovary, with surgery to remove gross tumour. This will almost always involve a total abdominal hysterectomy and bilateral salpingo-oophorectomy. Postoperative chemotherapy will be required with platinum analogues for all but the earliest cases. The treatment of carcinoma metastatic to the Fallopian tube is determined by the management of the primary tumour.

## Results

The overall 5-year survival rate is around 35 per cent. The prognosis is improved if the tumour is detected early. The 5-year survival for Stage Ia cases is in the region of 70 per cent, but in Stages Ib–IIIc survival falls to 25–30 per cent. Chemotherapy with platinum agents improves the survival.

### 🔑 Key Points

- Epithelial ovarian cancer is usually advanced at presentation and, except when the disease is confined to the ovaries and is well or moderately well differentiated, it has a poor prognosis.
- Oral contraceptive use protects against the development of ovarian cancer.
- Inheritance plays a significant role in approximately 5 per cent of epithelial ovarian cancers. The *BRCA1* gene is associated with 80 per cent of families with both breast and ovarian cancer. The risk of ovarian cancer in these families is less than the risk of breast cancer. *BRCA1* does not appear to be responsible for many sporadic cases of ovarian cancers.
- Population screening for ovarian cancer is not yet justified with the techniques evaluated so far.
- Standard treatment of epithelial carcinoma is surgery followed by a platinum agent in combination with paclitaxel. This approach allows many women to lead a relatively symptom-free life for periods of up to 3–4 years.
- A young woman with a solid ovarian tumour should be referred to a gynaecological oncologist, as she may have a curable germ cell tumour. If the diagnosis is made postoperatively, she should always be referred to a specialist team.
- Primary carcinoma of the Fallopian tube is treated like ovarian carcinoma.

## References

Kasprzak L, Foulkes WD, Shelling AN. Hereditary ovarian carcinoma. *BMJ* 1999; **318**: 786–9.

Oram DH, Jeyarajah AR. The role of ultrasound and tumour markers in the early detection of ovarian cancer. *Br J Obstet Gynaecol* 1994; **101**: 939–45.

Ponder B. Breast cancer genes – searches begin and end. *Nature* 1994; **371**: 279.

The Cancer and Steroid Hormone Study of the Centre for Disease Control and the National Institute of Child Health and Human Development. The reduction in risk of ovarian cancer associated with oral contraceptive use. *N Engl J Med* 1987; **316** : 650–5.

Van der Berg ME, van Lent M, Buyse M et al. The effect of debulking surgery after induction chemotherapy on the prognosis in advanced epithelial ovarian cancer. *N Engl J Med* 1995; **332**: 629–34.

Venn A, Watson L, Lumley J, Giles G, King C, Healy D. Breast and ovarian cancer incidence after infertility and in vitro fertilisation. *Lancet* 1995; **336**: 995–1000.

## Additional reading

Burger HG. Clinical utility of inhibin measurements. *J Clin Endocrinol Metab* 1993; **76**: 1391–6.

Cannistra SA. Cancer of the ovary. *N Engl J Med* 1993; **329**: 1550–9.

Eng C, Stratton M, Ponder B et al. Familial cancer syndromes. *Lancet* 1994; **343**: 709–13.

Gordon A, Lipton D, Woodruff JD. Dysgerminoma; a review of 158 cases from the Emil Novak ovarian tumor registry. *Obstet Gynaecol* 1981; **58**: 497–504.

Hellström AC, Silfverswärd C, Nilsson B, Pettersson F. Carcinoma of the fallopian tube. A clinical and histopathological review. The Radiumhemmet series. *Int J Gynecol Cancer* 1994; **4**: 395–400.

Hildreth NG, Kelsey JL, Li Volsi VA et al. An epidemiological study of epithelial carcinoma of the ovary. *Am J Epidemiol* 1981; **114**: 389–405.

Hird V, Maraveyas A, Snook D et al. Adjuvant therapy of ovarian cancer with radioactive monoclonal antibody. *Br J Cancer* 1993; **68**: 403–6.

Hunter RW, Alexander NDE, Soutter WP. Meta-analysis of surgery in advanced ovarian carcinoma: is maximum cytoreductive surgery an independent determinant of prognosis? *Am J Obstet Gynecol* 1992; **166**: 504–11.

Jacobs I, Davies AP, Bridges J et al. Prevalence screening for ovarian cancer in postmenopausal women by CA 125 measurement and ultrasonography. *BMJ* 1993; **306**: 1030–4.

McGuire WP, Hoskins WJ, Brady MF et al. Taxol and cisplatin (TP) improves outcome in advanced ovarian cancer (AOC) as compared to cytoxan and cisplatin (CP) [abstract]. *Proc ASCO* 1995; **14**: 275.

Newlands ES, Bagshaw KD. Advances in the treatment of germ cell tumours of the ovary. In: Bonnar J (ed.), *Recent advances in obstetrics and gynaecology*. Edinburgh: Churchill Livingstone, 1987, 143–56.

Potter ME, Partridge EE, Hatch KD, Soong S-J, Austin JM, Shingleton HM. Primary surgical therapy of ovarian cancer: how much and when? *Gynaecol Oncol* 1991; **40**: 195–200.

# Conditions affecting the vulva and vagina

## OVERVIEW

Space does not permit an exhaustive description of all of the many benign conditions which may affect the vulva. Instead, the emphasis is on common or important conditions (not always the same thing), with the intention of providing the reader with a sound framework upon which to build. Although cancer is rare and pre-invasive lesions very uncommon, both cause considerable distress but can usually be treated effectively.

## VULVA

### Anatomy

The vulva includes the mons pubis, the labia majora and minora, the clitoris, the vestibule of the vagina, the bulb of the vestibule and the greater vestibular glands (Bartholin's).

The mons pubis is a pad of fat anterior to the pubic symphysis and covered by hair-bearing skin. The labia majora extend posteriorly from the mons on either side of the pudendal cleft into which the urethra and vagina open. They merge with one another and the perineal skin anterior to the anus. They consist largely of areolar tissue and fat. The skin on their lateral aspects is pigmented and covered with crisp hairs. On the medial side, the skin is smooth and has many sebaceous glands. The labia minora are small folds of skin which lie between the labia majora and which divide anteriorly to envelop the clitoris. The medial surfaces contain many sebaceous glands. The clitoris is an erectile structure analogous to the glans penis. Partly hidden by the anterior folds of the labia minora, the clitoris consists of a body of two corpora cavernosa lying side by side and connected to the pubic and ischial rami, and a glans of sensitive, spongy erectile tissue. The vestibule is that area between the labia minora into which the urethra and vagina open. The bulbs of the vestibule lie on either side of the vaginal opening and are elongated masses of erectile tissue. The greater vestibular glands lie posterior to the bulbs of the vestibule and are connected to the surface by short ducts.

### Benign conditions of the vulva

Patients with vulval symptoms are encountered frequently in gynaecological practice. The complaint is often long-standing and distressing and often induces a feeling of despair in both patient and doctor. A careful, sympathetic approach and a readiness to consult colleagues in other disciplines are essential. Even when it seems that no specific therapy can be offered, many patients are helped by the knowledge that there is no serious underlying pathology and by a supportive attitude.

## History

The duration of the complaint, details of the onset and any precipitating factors must be elicited. Information about the treatments used so far is important, as many of these women will have already begun to use a variety of local preparations, some of which may be potentially harmful! The use of deodorants, bath gels, biological washing powders or shampoos may cause an allergic or irritation eczema. Wearing tight clothing, particularly nylon materials, may exacerbate the problem. Depression may be a result of the vulval condition rather than the cause, but it will still require treatment. A history of other illnesses or drug treatment may be relevant. The patient should be asked about other skin complaints. Sometimes a further line of enquiry is suggested by the findings on examination.

## Examination

An examination for evidence of systemic disease or of a generalized skin condition is advisable. Pelvic and vaginal examination should be performed unless the patient is too uncomfortable to allow it. Cervical cytology and colposcopic examination of the cervix and vagina may be useful and are mandatory if the vulval condition is thought to be premalignant. The vulva should be examined in a good light, preferably under low magnification. The colposcope is not ideal for this because of the narrow field of view, but it is often the best available option. Gentle pressure with a cotton-tipped applicator should be applied to erythematous areas to detect increased tenderness.

It is important to take biopsies whenever there is any doubt about the diagnosis. These can be performed readily under local anaesthesia (Fig. 14.1) using a disposable 4 mm Stiefel biopsy punch. Silver nitrate or Monsel's solution will control the small amount of bleeding which results.

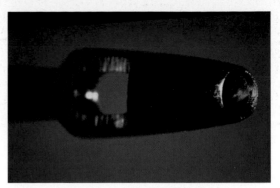

**Figure 14.1** Disposable 4 mm Stiefel biopsy punch.

## Symptoms of benign vulval conditions

### Pruritus vulvae

The term pruritus vulvae properly refers to vulval irritation for which no cause can be found. In practice, many gynaecologists use the term to describe this upsetting symptom regardless of whether or not a cause is evident. It should be distinguished from the burning sensation described by some women and discussed later.

Pruritus vulvae is commoner in older women and is most frequently encountered after the age of 40 years. The most common causes are lichen sclerosus and eczema due to an allergy or exposure to an irritant substance. Evidence of the latter is often obscured by the secondary effects of scratching – a thickening and whitening of the skin. The scratching initiates a vicious cycle, exacerbating the irritation and stimulating more scratching.

A vaginal discharge may give rise to vulval irritation. The discharge may be due to infection, but some women seem to experience a profuse physiological discharge. Cautery of the cervix often gives disappointing results in such cases. A bland barrier ointment like zinc and castor oil is sometimes useful in this situation. Threadworm infestation is very common in children and will cause pruritus ani and vulval irritation. Atrophic vaginitis responds to hormone replacement.

Occasionally, a systemic illness may cause pruritus vulvae. Diabetes, uraemia and liver failure and low ferritin levels are all possible causes to consider.

If no specific cause is found, steps must be taken to remove any possible source of irritation or allergy. Vulval deodorants and perfumed additions to the bath water must be avoided. Simple, unperfumed soap should be used for vulval hygiene and for washing underwear. After washing, the vulva must be dried carefully and gently – if necessary, a hair drier set at a low heat can be used. Loose-fitting cotton clothing should be worn to allow the evaporation of sweat. The patient would be well advised not to wear nylon tights.

Potent topical steroids, such as 0.1% diflucortolone valerate or 2.5% hydrocortisone may be used two to three times per day for a few weeks. Thereafter, 1% hydrocortisone will usually suffice to maintain the improvement and to treat relapses. A sedative at night, such as hydroxyzine hydrochloride, can be useful to break the cycle of nocturnal itching and scratching. An antihistamine taken during the day may help to relieve the itch without causing sedation.

It is important to treat depression appropriately. Even if the patient is not pathologically depressed, she can benefit greatly from sympathetic support and understanding, and time must be set aside for this when necessary.

## Vulval pain or burning

These symptoms cause considerable distress to the sufferers, who are often young women. The cause is frequently elusive and treatment is empirical. Steroid cream or ointment will help some of these women, but a multidisciplinary approach is required for many. Surgery is rarely helpful.

## Non-neoplastic disorders of the vulva

In few areas has there been as much confusion over the terminology used as in that of vulvar 'dystrophies'. The latest recommended scheme is shown in the box below. The non-neoplastic disorders have been separated from the potentially premalignant intraepithelial neoplasia. Only the non-neoplastic disorders will be discussed here.

---

### Classification of vulval disorders

**Non-neoplastic disorders**
- Lichen sclerosus
- Squamous cell hyperplasia (formerly hyperplastic dystrophy)
- Other dermatoses

---

### Vulval intraepithelial neoplasia (VIN)
- Squamous VIN
  - VIN I Mild dysplasia
  - VIN II Moderate dysplasia
  - VIN III Severe dysplasia or carcinoma in situ
- Non-squamous VIN
  - Paget's disease

---

## Lichen sclerosus

This is the commonest condition found in elderly women complaining of vulvar itch but may also be seen in children and, less commonly, in younger women. The cause is not known, but the condition is associated with autoimmune disorders.

Although it most commonly affects the vulva and peri-anal skin, lesions do appear elsewhere. The lesion is white and the skin looks thin, with a crinkled surface. The contours of the vulva slowly disappear and labial adhesions form. If the patient has been rubbing the area, the skin will become thickened (lichenified). The diagnosis can usually be made clinically but a biopsy should be performed whenever there is uncertainty. Even in a typical case, the histology may not be characteristic.

There is much uncertainty about the risk to patients with lichen sclerosus of developing vulval cancer. Vulval intraepithelial neoplasia (VIN) and lichen sclerosus can coexist in the same patient, and many patients with invasive carcinoma also have lichen sclerosus in the surrounding skin. About 4 per cent of women with lichen sclerosus develop invasive cancer.

Although there is a 9 per cent prevalence of thyroid disease, pernicious anaemia or diabetes in these patients, screening for these conditions may not be of value, as in most cases the diagnosis has already been made by the time the patient presents with her vulval complaint.

If the patient is asymptomatic, no treatment is required. Mild itching may be helped by aqueous cream or 1% hydrocortisone ointment applied three times daily. More potent steroids may be required for short periods. If the use of an ointment results in maceration, a cream base may be substituted. Some have suggested the long-term use of potent steroid creams such as clobetasol propionate. Some women benefit from 2% testosterone ointment, which should be applied twice or three times per day for 6 weeks; thereafter the frequency can be reduced to once or twice a week. Excessive dosage will result in clitoral hypertrophy and increased facial hair. There is virtually no place for vulvectomy for this condition, as the morbidity is not justified in the face of a high recurrence rate. The same may be said of laser vaporization.

## Squamous cell hyperplasia

Squamous cell hyperplasia is a term applied when there is histological evidence of hyperplasia without any clinical evidence of the cause. Chronic rubbing of otherwise normal skin (lichen simplex), psoriasis, condylomata acuminata and infection with *Candida albicans* are among the diagnoses that must be excluded before this term may be applied. This stipulation is likely to reduce to near zero the number of cases assigned to this category on clinical grounds.

## Other dermatoses

These problems are often seen by dermatologists, but knowledge of this area is important. The most common general diseases causing itching of the vulva are diabetes, uraemia and liver failure. In diabetes, the vulva, as well as being itchy, is swollen and dark red in colour.

In allergic dermatitis, the skin is usually red and swollen and may later become thickened. Secondary infection may occur. The commonest irritants are perfumed soap, synthetic materials and washing powders, although there are many other contact allergens or irritants.

Psoriasis, intertrigo, lichen planus and scabies may affect the vulva. In lichen planus, the lesion on the vulva is characteristically a purple-white papule with a shiny surface and regular outline. There is a variant of this condition that is erosive and can lead to pain and bleeding as well as itching. In this latter condition there is a slight risk of malignancy.

Although these are covered elsewhere (Chapter 15), vaginal infections are the most common cause of vulval itching, particularly in younger women. Candidiasis and trichomoniasis are the most frequent causes. Human papilloma virus is not thought to cause pruritis vulvae.

## Vulval ulcers

There are nearly a dozen causes of benign ulcers of the vagina. However, most of these are transient or very rare. Any persistent ulcer should be biopsied to exclude malignancy.

### Causes of benign vulval ulcers

- Aphthous ulcers
- Herpes genitalis
- Primary syphilis
- Crohn's disease
- Behçet's disease
- Lipschutz ulcers
- Lymphogranuloma venereum
- Chancroid
- Donovanosis
- Tuberculosis

## Benign tumours

### Cystic tumours

The commonest of these are the cysts that arise from the duct of Bartholin's gland, which lies in the subcutaneous tissue below the lower third of the labium majorum. When the duct becomes blocked, a tense retention cyst forms. The patient usually presents only after infection has supervened and a painful abscess has formed. Incision and marsupialization of the abscess and antibiotic therapy give excellent results. The pus from the abscess should be sent for culture in media suitable for the detection of gonococcal infection. In women aged over 40 years, a biopsy of the cyst wall should be sent for histological examination to exclude carcinoma.

A large variety of other cystic lesions may be found on the vagina. In most cases, surgical excision and histological examination will be required to determine their nature.

### Solid tumours

The commonest are condylomata acuminata presenting as small papules, which are sometimes sessile and often polypoid. They are due to infection with human papillomavirus, usually type 6 or 11. A great variety of other epithelial and non-epithelial tumours may be found. The commonest of these are squamous papillomata, skin tags, lipomas and fibromas. Very rarely, normal breast tissue may be found on the vulva, as may endometriosis.

## Premalignant conditions

Both squamous VIN and adenocarcinoma in situ (Paget's disease) occur on the vulva. The latter is very rare. The histological features and terminology of VIN are analogous to those of cervical intraepithelial neoplasia (CIN) and vaginal intraepithelial neoplasia (VAIN). In the same way, the histological appearance of Paget's disease is similar to the lesion seen in the breast. In a third of cases of Paget's disease, there is an associated invasive cancer, often an adenocarcinoma in underlying apocrine glands, and these carry an especially poor prognosis.

## Natural history of VIN

Forty per cent of women with VIN are younger than 41 years. Although histologically very similar to CIN and often occurring in association with it, VIN has been said not to have the same malignant potential. However, this opinion is based largely on studies of women who have been treated by excision biopsy or vulvectomy. This may not be true of untreated or inadequately treated patients.

## Diagnosis and assessment of VIN

Intraepithelial disease of the vulva often presents as pruritus vulvae, but 20–45 per cent are asymptomatic and are frequently found after treatment of pre-invasive or invasive disease at other sites in the lower genital tract, particularly the cervix.

These lesions are often raised above the surrounding skin and have a rough surface. The colour is variable: white, due to hyperkeratinization; red, due to thinness of the epithelium; or dark brown, due to increased melanin deposition in the epithelial cells (Fig. 14.2). They are very often multifocal.

However, the full extent of the abnormality is often not apparent until 5% acetic acid is applied (Fig. 14.3). After 2 minutes, VIN turns white and mosaic or punctation may be visible. Although these changes may be seen with the naked eye in a good light, it is much easier to use a hand lens or a colposcope. Toluidine blue is also used as a nuclear stain, but

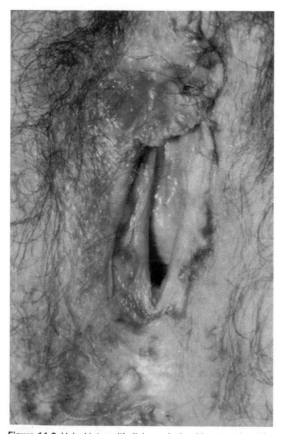

**Figure 14.2** Vulval intraepithelial neoplasia without acetic acid.

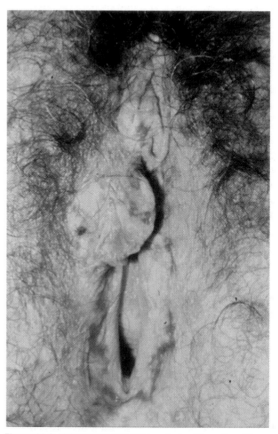

**Figure 14.3** Vulval intraepithelial neoplasia with acetic acid.

areas of ulceration give false-positive results and hyperkeratinization gives false negatives.

Adequate biopsies must be taken from abnormal areas to rule out invasive disease. These can usually be done under local anaesthesia in the outpatient clinic using a disposable 4 mm Stiefel biopsy punch.

## Treatment of VIN

The treatment of VIN is difficult. Uncertainty about the malignant potential, the multifocal nature of the disorder, and the discomfort and mutilation resulting from therapy suggest that recommendations should be cautious and conservative in order to avoid making the treatment worse than the disease. The youth of many of these patients is a further important consideration. Spontaneous regression of VIN III in women with the variant known as Bowenoid papulosis is well described. These women are young, often present in pregnancy, have dark skin and the lesions are usually multifocal, papular and pigmented. However, progression to invasion does occur in young women.

The documented progression of untreated cases of VIN III to invasive cancer underlines the potential importance of these lesions. If the patient has presented with symptoms, therapy is required. Asymptomatic patients, particularly under the age of 50 years, may be observed closely. Biopsies should be repeated if there are any suspicious changes.

Provided invasion has been excluded as far as possible, topical steroids offer symptomatic relief for many women. A strong, fluorodinated steroid is usually required. This may be applied twice or thrice daily for not more than 6 months because of the thinning of the skin that may result. Frequent review is necessary initially.

If the lesion is small, an excision biopsy may be both diagnostic and therapeutic. If the disease is multifocal or covers a wide area, a skin graft may improve the cosmetic result of a skinning vulvectomy. However, the donor site is often very painful and a satisfactory result can be obtained in most patients without grafting.

An alternative approach used to be to vaporize the abnormal epithelium with the carbon-dioxide laser. In practice, laser vaporization has proved to be disappointing in the UK and is now seldom used.

Assessment of the results of treatment should include a consideration of the length of follow-up. Surgical excision is associated with crude recurrence rates of 15–43 per cent. Close observation and re-biopsy are essential to detect invasive disease among those who relapse. Repeated treatments are commonly required.

## Conclusions

Vulval intraepithelial neoplasia is becoming more common, especially in young women. The treatment must be carefully tailored to the individual to avoid mutilating therapy whenever possible.

In view of the mutilating nature of treatment, the high recurrence rate and the uncertainty about the risk of invasion, there is a place for careful observation, especially of young women without severe symptoms. However, some of these untreated patients will develop vulval cancer, so the importance of close follow-up must be emphasized to the patient and her general practitioner.

## Paget's disease

This uncommon condition is similar to that found in the breast. Pruritus is the presenting complaint. It often presents as a red, crusted plaque with sharp edges. The diagnosis must be made by biopsy.

In approximately one-third of patients there is an adenocarcinoma in the apocrine glands, and concomitant genital malignancies are found in 15–25 per cent. These are most commonly vulval or cervical, but transitional cell carcinoma of the bladder (or kidney) and ovarian, endometrial, vaginal and urethral carcinomas have all been reported.

The treatment of Paget's disease is very wide local excision, usually including total vulvectomy because of the propensity of this condition to involve apparently normal skin. The specimen must be examined histologically, with great care to exclude an apocrine adenocarcinoma.

## Invasive disease of the vulva

Invasive vulvar cancer is an uncommon and unpleasant but potentially curable disease, even in elderly, unfit women if referred early and managed correctly from the outset. The surgical treatment appears deceptively simple, but few gynaecologists and their nursing colleagues acquire sufficient experience of this disease to offer the highest quality of care to these women. All too often, an inadequate initial attempt at surgery is made and the patient is referred for specialist care only after recurrent disease is evident.

There are about 800 new cases of carcinoma of the vulva each year in England and the annual incidence is approximately 3.2/100 000, making it about three times less common than cervical cancer. The majority of these women are elderly, and with increased life expectancy, this cancer will be seen more frequently. About 95 per cent of cases are squamous, and melanoma is the commonest of the remainder. Little is known of the aetiology of vulvar cancer.

## Natural history

After local invasion into the underlying and surrounding tissues and into the vagina, and the anus, vulval cancer spreads predominantly via the lymphatic system. The lymph drains from the vulva to the inguinal and femoral glands in the groin and then to the external iliac glands. Drainage to both groins occurs from midline structures – the perineum and the clitoris – but some contralateral spread may take place from other parts of the vulva. Spread to the contralateral groin occurs in about 25 per cent of those cases with positive groin nodes.

Only tumours with less than 1 mm of invasion carry a sufficiently low risk of lymphatic spread to be considered 'microinvasive'.

## Staging

The FIGO classification is shown in Table 14.1. In spite of the apparent limitations of this classification, it does give a reasonable guide to the prognosis. The main drawback was reliance on clinical palpation of the groin nodes, which is notoriously inaccurate. Now that the surgical findings are incorporated in the staging evaluation, the prognostic value of stage is greatly improved.

## Diagnosis and assessment

Most patients with invasive disease (71 per cent) complain of irritation or pruritus, and 57 per cent note a

**Table 14.1**   The FIGO staging of vulval cancer (1995)

| Stage | Definition |
|-------|------------|
| Ia | Confined to vulva and/or perineum, 2 cm or less maximum diameter |
| | Groin nodes not palpable |
| | Stromal invasion no greater than 1 mm |
| Ib | As for Ia but stromal invasion >1 mm |
| II | Confined to vulva and/or perineum, more than 2 cm maximum diameter |
| | Groin nodes not palpable |
| III | Extends beyond the vulva, vagina, lower urethra or anus; or unilateral regional lymph node metastasis |
| IVa | Involves the mucosa of rectum or bladder; upper urethra; or pelvic bone; and/or bilateral regional lymph node metastases |
| IVb | Any distant metastasis including pelvic lymph node |

vulvar mass or ulcer. It is usually not until the mass appears that medical advice is sought. Bleeding (28 per cent) and discharge (23 per cent) are less common presentations. One of the major problems in invasive vulvar cancer is the delay between the first appearance of symptoms and referral for a gynaecological opinion. This is only partly due to the patient's reluctance to attend. In many cases, the doctor fails to recognize the gravity of the lesion and prescribes topical therapy, sometimes without examining the woman.

Because of the multicentric nature of female lower genital tract cancer, the investigation of a patient with vulvar cancer should include inspection of the cervix and cervical cytology. The groin nodes must be palpated carefully and any suspicious nodes sampled by fine-needle aspiration. A chest X-ray is always required, but intravenous pyelography (IVP) or magnetic resonance imaging (MRI) of the pelvis may sometimes be helpful. Thorough examination under anaesthesia and a full-thickness, generous biopsy are the most important investigations. The examination should note particularly the size and distribution of the primary lesion, especially the involvement of the urethra or anus, and secondary lesions in the vulval or perineal skin must be sought. The groins should be re-examined under general anaesthesia when the diagnostic biopsies are taken, as previously undetected nodes may be palpated at that time.

## Treatment

Surgery is the mainstay of treatment. The introduction of radical vulvectomy reduced the mortality from 80 per cent to 40 per cent. However, to control lymphatic spread, these techniques removed large areas of normal skin from the groins and primary wound closure was rarely achieved. Modifications of this en-bloc excision were devised to allow primary closure and to reduce the considerable morbidity. Although these variations did reduce the rate of wound breakdown without any apparent loss of efficacy, the morbidity remained high and impaired psychosexual function was common.

In pursuit of an effective treatment with lower morbidity, the en-bloc dissection of the groin nodes in continuity with the vulva was replaced by an operation using three separate incisions. This depended on the principle that lymphatic metastases developed initially by embolization. Therefore, in the early stages of spread, there would be no residual tumour in the lymphatic channels between the tumour and the local lymph nodes in the groin. Many studies have since attested to the reduced morbidity of this method without loss of efficacy. Further refinements in technique have helped greatly to reduce the morbidity of surgery.

The most common complication is wound breakdown and infection. With the triple incision technique, this is seldom more than a minor problem. Osteitis pubis is a rare but very serious complication that requires intensive and prolonged antibiotic therapy. Thromboembolic disease is always a greatly feared complication of surgery for malignant disease, but the combination of preoperative epidural analgesia to ensure good venous return with subcutaneous heparin begun 12–24 hours before the operation seems to reduce this risk. Secondary haemorrhage occurs from time to time. Chronic leg oedema may be expected in about 15 per cent of women. Numbness and paraesthesia over the anterior thigh are common due to the division of small cutaneous branches of the femoral nerve. Loss of body image and impaired sexual function undoubtedly occur, but the patients' responses to surgery are enormously variable and

probably depend on the woman's age, upbringing and attitudes to life.

The role of radiotherapy is largely limited to treating the pelvic nodes when more than two groin nodes are found to be involved. It may have a place in reducing the size of very large lesions prior to surgery in cases where the anus is involved. Some have advocated a wider role but have failed to provide adequate evidence to support their view.

The survival rates after treatment are very good provided the lesion is confined to the vulva. Once spread has occurred, the outcome is less certain.

## VAGINA

### Introduction

Many of the disorders that affect the vagina are discussed in depth elsewhere in this book: congenital abnormalities in Chapters 2 and 3; infections in Chapter 15; psychosexual problems in Chapter 19; atrophic changes in Chapter 18; and prolapse in Chapter 17. The purpose of this short section is to discuss benign and malignant tumours of the vagina.

### Benign tumours

Tumours in the vagina are uncommon. Condylomata acuminata are by far the commonest seen. The frond-like surface is usually characteristic, but it is wise to await the result of a biopsy before instituting treatment, especially if the lesion is close to the cervix.

Endometriotic deposits may be seen in the vagina. They are most common in an episiotomy wound and may lie deep to the epithelium.

Simple mesonephric (Gartner's) or paramesonephric cysts may be seen, especially high up near the fornices. If asymptomatic, they are best not treated. If treatment is required, marsupialization is effective and safer than excision.

Adenosis – multiple mucus-containing vaginal cysts – is a rare condition, which even more rarely gives rise to symptoms. A variety of abnormalities are reported in the daughters of women who took diethylstilboestrol during their pregnancy. Most of these are of no significance.

## Vaginal intraepithelial neoplasia

The terminology and pathology of VAIN are analogous to those of CIN (VAIN I–III). The main difference is that vaginal epithelium does not normally have crypts, so the epithelial abnormality remains superficial until invasion occurs. The common exception to this is found following surgery – usually hysterectomy – when abnormal epithelium can be buried below the suture line or in suture tracks.

## Natural history of VAIN

VAIN is seldom seen as an isolated vaginal lesion. It is more usual for it to be a vaginal extension of CIN. In most cases it is diagnosed colposcopically prior to any treatment during the investigation of an abnormal smear. However, it may not be recognized until after a hysterectomy has been performed. When this happens, abnormal epithelium is likely to be buried behind the sutures used to close the vault. Consequently a portion of the lesion will remain invisible and unevaluable. These often prove to have unexpected invasive disease. Untreated or inadequately treated VAIN may progress to frank invasive cancer. Very rarely, VAIN may be seen many years after radiotherapy for cervical carcinoma, when it is probably a new lesion. Care must be taken in these women to ensure that post-radiotherapy changes are not being misinterpreted as VAIN.

## Treatment of VAIN

If the cervix is still in situ, local ablation or excision of VAIN is very effective. After hysterectomy, if the lesion involves the suture line, a partial vaginal colpectomy that removes the vaginal vault is usually recommended to younger women. The results of this approach are good, and early invasion may be identified. In older women or when access is poor, local radiotherapy produces excellent results.

## Vaginal cancer

Invasive vaginal cancer is rare. With 184 cases in England and Wales in 1997, the incidence was 0.7/100 000 women.

There is little firm evidence of aetiological agents. Three small studies raised a concern that women below the age of 40 treated with radiotherapy for cervical cancer may be at a high risk of subsequently developing vaginal cancer 10–40 years later. However, two enormous retrospective studies contradicted this meagre evidence.

For some time, the prevalence of clear cell adenocarcinoma of the vagina was thought to be increased by intrauterine exposure to diethylstilboestrol. With the accrual of more information, the risks now seem to be very low and to lie between 0.1 and 1.0 per 1000. Whereas vaginal adenosis and minor anatomical abnormalities of no significance (e.g. cervical cockscomb) are common following intrauterine diethylstilboestrol exposure, the only lesion of any significance that is seen more commonly is CIN. Uterine malformations may be more common and may result in impaired fecundity in a small minority of cases.

## Pathology

The great majority (92 per cent) of primary vaginal cancers are squamous. Clear cell adenocarcinomas, malignant melanomas, embryonal rhabdomyosarcomas and endodermal sinus tumours are the commonest of the small number of other tumours seen very rarely in the vagina.

## Natural history

The upper vagina is the commonest site for invasive disease. Squamous vaginal cancer spreads by local invasion initially. Lymphatic spread occurs to the pelvic nodes from the upper vagina and to both pelvic and inguinal nodes from the lower vagina.

## Clinical staging

The FIGO clinical staging is shown in Table 14.2.

## Diagnosis and assessment

The most common presenting symptom is vaginal bleeding (53–65 per cent), with vaginal discharge (11–16 per cent) and pelvic pain (4–11 per cent)

**Table 14.2** FIGO staging for vaginal cancer (1995)

| Stage | Definition |
|---|---|
| 0 | Intraepithelial neoplasia |
| I | Invasive carcinoma confined to vaginal mucosa |
| II | Subvaginal infiltration not extending to pelvic wall |
| III | Extends to pelvic wall |
| IVa | Involves mucosa of bladder or rectum |
| IVb | Spread beyond the pelvis |

**Table 14.3** Survival by FIGO stage (1988)

| FIGO stage | Corrected 5-year survival (%) |
|---|---|
| I | 97 |
| II | 85 |
| III | 46 |
| IV | 50 |

being less common. Some are detected when asymptomatic by cervical cytology.

High-definition MRI has become the most important part of the pre-treatment assessment of invasive cancer of the vagina. A careful examination under anaesthesia combined with colposcopy will identify coexisting VAIN and help to define the location of the lesion. A chest X ray and an IVP are the only radiological investigations required routinely.

## Treatment and results

Invasive vaginal cancer is usually treated with radiotherapy. Early cases, Stage I–IIa, may be treated entirely with interstitial therapy, but external beam therapy is used more commonly. Cases with parametrial involvement receive teletherapy to the pelvis as for carcinoma of the cervix, with a tumour dose of 45 Gy followed by interstitial or intracavitary therapy to a total dose of 70–75 Gy. The field may be extended to include the groins if the tumour involves the lower half of the vagina.

A Stage I lesion in the upper vagina can be adequately treated by radical hysterectomy (if the uterus is still present), radical vaginectomy and pelvic lymphadenectomy. Exenteration is required for more advanced lesions and carries the problems of stomata. However, surgery may be the treatment of choice for women who have had prior pelvic radiotherapy.

The 5-year survival figures described for Stage I are generally good, but the results of therapy in more advanced disease are much less satisfactory (Table 14.3).

### 🔑 Key Points

- Vulval itch is most commonly due to lichen sclerosus but may be caused by any of a large number of different disorders. Frequently no obvious cause is found.
- Strong steroid creams are often helpful in relieving the symptoms, but repeated courses of treatment are commonly required.
- Vulval intraepithelial neoplasia is difficult to treat satisfactorily and care must be taken not to make the treatment worse than the disease.
- Vulval cancer is very rare and is most commonly found in the elderly.
- The prognosis for vulval cancer is good if the lesion is treated adequately at an early stage.
- Even elderly and relatively unfit women should be treated surgically.
- The risks of vaginal cancer in diethylstilboestrol-exposed women now appear to be very low indeed.
- Early vaginal cancer may be treated with surgery or interstitial brachytherapy, but more advanced cases are better treated with radiotherapy.

# Infections in gynaecology

## OVERVIEW

Most women experience an infection of the urogenital tract at some time. The most common symptomatic infections are vulvo-vaginal candidiasis (thrush) and urinary tract infections. The sexually transmissible bacterial infections chlamydia and gonorrhoea can be carried asymptomatically for months or even years. Viral infections such as human papillomavirus (HPV) and herpes simplex virus (HSV) may persist for life. Upper genital tract infection is a threat to a woman's future fertility. The long-term sequelae of damage to the Fallopian tubes include ectopic pregnancy and tubular factor infertility.

Worldwide, human immunodeficiency virus (HIV) infection is predominantly acquired sexually and in some parts of the world as many as 25–30 per cent of pregnant women are now infected. Clinicians need to be aware of the way that HIV alters the manifestations of, and host susceptibility to, other infections.

## Principles of management of sexually transmissible infections

Many gynaecological infections are sexually transmissible. Others, such as *Candida* and urinary tract infection, are frequently triggered by sexual intercourse although the organism is colonizing the woman beforehand. It takes practice to be comfortable taking a sexual history from a patient. If the clinician is embarrassed, this is quickly transmitted to the patient. It is also difficult to take a sexual history if the patient's friends or relatives are present, or in a ward or cubicle in which there is inadequate privacy and soundproofing. It is sometimes necessary, therefore, to postpone seeking a detailed history until the right atmosphere can be provided. In order to assess the risk of an individual having acquired a sexually transmitted disease (STD), it is necessary to find out:

- when sexual intercourse last took place,
- whether this was oral, vaginal or anal,
- what contraception was used,
- when the woman last had a different sexual partner,
- a travel history and knowledge about the origin of partners which may indicate a risk of a tropical infection seldom seen in the UK,
- information concerning any previous pregnancies and menstruation.

Enquire about intravenous drug use in the patient and her partners. Do not assume that a woman is heterosexual until you have ascertained the sex of her partners.

**Table 15.1** Differential diagnosis of vaginal discharge

| Symptoms and signs | Candidiasis | Bacterial vaginosis | Trichomoniasis | Cervicitis |
|---|---|---|---|---|
| Itching or soreness | ++ | − | +++ | − |
| Smell | May be 'yeasty' | Offensive, fishy | May be offensive | − |
| Colour | White | White or yellow | Yellow or green | Clear or coloured |
| Consistency | Curdy | Thin, homogeneous | Thin, homogeneous | Mucoid |
| pH | <4.5 | 4.5–7.0 | 4.5–7.0 | <4.5 |
| Confirmed by | Microscopy and culture | Microscopy | Microscopy and culture | Microscopy, tests for *Chlamydia* and gonorrhoea |

If one sexually transmissible infection is present, there may be others. Ideally, therefore, a full screen should be performed for *Chlamydia*, gonorrhoea, vaginal infections and serological tests for syphilis, hepatitis B, HIV and hepatitis C if indicated. If facilities are not available for such a screen, the patient should be referred to a genitourinary medicine (GUM) clinic.

To break the chain of infection and prevent re-infection, it is essential that the patient avoids intercourse until she is sure that her partner(s) has been screened and received appropriate treatment. Follow-up evaluation and tests of cure are essential for individuals infected with *Neisseria gonorrhoeae* and are advisable for other infections.

## Lower genital tract infections

At birth, the neonate has been exposed to high levels of oestrogen and progesterone from her mother and the vagina is lined with stratified squamous epithelium. Sometimes a baby girl has a withdrawal bleed, analogous to a period, as the effect of maternal oestrogen wanes. It is possible for *Trichomonas vaginalis* to be transmitted at birth, but the infection usually clears spontaneously.

In young females the vagina is lined with a simple cuboidal epithelium. The pH is neutral and it is colonized by organisms similar to skin commensals. Under the influence of oestrogen at puberty, stratified squamous epithelium develops and lactobacilli become the predominant organisms. A drop in the pH accompanies this change to a level of approximately 3.5–4.5. Following the menopause, atrophic changes occur,

with a return to bacterial flora similar to that of the skin. The pH again rises to 7.0.

Vaginal discharge can originate from anywhere in the upper or lower genital tract (Table 15.1). Discharge arising from the vagina itself can be physiological or due to bacterial vaginosis (BV), candidiasis or *Trichomonas* infection (Fig. 15.1). Its presence can be very alarming for a woman, particularly if she is concerned that she might have caught a serious sexually transmitted infection (STI).

## Physiological discharge

Normal vaginal discharge is white, becoming yellowish on contact with air, due to oxidation. It consists of desquamated epithelial cells from the vagina and cervix, mucus originating mainly from the cervical glands, bacteria and fluid, which is formed as a transudate from the vaginal wall. More than 95 per cent of the bacteria present are lactobacilli. The acidic pH is maintained by the lactobacilli and through the production of lactic acid by the vaginal epithelium metabolizing glycogen. Physiological discharge increases due to increased mucus production from the cervix in mid-cycle. It also increases in pregnancy and sometimes when women begin using a combined oral contraceptive pill.

## Vaginal candidiasis

Over three-quarters of women have at least one episode of vaginal candidiasis. A few women have frequent recurrences. The organism is carried in the gut, under the nails, in the vagina and on the skin.

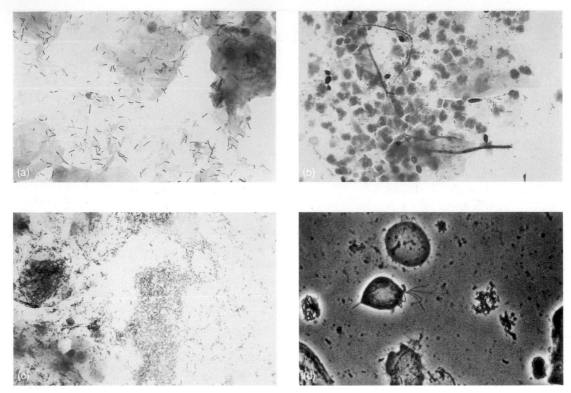

**Figure 15.1** Vaginal and cervical flora (all 1000 × magnified).
(a) Normal: lactobacilli – seen as large Gram-positive rods – predominate. Squamous epithelial cells are Gram negative with a large amount of cytoplasm. (b) Candidiasis: there are speckled Gram-positive spores and long pseudohyphae visible. There are numerous polymorphs present and the bacterial flora is abnormal, resembling bacterial vaginosis. (c) Bacterial vaginosis: there is an overgrowth of anaerobic organisms, including *Gardnerella vaginalis* (small Gram-variable cocci), and a decrease in the numbers of lactobacilli. A 'clue cell' is seen. This is an epithelial cell covered with small bacteria so that the edge of the cell is obscured. (d) Trichomoniasis: an unstained 'wet mount' of vaginal fluid from a woman with *Trichomonas vaginalis* infection. There is a cone-shaped, flagellated organism in the centre, with a terminal spike and four flagella visible. In practice, the organism is identified under the microscope by movement, with amoeboid motion and its flagella waving.

The yeast *Candida albicans* is implicated in more than 80 per cent of cases; *C. glabrata*, *C. krusei* and *C. tropicalis* account for most of the rest. Sexual acquisition is rarely important, although the physical trauma of intercourse may be sufficient to trigger an attack in a predisposed individual.

The classical presentation is with itching and soreness of the vagina and vulva, with a curdy, white discharge, which may smell yeasty, but in some cases there may be itching and redness with a thin, watery discharge. The pH of vaginal fluid is usually normal, between 3.5 and 4.5. Microscopy and culture of the vaginal fluid can confirm a diagnosis (Fig. 15.1b). Asymptomatic women from whom *Candida* is grown on culture do not require treatment.

## Factors predisposing to vaginal candidiasis

- Immunosuppression
- HIV
- Immunosuppressive therapy, e.g. steroids
- Diabetes mellitus
- Vaginal douching, bubble bath, shower gel, tight clothing, tights
- Increased oestrogen
- Pregnancy
- High-dose combined oral contraceptive pill
- Underlying dermatosis, e.g. eczema
- Broad-spectrum antibiotic therapy

Recurrent *Candida*, or *Candida* not responding to treatment, is relatively uncommon. If this appears to be the case, it is important to consider other diagnoses, particularly herpes simplex, which causes localized ulceration and soreness, and dermatological conditions such as eczema and lichen sclerosus et atrophicus.

As a general rule, it is better to use a topical rather than a systemic treatment. This minimizes the risk of systemic side effects. Vaginal creams and pessaries can be prescribed at a variety of doses and durations of treatment. For uncomplicated *Candida*, a single-dose treatment, such as clotrimazole 500 mg, is adequate. Some women have a preference for oral therapy, particularly if treatment is required at the time of menstruation. A single 150 mg tablet of fluconazole is usually effective, but its activity is limited to *C. albicans* strains. Longer courses of treatment are needed when there are predisposing factors that cannot be eliminated, such as steroid therapy. If recurrences occur frequently, it is worth performing a full blood count to check for anaemia and checking thyroid function, but usually these are normal. Many clinicians prescribe treatment to be taken once or twice a month for 6 months to suppress recurrences.

## Bacterial vaginosis

Bacterial vaginosis is the commonest cause of abnormal vaginal discharge in women of childbearing age. Studies in antenatal clinics and gynaecology clinics show a prevalence of approximately 12 per cent in the UK. It is commoner in women of Afro-Caribbean origin and in those who have an intrauterine device (IUD). Higher prevalence is generally reported in women undergoing elective termination of pregnancy. It is probably commoner in women with STIs, but has been reported in virgins, and it may be particularly common in lesbian women. The condition often arises spontaneously around the time of menstruation and may resolve spontaneously in mid-cycle.

When BV develops, the predominantly anaerobic organisms that are usually present in the vagina at low concentration increase in concentration up to a thousand-fold. This is accompanied by a rise in vaginal pH to between 4.5 and 7.0, and ultimately the lactobacilli may disappear. The organisms most commonly associated with BV are *Gardnerella vaginalis*, *Bacteroides (Prevotella)* spp., *Mobiluncus* spp. and *Mycoplasma hominis*. At present we do not know what triggers these dramatic changes in the vaginal ecology.

The principal symptom of BV is an offensive fishy smelling discharge; it is characteristically thin, homogeneous and adherent to the walls of the vagina and may be white or yellow. The smell is particularly noticeable around the time of menstruation or following intercourse; however, semen itself can give off a weak fishy smell.

The diagnosis is commonly made in clinical practice using the composite (Amsel) criteria:
- vaginal pH > 4.5,
- release of a fishy smell on addition of alkali (10% potassium hydroxide),
- a characteristic discharge on examination,
- presence of 'clue cells' on microscopy.

'Clue cells' are vaginal epithelial cells so heavily coated with bacteria that the border is obscured. BV can also be diagnosed from a Gram-stained vaginal smear. Large numbers of Gram-positive and Gram-negative cocci are seen, with reduced or absent large Gram-positive bacilli (lactobacilli). Culture of a high vaginal swab yields mixed anaerobes and a high concentration of *Gardnerella vaginalis*. However, *Gardenella vaginalis* can be grown from cultures taken from up to 50 per cent of women with normal vaginal flora. Its presence is not, therefore, diagnostic of BV.

The simplest and cheapest treatment for BV is metronidazole 400 mg twice a day for 5 days, or 2 g as a single dose. Topical preparations are available in the form of metronidazole gel 0.75% or clindamycin cream 2%. Initial cure rates are over 80 per cent, but up to 30 per cent of women relapse within 1 month of treatment.

It is now established that women with BV are at a greater risk of second trimester miscarriage and preterm delivery during pregnancy, which may result in perinatal mortality or cerebral palsy. Women with a prior history of second trimester loss or idiopathic preterm birth should be screened for BV and treated with metronidazole early in the second trimester. It has also been demonstrated that treating women with BV with metronidazole prior to termination of pregnancy reduces the subsequent incidence of endometritis and pelvic inflammatory disease (PID). Women with BV are also at increased risk of infections after surgery.

In some women the vaginal flora is in a dynamic state, with BV developing and remitting spontaneously. Symptomatic women with recurrent BV can become frustrated as the condition responds rapidly to treatment with antibiotics but may also relapse rapidly. Regular treatment once or twice a month with oral or topical metronidazole is sometimes helpful.

## Trichomoniasis

This sexually transmissible infection can be carried asymptomatically for several months before causing symptoms. The incidence has been falling in the UK over the last 20 years. In men it is often carried asymptomatically, but may present as non-gonococcal urethritis (NGU). In women it causes a vulvovaginitis that can be severe, accompanied by a purulent, sometimes offensive, vaginal discharge. In many cases BV develops as well.

Examination shows a yellow or green vaginal discharge with inflammation sometimes extending out onto the vulva and adjacent skin. Punctate haemorrhages can occur on the cervix, giving the appearance of a 'strawberry cervix'.

The diagnosis is confirmed by culture, preferably in a specific medium such as Fineberg–Whittington. Microscopy of vaginal secretions mixed with saline has 60 per cent sensitivity for detecting the organism. Numerous polymorphonuclear cells are seen and the motile organism is identified from its shape and four moving flagellae.

Treatment is with metronidazole, either 2 g as a single dose or 400 mg twice a day for 5 days. The woman should be advised to send her sexual partner(s) for treatment before resuming intercourse together.

Trichomoniasis has occasionally been identified in the upper genital tract of women with PID but is probably not an important cause of genital tract pathology. It can be isolated from the bladder. Occasionally persistent trichomoniasis is seen. This may be due to poor compliance with medication, poor absorption or a resistant organism. Review the history to rule out re-infection from an untreated partner. The usual approach is to use higher doses of metronidazole, initially 400 mg three times a day, increasing to 1 g per rectum or intravenously twice a day. Neurological toxicity may be encountered with high doses. Unfortunately, alternative treatments are limited, but include arsphenamine pessaries and clotrimazole, which has an inhibitory effect on *Trichomonas vaginalis*.

## Vaginal discharge in children

Vaginal infections are common in childhood and mostly not related to sexual abuse. Streptococcal infections are the commonest cause. *Shigella* spp. can cause a haemorrhagic chronic vaginitis, often with no history of diarrhoea. Recurrent vaginal infections should lead to suspicion of a foreign body. An examination under anaesthesia may be necessary to exclude or remove the cause.

Pinworms (*Enterobius vermicularis*) are common and migrate from the anus at night, causing intense irritation and inevitable scratching by the child. The clue to the diagnosis is the nocturnal pattern. A Selotape test can be performed to look for eggs if the worms have not been witnessed at night.

If sexual abuse occurs leading to infection with *Chlamydia* or gonorrhoea, a generalized vaginitis occurs. Adequate testing can therefore be performed from vaginal swabs, negating the need to observe the cervix with the aid of a speculum.

## Other conditions affecting the vagina

Other causes of discharge include atrophic vaginitis, toxic shock syndrome, Bartholin's abscess and infestations.

Atrophic vaginitis is common in postmenopausal women. Over the 5 years following the cessation of menstruation, the vaginal epithelium atrophies and the lactobacilli are once again replaced by typical skin commensal organisms. This can lead to superficial dyspareunia and vaginal soreness. The treatment of choice is oestrogen replacement with either topical dienoestrol cream or systemic therapy.

Occasionally a true bacterial vaginitis is encountered due to a *Streptococcus* or other organism. It responds to appropriate antibiotic therapy. Toxic shock syndrome is a rare condition associated with the retention of tampons or foreign bodies in the vagina. An overgrowth of staphylococci producing a toxin causes systemic shock with fever, diarrhoea, vomiting and an erythematous rash. There is a 10 per cent mortality rate. More frequently a foreign body or retained tampon merely causes an offensive discharge.

## Bartholin's abscess

Bartholin's glands are situated on either side of the vagina, opening into the vestibule. Cysts can develop if the opening becomes blocked; these present as painless swellings. If they become infected, a Bartholin's abscess develops. Examination reveals a hot, tender abscess adjacent to the lower part of the vagina. Surgical treatment is required. This is usually done by marsupialization. Culture may yield a variety of organisms, including *Neisseria gonorrhoeae*, streptococci, staphylococci, mixed anaerobic organisms or *Escherichia coli*.

## Infestations

Pubic lice and scabies are transmitted by close bodily contact. Pubic lice (*Phthirus pubis*) attach their eggs to the base of pubic hair. Their claws only attach to thick body hair, so they can also colonize the axillae and eyelashes. Infected individuals may report small itchy papules, or notice debris from the lice in their underwear. Lice are treated by the application of topical agents such as malathion, carbaryl or permethrin. Treatment should be repeated after 7 days, and be supplied for partners to use simultaneously.

Scabies (*Sarcoptes scabiei*) causes an intensely itchy papular rash. If acquired during intercourse, it may be initially confined to the genital area. It responds to applications of malathion or permethrin; however, symptoms may take up to 6 weeks to resolve completely.

### Key Points: vaginal infections

- Vaginal candidiasis is an opportunistic infection, not an STD.
- Women with asymptomatic candidal colonization do not require treatment.
- Bacterial vaginosis is a common, relapsing condition, with half of those affected being asymptomatic.
- Bacterial vaginosis is associated with preterm birth, and upper genital tract infection following termination of pregnancy (TOP), gynaecological surgery and Caesarean section.
- *Trichomonas vaginalis* is sexually transmitted. Partners must be treated to prevent re-infection.

## Upper genital tract infections

Pelvic inflammatory disease is a broad term used to cover upper genital tract infection, i.e. endometritis, parametritis, salpingitis and oophoritis. These infections usually spread from the vagina or cervix through the uterine cavity. Lymphatic spread may occur, either parametrially or along the surface of the uterus. Although rare, salpingitis has occurred in women who have been sterilized. Infection can also spread from the bowel or can be blood borne. Many different organisms have been cultured from women with PID, but 80 per cent of cases are triggered by a sexually transmissible infection – either *Chlamydia* or gonorrhoea. *Mycoplasma genitalium* is probably sexually transmitted and has been implicated in PID in women and in NGU in men. It is difficult to detect, requiring special culture medium or a polymerase chain reaction (PCR) test. Endogenous anaerobes, such *Bacteroides* spp. or *Mycoplasma hominis*, often come in as secondary invaders and are responsible for subsequent tubal abscess formation.

Pelvic inflammatory disease is an important condition because it results in tubal damage leading to ectopic pregnancy and tubal factor infertility. As many as 20 per cent of women may be left with chronic pelvic pain. The symptoms and signs may be mild and subtle, with many women unaware of the significance of mild pelvic pain and possible future fertility. On the other hand, many women are now aware of these complications and seek reassurance about their future fertility when they receive a diagnosis of PID.

### Chlamydia trachomatis

*Chlamydia trachomatis* is the commonest bacterial STI in industrialized countries. As many as 10 per cent of women of childbearing age are infected in inner cities in the UK. Women under 25 years of age have the highest prevalence. Many infections are asymptomatic: approximately 50 per cent in men and 80 per cent in women. In men it is the most important cause of NGU. In women it causes cervicitis and PID. Genital strains can colonize the throat and also cause conjunctivitis. It can infect the rectum, although only lymphogranuloma venereum (LGV) strains of *Chlamydia* cause a severe proctitis.

*Chlamydia trachomatis* is a small bacterium that is an obligate intracellular pathogen. Serovars A–C cause trachoma, infecting the conjunctiva. Serovars D–K cause genital infections. Specific LGV serovars (L1–L3) cause LGV. The infectious particle are the elementary bodies that infect columnar epithelial cells in the genital tract. They gain entry to the cells by binding to specific surface receptors. Once inside the cell, inclusion bodies form, which contain the metabolically active reticulate bodies. These divide by binary fission. After a 48-hour life cycle, reticulate bodies condense into elementary bodies which are released from the cell surface. Heavily infected cells die but it is the inflammatory response to infection that contributes most to damaging the epithelial surface.

Humoral immunity may protect from re-infection, but antibodies are serovar specific and the protection is short lived. Cell-mediated immunity, with activation of cytotoxic T cells and production of interferon-gamma, is more important for controlling established infection.

Chlamydial infection is diagnosed by specific tests. Initially, cell culture techniques were used. Enzyme-linked immunosorbent assay (ELISA) tests are now used more commonly, but their sensitivity is limited. It is essential that samples are collected from the endocervix and areas of cervical ectropion so that columnar epithelial cells are harvested. Tests that detect DNA, such as the PCR and the ligase chain reaction (LCR), are much more sensitive. They can be applied to urine samples or vaginal swabs and have detection rates superior to ELISA tests on cervical swabs. This means that non-invasive screening for *Chlamydia* is now possible. Unfortunately, higher cost has limited the availability of such tests in the UK. A direct fluorescent antibody (DFA) test can be performed on cervical smears rolled onto a specific collecting slide and fixed in alcohol. ELISA tests cannot be used reliably on rectal or conjunctival swabs, for which DFA is more appropriate.

In Scandinavian countries, nationwide screening programmes have reduced the incidence of chlamydial infection, with concomitant reductions in the incidence of PID and ectopic pregnancy. A national screening programme is starting in the UK.

Serological tests are not performed routinely in the diagnosis of chlamydial infections. Micro-immuno-fluorescence can be used to detect serum antibodies, which are not present in all infected individuals. The highest antibody titres are found in women with PID or disseminated infection. These highest titres are present in 60 per cent of women with tubal factor infertility.

The following treatments are effective for uncomplicated chlamydial infection:
- doxycycline 100 mg twice a day for 7 days
- azithromycin 1 g as a single dose
- ofloxacin 400 mg daily for 7 days.

The following are used in pregnancy:
- azithromycin 1 g as a single dose
- erythromycin 500 mg twice a day for 14 days.

It is essential that sex partners are screened fully for STIs and prescribed treatment for *Chlamydia* before sexual intercourse is resumed.

## Gonorrhoea

The incidence of gonorrhoea has declined in developed countries in the last two decades. The prevalence is less than 1 per cent in women of childbearing age. Chronic asymptomatic infection is common: 50 per cent of women have no symptoms or signs of infection. Approximately 70 per cent of men, however, are symptomatic. In men, gonorrhoea causes a severe urethritis, with green urethral discharge and dysuria. In women, the spectrum of disease is similar to that of *Chlamydia*. *Neisseria gonorrhoeae* may be carried in the throat or cause an exudative tonsillitis. It occasionally causes conjunctivitis in adults. It also causes proctitis in women and homosexual men, who may present with purulent discharge, bleeding and rectal pain.

*Neisseria gonorrhoeae* is a Gram-negative diplococcus, which colonizes columnar or cuboidal epithelium. In chronic infection there is a complex interaction with the host immune system. The expression of antigenic surface proteins changes over time in the face of an effective antibody response. Protective immunity does not appear to develop. There are no reliable serological tests for gonorrhoea. Where antibiotic use is not controlled adequately, resistant strains emerge rapidly. Chromosomal mutations conferring reduced sensitivity to penicillin emerge slowly in an incremental way. High-level resistance to penicillin is mediated by a plasmid; the first one described encoded a penicillinase enzyme (PPNG [penicillinase-producing *Neisseria gonorrhoeae*] strains). Chromosomal mutations conferring resistance to quinolone antibiotics have emerged in developing countries in the last two decades.

In GUM clinics, the diagnosis is made presumptively by observing typical Gram-negative intracellular diplococci on Gram-stained smears of urethral, cervical and rectal swabs (Fig. 15.2). It is a fastidious organism, requiring a carbon dioxide concentration of 7 per cent, specific media such as blood agar and antibiotics to inhibit the growth of other organisms. It may fail to grow on culture, particularly if transport to the laboratory is delayed. DNA-based detection tests are available for screening, but culture remains essential to allow antibiotic sensitivity testing.

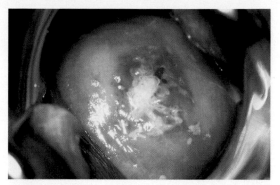

**Figure 15.3** Cervicitis. The cervix is inflamed with erythema and contact bleeding from the columnar epithelium. This can be associated with gonorrhoea, *Chlamydia* or non-specific infections.

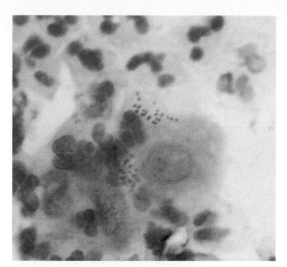

**Figure 15.2** Vaginal and cervical flora (1000× magnified.) A Gram-stained smear of cervical secretions showing polymorphs and Gram-negative intracellular diplococci. This appearance is highly suggestive of gonorrhoea.

The following treatments are effective for sensitive strains of gonorrhoea infection:

- amoxycillin 1 g with probenecid 2 g as a single dose,
- ciprofloxacin 500 mg as a single dose,
- spectinomycin 2 g as a single dose (intramuscularly),
- azithromycin 1 g as a single dose,
- ceftriaxone 250 mg as a single dose (intramuscularly),
- cefixime 400 mg as a single dose.

The choice of treatment is dictated by local sensitivity patterns, a history of recent travel and cost. It is essential that sex partners are screened fully for STIs and prescribed treatment for gonorrhoea before sexual intercourse is resumed. More than 50 per cent of women infected with gonorrhoea have a concomitant chlamydial infection. Therefore, chlamydial treatment is prescribed routinely for all women with gonorrhoea and their partners.

Because of the possibility of antibiotic resistance and occasional treatment failures, women should have two sets of cultures performed following treatment, as tests of cure. These should include rectal swabs, as infection can spread to the rectum from vaginal secretions.

## Cervicitis

Mucopurulent cervicitis is a clinical diagnosis based on detecting purulent mucus at the cervical os and is often accompanied by contact bleeding (Fig. 15.3). It can be confused with a benign ectropion, but the latter does not usually bleed heavily unless swabbed very vigorously. Women with cervicitis may present with postcoital bleeding or complain of a purulent vaginal discharge. Many, however, are asymptomatic. Cervicitis is often caused by a sexually transmissible agent, with the male partner having NGU. Tests for *Chlamydia* and gonorrhoea should be performed. If ulceration is present, test for herpes simplex.

The treatment is the same as for *Chlamydia*. Chronic cervicitis produces scarring. Nabothian follicles are mucus-containing cysts up to 1 cm in diameter, which are often present following chronic cervicitis.

## Pelvic inflammatory disease

As infection ascends into the uterus, endometritis develops. Plasma cells are seen on endometrial biopsy, and germinal centres may develop with chronic chlamydial infection. It may be associated with intermenstrual bleeding.

The first stage of salpingitis involves mucosal inflammation with swelling, redness and deciliation. Polymorphonuclear cells invade the submucosa, followed by mononuclear cells and plasma cells. Inflammatory exudate fills the lumen of the tube, and adhesions develop between mucosal folds. Inflammation extends to the serosal surface and pus exudes from the fimbriae to the ovaries and adnexae. At laparoscopy the tubes are swollen and red in mild cases. In more severe cases, the tubes are fixed to adjacent

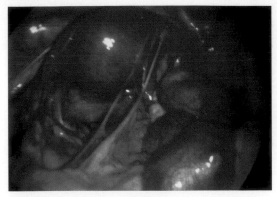

**Figure 15.4** Laparoscopic view of uterus and right Fallopian tube. The tube is dilated (hydrosalpinx or pyosalpinx) and there are bands of adhesions running from the uterine fundus to the omentum. The part of the left Fallopian tube that is visible is also dilated.

**Table 15.2**  Findings at laparoscopy in women undergoing laparoscopy for suspected pelvic inflammatory disease (PID)

| Diagnosis at laparoscopy | Percentage of women |
| --- | --- |
| Salpingitis/PID | 65 |
| Normal findings | 22 |
| Appendicitis | 3 |
| Endometriosis | 2 |
| Bleeding corpus luteum | 2 |
| Ectopic pregnancy | 2 |
| Miscellaneous | 4 |

structures by fibrin exudate and adhesions. With pelvic peritonitis, all the organs are congested, with multiple adhesions producing an inflammatory mass. The omentum usually confines the infection to the pelvis. The infection causes considerable tissue destruction; tubal or tubo-ovarian abscesses may develop.

Subsequent scarring may lead to the fimbriae being drawn into the ends of the Fallopian tubes, adhering and sealing the ends of the tubes. The uterus and tubes may be pulled back into the pelvis by adhesions, becoming fixed and retroverted. A hydrosalpinx is caused by accumulation of fluid within the tube, which expands and swells. If infected, a pyosalpinx results. Pelvic adhesions organize, matting together the pelvic organs. Some recovery of the ciliated epithelium within the tubes usually occurs.

### Clinical features

As infection ascends into the uterus, Fallopian tubes and ovaries, pelvic pain and deep dyspareunia develop. Intermenstrual bleeding may be caused by endometritis. It is not uncommon for women to have an associated urinary tract infection. An abnormal urine dipstick test should not distract one from the diagnosis of PID. The diagnosis of PID is based on the following.
- A history of pelvic pain and deep dyspareunia.
- On examination: cervical motion tenderness (often called cervical excitation) with or without uterine and adnexal tenderness.
- Lower genital tract infection: BV, trichomoniasis or cervicitis.

- In more severe cases: pyrexia, a raised neutrophil count and a raised erythrocyte sedimentation rate (ESR).
- An adnexal mass may be present in 20 per cent of women, usually those who are most systemically unwell.

At best, the clinical diagnosis is 70–80 per cent accurate. Laparoscopy is regarded as the 'gold standard' for diagnosis (Fig. 15.4). In early salpingitis, however, the inflammation may not be visible from the serosal surface of the tubes. The important differential diagnoses are shown in Table 15.2. The most important diagnosis to exclude acutely is ectopic pregnancy. If there is any doubt about the possibility of pregnancy, a urine pregnancy test should be performed. If early pregnancy is established, an ultrasound scan to look for evidence of an intrauterine pregnancy is essential.

### 🔑 Key Points: pelvic inflammatory disease

- Most episodes of PID are associated with traditional STD pathogens: *Chlamydia* and *Neisseria gonorrhoeae*.
- Secondary invasion with anaerobes is common, so that combinations of antibiotics are required to cover the spectrum of likely pathogens.
- Partner notification is an important part of management.
- PID is associated with tubal damage leading to ectopic pregnancy and tubal factor infertility.
- Most chlamydial amd gonococcal infections are asymptomatic: 'safer sex' and screening are the best means of prevention.

When PID is suspected, endocervical swabs should be taken for the detection of *C. trachomatis* and *N. gonorrhoeae*. A high vaginal swab should be taken for the detection of *Trichomonas vaginalis* and BV. Laparoscopy should be performed if the clinical diagnosis is uncertain, drainage of an abscess might be required, or there is no improvement after 24–48 hours of intravenous antibiotic treatment in a systemically unwell woman.

Ambulant patients with mild symptoms can be treated as outpatients. The antibiotic regimen should cover both *Chlamydia* and gonorrhoea, as well as an anaerobic organism. It is usual to prescribe doxycycline 100 mg twice a day for 14 days with 5 days of metronidazole 400 mg twice a day. If gonorrhoea is suspected, prescribe ciprofloxacin 500 mg as a single dose in addition. An alternative is to use ofloxacin 400 mg daily for 2 weeks with 5 days of metronidazole 400 mg twice a day. Patients who are systemically unwell, or in whom a tubal abscess is suspected, should be admitted for intravenous antibiotic treatment and may require laparoscopy definitely to establish the diagnosis. Intravenous cephalosporin and metronidazole can be used initially, but it is essential that a 2-week course of doxycycline is prescribed to eradicate any possible chlamydial infection.

It is essential that sexual partners are screened for *Chlamydia* and gonorrhoea and prescribed appropriate antibiotic treatment before intercourse is resumed (Fig. 15.5).

## Other complications of Chlamydia *and gonorrhoea*

Intra-abdominal spread of *Chlamydia* or gonorrhoea can cause peri-appendicitis or perihepatitis. The latter is termed the Fitz–Hugh Curtis syndrome. Women and, rarely, men present with right hypochondrial pain and tenderness and pyrexia. They are frequently misdiagnosed as having cholecystitis. Careful examination usually elicits signs of salpingitis. At laparoscopy, fine 'violin string' adhesions are seen between the liver capsule and visceral peritoneum. Perihepatitis is cured by a 3-week course of appropriate antibiotics.

Disseminated infection with *Chlamydia* may cause Reiter's syndrome or sexually acquired reactive arthritis (SARA). This probably occurs in less than 1 per cent of cases. There is usually an asymmetrical oligoarthritis, affecting large joints of the lower limb. In Reiter's syndrome, the arthritis is accompanied by uveitis and a rash that, if florid, may be similar to psoriasis. It is associated with the presence of human leukocyte antigen (HLA) B27 haplotype, and there is overlap with other seronegative spondarthritides.

Disseminated infection with gonorrhoea occurs rarely (more often in women than men), but presents as a septic oligoarthritis, usually affecting the small joints of the hand or wrist, with a scanty papular rash.

## Pregnancy and vertical transmission
See *Obstetrics by Ten Teachers*, 18th edition, Chapter 15.

## Other causes of endometritis

### Tuberculosis
*Mycobacterium tuberculosis* can spread through the genital tract via the blood or lymphatics. There is nearly always tuberculosis elsewhere, usually pulmonary. Granulomata develop in the Fallopian tubes and subsequently the other genital organs. Infection may remain subclinical, presenting ultimately with amenorrhoea, infertility or, in a similar fashion to PID, with chronic, low-grade pelvic pain. The endometrium is involved in up to 80 per cent of cases and the ovaries in 20–30 per cent. Abnormal uterine bleeding is a presenting symptom in 10–40 per cent of patients.

Examination findings are normal in many women, but an adnexal mass or fixing of the pelvic organs may be detected. Diagnosis can be confirmed by obtaining endometrial tissue from biopsy or dilatation and curettage. The detection rate is greatest towards the end of the menstrual cycle. Even so, endometrial biopsy does not have 100 per cent sensitivity.

Because the presentation may be subtle, a high index of suspicion is essential. A Mantoux or Heaf test should be reactive in a woman with active tuberculosis unless she is immunosuppressed. A chest X-ray should be

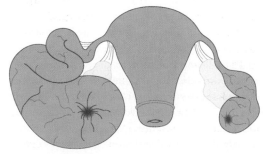

**Figure 15.5** Large hydrosalpinx of left Fallopian tube with a smaller hydrosalpinx on the right side.

performed to look for evidence of pulmonary tuberculosis. After chronic infection, bilateral tubal calcification may be seen on abdominal X-rays.

### Actinomycosis

This infection is almost exclusively seen in women with an IUD. It can be detected on cervical cytology and, if there are no clinical features to suggest PID, careful monitoring is required. If there is any history of pelvic pain, the IUD should be removed and antibiotic treatment with penicillin initiated. If undetected, actinomycosis can progress to widespread pelvic involvement with an inflammatory mass and fixing of the pelvic organs.

## Genital ulcer disease

The diagnosis of genital ulcers can be a considerable challenge for the clinician. In the UK, herpes simplex infection is by far the commonest cause. It is essential, however, to take adequate sexual and travel histories, as there are many other sexually transmissible causes of genital ulcers that are common in tropical countries.

## Herpes simplex virus

Most women experience considerable psychological distress upon receiving a diagnosis of genital herpes. They feel contaminated by acquiring an incurable STD that will inevitably be transmitted to future partners, making it difficult to initiate future relationships. Many are also aware that it can be transmitted to neonates, with disastrous consequences. Sensitive discussion and counselling are essential and several follow-up consultations may be required.

### Microbiology and diagnosis

Traditionally, herpes simplex virus type I (HSV-I) causes oral lesions (cold sores) and type II (HSV-II) causes genital herpes. Currently, cold sores caused by HSV-I infection are becoming less common in the UK, but they occur more often in lower socio-economic groups. Fewer adults are infected orally before they become sexually active, and more are therefore susceptible to the virus. Accordingly, 50 per cent of genital lesions are now caused by HSV-I. At present, approximately 20 per cent of GUM clinic attendees have antibodies to HSV-II, and 50–60 per cent have antibodies to HSV-I. Less than half those with antibodies to HSV-II are aware that they have herpes, or even report genital ulcers when questioned. Infection is frequently subclinical, so that an individual presents many years after acquisition with what is apparently a newly acquired infection. Individuals with one type of HSV infection can develop symptomatic infection from the other type, although there is some partial immunity.

---

**Classification of genital ulcers**

- Infective
- HSV
- Primary syphilis
- LGV
- Chancroid
- Donovanosis
- Human immunodeficiency virus (HIV)
- Non-infective
- Aphthous ulcers
- Trauma
- Skin disease, e.g. lichen sclerosis et atrophicus
- Behçet's syndrome
- Other multisystem disorders, e.g. sarcoidosis
- Dermatitis artefacta

---

The diagnosis is made by collecting serum from a vesicle with a small-gauge needle and syringe or by applying a cotton-tipped swab to ulcers. The virus is demonstrated by electron microscopy or culture in a tissue monolayer. Monoclonal antibodies are used to type the virus once cultured. Serological tests that can distinguish between HIV type 1 and type 2 antibodies are becoming available. A demonstration of HSV-II antibody usually indicates genital infection, whilst type I antibody could be either oral or genital.

### Primary herpes

Primary herpes presents up to 3 weeks after acquisition. There is usually widespread involvement of the vulva, and the vagina and cervix can also be affected (Fig. 15.6). Primary pharyngeal or rectal infections are seen following orogenital contact or anal intercourse.

Painful vesicles develop which coalesce into multiple ulcers. Peri-urethral involvement may cause severe pain, and urinary retention can result; this may also be partly due to involvement of the sacral nerves. If seen very early, primary herpes may only affect a small part of the vulva, appearing to be a recurrent

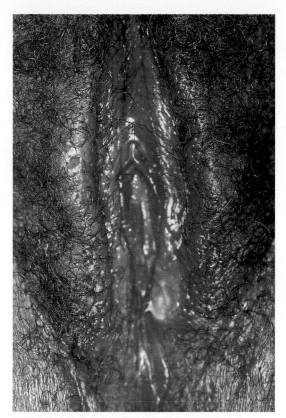

**Figure 15.6** Genital herpes. Several ulcers are seen on the vulva. Widespread lesions are seen in primary herpes and in recurrent herpes affecting pregnant or immunosuppressed women.

when virus particles are produced and track down the axons to the skin. Vesicles and ulcers then occur, usually in the same area. Sometimes distant anatomical sites are affected, if supplied by the same dermatomal nerve root. The spectrum of severity varies.

- Asymptomatic shedding of virus.
- Apparently trivial ulcers, resembling small abrasions on the vulva.
- Localized clusters of vesicles and ulcers over an area of 1–2 cm diameter.
- Widespread or chronic ulceration resembling a primary infection can be seen in pregnant women.
- If a woman is immunosuppressed, large atypical chronic ulcers may develop. A herpetic ulcer persisting for more than 1 month is acquired immunodeficiency syndrome (AIDS) defining in an individual with HIV infection.

A diagnosis of herpes can often be made by swabbing small ulcers in women who may present with an unrelated condition or who think they have recurrent thrush. It is important to advise such patients that herpes is likely, even if the initial swab is negative. The woman should return for a further culture as soon as any similar lesions occur, so that the diagnosis can be confirmed.

Patients with an established history of genital herpes may present with a recurrent episode requesting treatment. Antiviral agents are usually ineffective in treating an established attack, which will resolve just as quickly without specific treatment. It is usual to advise patients to keep the area clean by washing with salt water and to avoid sexual intercourse until fully healed.

A small proportion of individuals with genital herpes develop frequent recurrences (more than six to eight attacks a year) or are considerably incapacitated during attacks. It is then appropriate to prescribe long-term suppression with aciclovir 400 mg twice a day. This considerably reduces the frequency of attacks, although they can still occur and the infection can still be transmitted to partners. Many individuals experience a prodrome before the onset of vesicles and ulceration. This is usually a tingling sensation, but may include neuralgic symptoms, with pain in the thigh or perineum. An alternative strategy for these patients is episodic treatment. Prescribe a 5-day treatment pack to keep at home. The patient can then initiate treatment when prodromal symptoms arise. This may abort a developing attack of symptomatic herpes.

If individuals with a history of herpes take swabs every day, herpes can be detected on occasions, usually

episode. It is sensible therefore routinely to prescribe a course of antiviral medication for 5 days for all patients presenting with the first attack, even if the clinical suspicion is of a secondary episode. Diagnosis should always be confirmed by culture, or electron microscopy of a swab taken from the lesion. In primary herpes, partners should be advised to attend, although often the infecting lesion has healed.

Treatment includes analgesics and bathing in salt water. Lignocaine gel can be applied to particularly sore areas. Antiviral treatment stops viral replication, and healing occurs over the following week. Aciclovir 200 mg five times a day for 5 days is the cheapest and most established treatment. Famciclovir and valaciclovir have greater bio-availability, but are considerably more expensive.

### Recurrent herpes

Following a primary infection, herpes colonizes the neurones in the dorsal root ganglia, establishing a latent infection. Productive infection occurs intermittently for several consecutive days, even though there are no symptoms. Such asymptomatic shedding can transmit infection to a sexual partner. It is important, therefore, that people with herpes use condoms to reduce the likelihood of transmitting infection. If both partners have a history of genital herpes this is probably not necessary.

### Complications

There may be considerable psychological distress associated with a diagnosis of herpes. Counselling may help an individual to come to terms with the diagnosis. Occasionally, referral to a psychologist or psychiatrist is indicated. Self-help organizations such as The Herpes Association provide useful support.

Neurological involvement during primary herpes infection is uncommon. It may present as aseptic meningitis, transverse myelitis or autonomic neuropathy. Resolution usually takes 1–2 months. Although HSV-II is more frequently implicated in aseptic meningitis, HSV-I more often causes encephalitis in adults.

Herpes keratitis is a serious condition that can produce corneal scarring and blindness, particularly if treated inappropriately with steroids in the absence of antiviral agents. Both HSV-I and HSV-II can infect the eye, and direct inoculation from an infected site is the route of spread. The presence of a branching 'dendritic' ulcer visible with fluorescein drops is diagnostic. Recurrent episodes may occur.

### Pregnancy and vertical transmission

See *Obstetrics by Ten Teachers*, 18th edition, Chapter 15.

## Non-herpes genital ulcers

The differential diagnosis of genital ulcers is wide ranging from a variety of infections. Malignancy, particularly squamous cell carcinoma, may arise on a background of lichen sclerosis et atrophicus or vulval intraepithelial neoplasia. Multisystem disorders, such as Behçet's syndrome, systemic lupus erythematosus and sarcoidosis, may be associated with genital ulceration. It is advisable to arrange for a biopsy if there is any doubt about the diagnosis.

Simple aphthous ulcers can occur on the genital mucosa in the same way as in the mouth. HIV infection may present with genital ulceration, particularly persistent atypical herpetic ulcers. The presentation of other infections is modified by immunosuppression.

### Infective genital ulcers

These are more common in tropical countries but can be imported into the UK. At present, the incidence of syphilis is rising in European countries. The correct microbiological diagnosis can be difficult, and referral to an appropriate specialist may be appropriate.

## Syphilis

Syphilis is a systemic STI caused by *Treponema pallidum*. In vitro, *T. pallidum venereum* causing venereal syphilis cannot be distinguished from *T. pertenue*, which causes yaws, *T. pallidum endemicum*, which causes endemic syphilis, and *T. carateum*, which causes pinta. These three tropical treponematoses are not sexually transmitted but pass between children and household contacts. A description of them is beyond the scope of this chapter. Clinicians in the UK must be aware that they occur in sub-Saharan Africa, the Caribbean and most of the humid tropics (yaws), in desert regions (endemic syphilis), and isolated parts of Central and South America (pinta). Following such an infection, the serological tests for syphilis may remain positive for life, causing diagnostic confusion. The tropical treponematoses have become less common following mass treatment campaigns in the 1950s and 1960s, but they still occur.

The first manifestation of venereal syphilis is a painless ulcer (chancre) at the site of inoculation. These are usually single but can occasionally be multiple. The regional lymph nodes become enlarged. In women, the commonest site for a chancre is on the cervix; it may therefore pass unnoticed. A chancre usually arises 3–6 weeks after infection (Fig. 15.7), is painless and will resolve spontaneously without treatment after a few weeks. Chancres usually have a rubbery consistency and are accompanied by inguinal lymphadenopathy.

Secondary syphilis can arise as the chancre disappears or up to 6 months later. This is manifested by a systemic eruption, most often a non-itchy maculopapular rash. It is symmetrical and involves the palms of the hands and soles of the feet. More florid lesions resembling warts (condylomata lata) are seen in intertriginous areas, particularly peri-anally. Mucous patches and linear (snail track) ulcers are seen on the mucosal surfaces. There may be generalized lymphadenopathy. Other manifestations include alopecia, arthritis and meningitis. A sensorineural deafness can

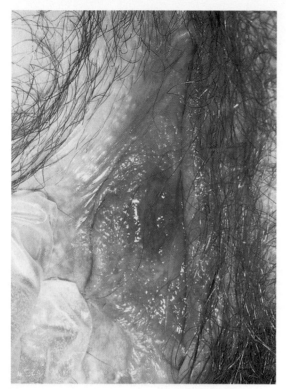

**Figure 15.7** Primary syphilitic chancre. A painless rubbery ulcer is seen on the vulva. In many women the chancre is sited on the cervix, in which case the infection may pass asymptomatically. (Courtesy of Dr Raymond Maw, Royal Victoria Hospital, Belfast.)

occur early in the infection, due to destruction of the hair cells in the inner ear.

The diagnosis of primary syphilis is made by demonstrating the organism by dark-field microscopy. The lesion is cleaned and mildly abraded so that clear serum exudes from the base. This is then collected and mixed with a drop of saline on a microscope slide. The slide is viewed under high power (38003) using dark-field illumination. *Treponema pallidum* can be seen as tightly wound spiral organisms, which move and bend in a characteristic fashion. Inexperienced observers can be misled by other spirochaetes that may be present on mucosal surfaces but are less tightly coiled.

Serological tests for syphilis should be requested, including a fluorescent treponemal antibody (FTA) test. This is the most sensitive and specific test for syphilis, but is time consuming to perform, requiring skilled interpretation. Most laboratories routinely perform a specific treponemal test such as the *Treponema pallidum* haemagglutination assay (TPHA) or *Treponema pallidum* particle agglutination (TPPA). A reaginic or

non-specific test such as the Venereal Disease Reference Laboratory (VDRL) test or rapid plasma reagin (RPR) test is used in addition. These are diluted down serially to give a titre such as 1 in 64, at the threshold of reaction of the test. In early primary syphilis, however, the serological tests may all be negative. Chancres on the cervix may be misdiagnosed clinically as cervical carcinomas. If there is any doubt, biopsies must be taken. An extensive infiltrate of lymphocytes and plasma cells is seen histologically. Specialized stains, such as silver, reveal the presence of spirochaetes.

In secondary syphilis, the serological tests are positive with a VDRL titre of usually 1 in 32 or greater. Dark-ground examination can be performed from mucosal lesions or condylomata lata. Following treatment of primary or secondary syphilis, the titre of VDRL should fall twofold every 3 months, becoming negative within 2 years.

Following the resolution of secondary syphilis, a period of latency occurs. There are no outward manifestations of infection, which is only detected on serological testing. There is a potential for lesions of secondary syphilis to relapse for up to 2 years, during which time infection can be transmitted to a sexual partner. This is called early latent syphilis.

Primary and secondary syphilis are not life threatening. The importance of the diagnosis rests on the risk of late tertiary syphilis. Neurosyphilis can be manifest within 5 years of infection in the form of meningovascular syphilis presenting with a stroke. This may subsequently progress to tabes dorsalis, or general paresis of the insane. Approximately 10 per cent of men and 5 per cent of women develop neurosyphilis if not treated in the early stages. Approximately 20 per cent will develop cardiovascular syphilis manifesting as thoracic aortic aneurysm or aortic regurgitation, which can present many years later.

Syphilis is also important because of the risk of vertical transmission. At its most severe, this will cause intrauterine death or a severely affected neonate. Neonates at risk should be fully evaluated, including a lumbar puncture, and receive intravenous penicillin. Less severe infection may present during late childhood with the stigmata of congenital syphilis, including eighth nerve deafness, interstitial keratitis and abnormal teeth. The risk of congenital infection is greatest, as high as 70 per cent, with primary and secondary syphilis, but can occur even 5–10 years later. The effects of late congenital syphilis are not prevented unless the mother is treated before 20 weeks' gestation.

## Treatment

*Treponema pallidum* replicates slowly, with an estimated doubling time of 20 hours. Sustained treponemicidal levels of antibiotic are needed for a minimum of 12 days in early syphilis. The treatment of choice is penicillin. A variety of regimens is used (Table 15.3):

- procaine penicillin 1.2 MU daily by intramuscular injection for 12 days,
- benzathine penicillin 2.4 MU by intramuscular injection, repeated after 7 days,
- doxycycline 100 mg two times a day for 14 days,
- erythromycin 500 mg four times a day for 14 days.

In the UK, administration of procaine penicillin 1.2 MU daily is prescribed commonly. If the infection has been present for more than 1 year, treatment is extended to 21 days for penicillin regimens and 28 days for oral regimens. Only intravenous penicillin or high doses of procaine penicillin (2.4 MU daily) combined with probenecid (500 mg four times/day) produce acceptable levels of penicillin in the cerebrospinal fluid to treat neurosyphilis. In pregnancy, the absorption of erythromycin is unreliable. Consider intravenous treatment for penicillin-allergic pregnant women, or desensitization to penicillin.

Partner notification is essential: the sexual history should be reviewed. In some cases, partners from a few years previously should be contacted when possible. Children may need to be tested, as well as siblings if congenital infection is possible. This may be arranged most easily with the help of a GUM clinic.

## Tropical genital ulcer disease

Sexually transmitted infections causing genital ulcer disease present considerable diagnostic difficulty. In some cases more than one infecting agent may be present. Most of the aetiological agents cannot be cultured in standard microbiological media, and histological examination of tissue is sometimes the only means of confirming the diagnosis. In many tropical countries where resources are poor, a syndromic approach is taken to the treatment of genital ulcers. Recommended treatments are shown in Table 15.3.

**Table 15.3**   Treatment for bacterial genital ulcers

| Antibacterial agent | Primary syphilis | Lymphogranuloma venereum | Chancroid | Donovanosis |
|---|---|---|---|---|
| Azithromycin | Active, but not fully evaluated | Active, but not fully evaluated | 1 g stat | |
| Ceftriaxone | Active, but not fully evaluated | | 250 mg stat i.m. | |
| Ciprofloxacin | Not active | Not reliable | 500 mg twice/day for 3 days | 750 mg twice/day for 21 days minimum |
| Cotrimoxazole | Not active | | May be used, but resistance is common in some areas | 960 mg twice/day for 21 days minimum |
| Doxycycline | 100 mg twice/day for 14 days | 100 mg twice/day for 21 days | | 100 mg twice/day for 21 days minimum |
| Erythromycin | 500 mg four times/day for 14 days | 500 mg four times/day for 21 days | 500 mg four times/day for 7 days | 500 mg four times/day for 21 days minimum |
| Penicillin | Procaine penicillin 1.2 MU/day for 12 days | | | |

i.m., intramuscularly.

## Lymphogranuloma venereum

Lymphogranuloma venereum is caused by specific serovars (L1–L3) of *Chlamydia trachomatis*. It is found in the Far East, sub-Saharan Africa and South America. In the early stages there is often a small superficial ulcer that can slowly increase in size but often goes unnoticed. More obvious are the enlarged nodes, which become compressed by the inguinal ligament leading to the 'groove sign'. The nodes can become matted together and discharge pus, forming a bubo. In women, a severe proctocolitis can progress to fistulae and strictures. The diagnosis can be confirmed serologically by a complement fixation test.

## Chancroid

Chancroid is an infection caused by *Haemophilus ducreyi*. The geographical distribution is similar to that of LGV. It starts with small, shallow ulcers, which are usually multiple and painful. The edges are irregular and there is localized lymphadenopathy. The sores may persist for several months and the glands can suppurate through the skin. The organism can only be grown on specialized culture medium and, ideally, the medium should be inoculated directly from the patient. Even so it may be difficult to obtain a positive culture. There is a characteristic appearance on biopsy, when Ducrey's bacillus may be seen.

## Granuloma inguinale (Donovanosis)

Granuloma inguinale is an infection caused by *Klebsiella granulomatis* (previously known as *Calymmatobacterium granulomatis*). It is endemic in India, Papua New Guinea and southern Africa. It is usually a slowly progressive infection starting with discrete papules on the skin or vulva which can enlarge to form 'beefy red' painful ulcers. These spread slowly around the genitalia and perineum. As they heal, fibrosis can develop, which may lead to lymphoedema and elephantiasis. Diagnosis is best confirmed by biopsy or a crush preparation in which Donovan bodies are visible.

### 🔑 Key Points: genital ulcers

- The commonest cause of genital ulceration in the UK is HSV.
- Many women with serological evidence of herpes infection have subclinical infection, or are not aware of the significance of occasional ulceration.
- Syphilis is currently uncommon in the UK. It presents with painless ulcers and inguinal lymphadenopathy.
- Atypical manifestations of infections occur in the immunosuppressed, such as those with HIV infection.

## Other viral infections

## Human papillomavirus

More than 70 different types of HPV have been described. Although strains causing hand warts occasionally spread to the genital area, certain genital strains preferentially infect the genital mucosa. These are thought to be sexually transmitted. Infection is often established asymptomatically and may be carried for years, probably lifelong. In one study, genital warts developed in nearly two-thirds of contacts of patients with visible genital warts within 3 months of starting the relationship. There is less information on the role of asymptomatic shedding of wart virus in those with subclinical lesions. The virus can infect the skin of the vulva and perineum, the vagina, cervix and rectum (Fig. 15.8); possibly orogenital contact leads to warts developing in the mouth or lips. Warts are frequently multiple and slowly increase in size.

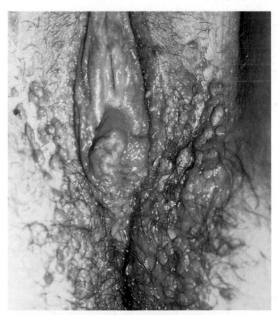

**Figure 15.8** Genital warts. Multiple warts are seen over the lower vulva. (Courtesy of Dr Richard Lau, St George's Hospital, London.)

They can spread directly to the peri-anal skin without anal intercourse being practised. The same strains can affect the larynx of a neonate (rarely) but do not usually spread to normal skin.

The majority of genital warts are caused by HPV types 6 and 11 – viruses that have little oncogenic potential. HPV types 16 and 18 may cause flat warts and have been linked with the development of cervical carcinoma. The majority of squamous cell carcinomas of the cervix contain DNA sequences from oncogenic HPV strains. It is thought that viral proteins, called E6 and E7, bind to p53 and pRB proteins produced by anti-oncogenes. This leads to dysregulation of the cell cycle and cell proliferation. Carcinomas that lack HPV sequences usually have other mutations that affect *P53* gene expression. Several other events need to occur at the molecular level to initiate a cancer cell. Most women infected with HPV 16 or 18 do not develop cancer. Smoking is an important risk factor that should be discouraged.

Visible genital warts are usually treated with physical methods such as cryotherapy. Application of podophyllin once or twice a week for up to 6 weeks will produce cure in 50–60 per cent of women. A purified extract of podophyllotoxin has the advantage of self-application at home: twice a day for 3 days. Healing may be followed by ulceration, so patients should be instructed on its use with care. Petroleum jelly can be applied to adjacent normal skin to protect it. Surgical treatment is used for intractable cases, employing lasers, electrocautery or scissor excision.

Many women have heard of a link between genital warts and cervical cancer. It is important to explain that most visible genital warts are not caused by oncogenic strains of virus and that the risk of cervical cancer is not greatly increased. If cervical cytology has not been performed within 3 years, it should be done, but there is no need to advocate yearly smears or any other enhanced surveillance. Women with warts on the cervix should, however, be referred for expert colposcopic assessment. Recent sexual partners should be examined for evidence of genital warts and other infections. Traditionally, patients with warts have been advised to use barrier methods of contraception during treatment and for the subsequent 3 months. Not enough is known about the risks of transmission of asymptomatic wart virus carriage to allow evidence-based recommendations to be made. Discuss the role of condoms in the general context of protecting against both the acquisition and transmission of STIs with new partners.

Whatever treatment is used, the warts will recur until the immune response controls the growth of the wart virus. This can take several weeks or even months in some patients, who may become frustrated by such persistence. Patients who are immunosuppressed, such as those with HIV infection or underlying malignancies, are particularly difficult to treat. Immune-based therapies with interferon or topical application of imiquimod (a cream that stimulates local cytokine release) may be helpful for such patients. A new class of antiviral drugs based on nucleotide analogues is active against HPV and may become useful for its treatment.

### ⚷ Key Points: genital warts

- Most genital warts are caused by sexually transmitted strains of HPV.
- Long-lasting resolution of visible warts requires a good cell-mediated immune response.
- Infections persist for many years, and relapse can occur at any time.
- Several types of HPV, particularly 16 and 18, are associated with cervical cancer.
- Attention should be paid to reversible risk factors such as smoking.

## Molluscum contagiosum

This poxvirus produces painless, pearly lesions with a dimple, up to 5 mm in diameter. These are common in childhood and clear after a few months. Adults may acquire infection during sexual intercourse, and the lesions can be mistaken for genital warts. Infection resolves with cryotherapy or following curettage and the application of phenol. The fluid from the vesicles is infectious, and patients should be warned not to pick at them. In immunosuppressed individuals, widespread, large, confluent lesions may develop. These are currently almost untreatable, as resolution requires an immune response. Nucleotide analogue drugs show in-vitro activity against the virus, offering the prospect of antiviral treatment.

## HIV infection

Acquired immunodeficiency syndrome was first described in San Francisco in 1983. It is caused by infection with HIV. More than 20 million individuals are now infected worldwide, and in countries with a high prevalence it is the leading cause of death in young adults. It is a particularly devastating disease because of the stigma of sexual transmission and the risk of vertical transmission to children. Even for children who are not infected, the death of one or both parents threatens their development and survival in many parts of the world. The prevalence is greatest in sub-Saharan Africa, where in several cities as many as a third of pregnant women are infected. A resurgence in tuberculosis has occurred hand in hand with the AIDS epidemic.

The onset of immunodeficiency can be manifest in any organ system, so a high index of suspicion is required to recognize the way in which other disease processes are altered. This section focuses on the gynaecological aspects of HIV infection.

## Natural history and principles of treatment

Twenty per cent of those infected with HIV experience an acute seroconversion illness a few weeks after acquisition. Clinical features include fever, generalized lymphadenopathy, a macular erythematous rash, pharyngitis and conjunctivitis. A steady decline in immune function over the first few years may manifest as non-life-threatening opportunistic conditions such as recurrent oral and vaginal candidiasis, single dermatome herpes zoster (shingles), frequent and prolonged episodes of oral or genital herpes or persistent warts. Furry white patches on the sides of the tongue, termed hairy oral leukoplakia (HOL) (Fig. 15.9), may come and go and are pathognomonic of immunodeficiency. Persistent generalized lymphadenopathy may be present. Skin problems include seborrhoeic dermatitis, folliculitis, dry skin, tinea pedis and a high frequency of allergic reactions.

### Common manifestations of AIDS

**Pulmonary**
- *Pneumocystis carinii* pneumonia
- Tuberculosis – pulmonary or extrapulmonary

**Neurological**
- Cerebral toxoplasmosis
- Cryptococcal meningitis
- AIDS dementia

**Gastrointestinal**
- Diarrhoea and wasting syndrome, which may be due to infection with *Cryptosporidium*, *Microsporidium*, *Isospora*
- Oesophageal candidiasis

**Ophthalmic**
- Cytomegalovirus retinitis

**Malignancy**
- Kaposi's sarcoma (Fig. 15.10)
- Non-Hodgkin's lymphoma

**Systemic**
- *Mycobacterium avium intracellulare* complex infection

Without antiretroviral treatment, the median time to the development of AIDS is 10 years. Essentially AIDS is defined by the onset of life-threatening opportunistic infections or malignancies associated with immunodeficiency. The commonest presentations are listed in the box above. There are two strategies used in treatment. Combinations of antiretroviral drugs are prescribed. These may include two or more nucleoside analogue reverse transcriptase inhibitors, such as zidovudine or didinasine, a non-nucleoside reverse transcriptase inhibitor, such as nevirapine, and one or more protease inhibitors, such as nelfinavir. If successful, the immune system improves after a few months. These drugs, particularly some of the protease

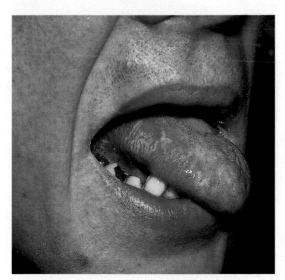

**Figure 15.9** Hairy oral leukoplakia. Filliform white ridges are seen on the lateral border of the tongue. This is almost pathognomonic of HIV infection, but may be seen in immunosuppression due to other causes. It can appear early in the course of the disease and is not AIDS defining.

inhibitors, have many potential interactions with other drugs through effects on the cytochrome P-450 enzymes. One effect is to increase the rate of breakdown of synthetic oestrogens in oral contraceptive pills.

If immunodeficiency has already occurred, treatment and prevention of opportunistic infections are needed. This may include cotrimoxazole to prevent *Pneumocystis carinii* pneumonia (PCP) and, in severely immunosuppressed individuals with CD4 counts below 0.005/L, azithromycin to prevent disseminated *Mycobacterium avium intracellulare* complex (MAC) infection, and ganciclovir to prevent cytomegalovirus (CMV) infection. Regular administration of antifungal agents may be necessary to control oral and vaginal candidiasis.

## Virology

Human immunodeficiency virus is a retrovirus with its genetic code in a single strand of RNA. Reverse transcriptase is carried within the core to enable proviral DNA to be produced in an infected cell. The outer membrane protein, gp-120, binds to CD4 receptors, which are present on T-helper lymphocytes, macrophages, dendritic cells and microglia. Co-receptors, such as the CCR-5 chemokine receptor, are also used to enhance viral entry. Approximately 1 per cent of Caucasians have a homozygous mutation in the receptor, which is associated with resistance to acquiring infection. Another viral protein, p24, surrounds the RNA and enzymes present within the core of the virus, which enters the cytoplasm of an infected cell. Once proviral DNA has been integrated into the host genome, viral peptides are transcribed. These peptides are cleaved by specific viral protease enzymes before the daughter virus particles are assembled.

Current antiretroviral drugs target reverse transcriptase or viral proteases. The aim of therapy is to reduce the level of virus in the plasma to zero with a combination of antiretroviral agents. If total suppression of viral replication is not achieved, resistant strains of virus will inevitably arise within the patient over the course of a few months. This is because reverse transcription is inherently inaccurate, leading to a high rate of mutation. With each cycle of replication of virus, which takes 48 hours, single point mutations arise, which will confer reduced sensitivity to antiviral agents.

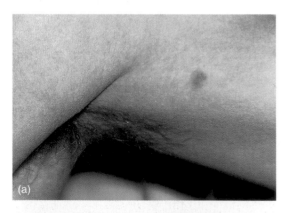

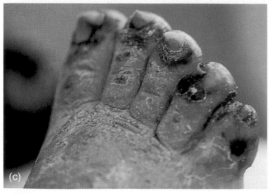

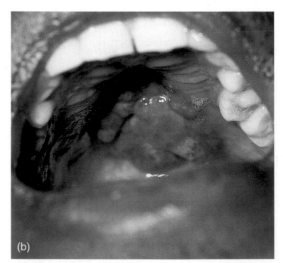

**Figure 15.10** Kaposi's sarcoma. (a) The early lesion is red/purple and palpable. (b) Advanced Kaposi's sarcoma with extensive involvement of the palate. This is usually accompanied by visceral involvement elsewhere, e.g. gut and lung. (c) Advanced Kaposi's sarcoma of the foot producing lymphoedema of the leg and gangrene of the toes. This was a pre-terminal event.

If therapy is effective, the CD4 lymphocyte count rises progressively, and at least partial immune restoration occurs. Unfortunately, HIV infects long-lived memory cells from which the virus can rapidly reseed the body on cessation of therapy. Eradication, and thus cure, is unlikely, even after several years of treatment.

## Diagnosis

Human immunodeficiency virus infection is diagnosed by finding antibodies to gp-120. During seroconversion, p24 antigen is detectable in the serum before antibodies are produced. We monitor the disease by measuring the level of CD4 lymphocytes in peripheral blood; a normal level is >0.5/L. There is a 10 per cent risk of AIDS developing within 1 year when the CD4 lymphocyte count drops to 0.2/L. This is the level at which primary prophylaxis against PCP is recommended. Using PCR technology, we can also measure the concentration of viral RNA in the plasma. A high level (>100 000 particles/mL) predicts rapid disease development.

As the consequences of receiving a diagnosis of HIV are serious, a test should only be performed with informed consent from the patient, who may wish to discuss it with a partner, for whom the test may have major implications. If you suspect an individual has HIV, look for HOL, generalized lymphadenopathy and skin rashes. There is often lymphopenia or thrombocytopenia on a full blood count. Polyclonal immunoglobulin G (IgG) production produces a raised total protein level. Kaposi's sarcoma (Fig. 15.10) may be evident, with multiple red or purple tumours anywhere on the body.

## Transmission

In most developing countries, HIV is principally spread through vaginal intercourse, with approximately equal numbers of men and women infected. In developed countries, the majority of infections have been acquired through homosexual sex or intravenous drug use, although the incidence of heterosexual transmission is increasing. Genital infections are risk factors for HIV transmission and acquisition, including genital ulcer disease, *Chlamydia* and gonorrhoea. BV may also be a risk factor and is very common in some African countries, with a prevalence of 50 per cent or greater. Good control of STIs should reduce the incidence of HIV infection.

*Vertical transmission*
See *Obstetrics by Ten Teachers*, 18th edition, Chapter 15.

## Gynaecological manifestations

Human papillomavirus infection flourishes in immunosuppressed individuals. Genital warts often persist despite aggressive surgical treatment. Chronic HPV infection can result in the development of cervical carcinoma, vulval intraepithelial neoplasia and Bowen's disease. Because of this, most physicians perform cervical cytology annually in women with HIV infection. Persistent atypical warty lesions of the skin or vulva should be biopsied.

Other infections can also be more persistent in HIV-infected individuals. There is limited evidence that PID requires longer courses of antibiotics in women with HIV. Careful follow-up is certainly indicated. Postpartum endometritis is common in this group of women, and HSV has been implicated occasionally. Eruptions of secondary genital herpes may become widespread, severe and persist for weeks if not diagnosed and treated. Genital herpes often presents as deep, painful ulceration (Fig. 15.11).

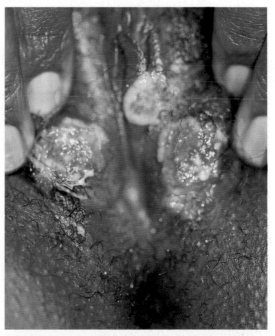

**Figure 15.11** Large multiple ulcers due to recurrent herpes simplex in a woman with HIV infection. An ulcer that persists for more than 1 month is clinically AIDS defining.

Although all HIV-infected women are urged to use condoms to prevent them transmitting the infection to others, they should also be advised to use a more reliable form of contraception if they do not wish to become pregnant. Medication prescribed for HIV may interact with the metabolism of synthetic oestrogens.

If an HIV-infected woman plans to become pregnant, the means of reducing the risk of vertical transmission should be discussed with her, as should the consequences for the child of possibly losing his or her mother in childhood. If the partner is HIV negative, the couple should be assisted to perform artificial insemination by providing information and syringes or pipettes. At present, the provision of infertility treatments to HIV-infected women is controversial, but has been offered by some gynaecologists.

## New developments

DNA-based tests such as PCR or LCR offer the possibility of non-invasive sample collection to screen for infections such as *Chlamydia* and gonorrhoea. A national screening programme will reduce the incidence of *Chlamydia*, PID and subsequent ectopic pregnancy and infertility.

Screening for and treating genital infections such as BV in pregnancy may significantly reduce the incidence of

miscarriage, preterm birth and subsequent neurological impairment.

The development of antiviral drugs continues. New agents are being developed that are likely to be effective against HPVs, herpes viruses and HIV. Novel immune stimulators that can be applied topically are also being evaluated.

Vaccines are being developed for the same chronic infections. If successful, this approach should reduce the incidence of carcinoma of the cervix related to HPV infection.

### 🔑 Key Points: HIV infection

- The incidence of HIV is increasing rapidly worldwide.
- A high index of suspicion is needed, as risk factors are not always apparent in affected individuals, some of whom might remain well for 15–20 years without specific treatment.
- Treatment with combination antiretroviral therapy can improve life expectancy and reduce hospital admissions, but it is expensive and complex to manage and there is considerable drug-associated toxicity.
- Some of the antiretroviral drugs have major pharmacokinetic interactions, including effects on the combined oral contraceptive pill, some antihistamines and antituberculous medication.

## CASE HISTORY

A 25-year-old single woman presented with a history of increased non-offensive vaginal discharge, postcoital bleeding, right hypochondrial pain and feeling generally unwell. She had been in a new relationship for 1 month, having separated from her previous boyfriend 3 months earlier. On enquiry, she reported mild deep dyspareunia. She was taking the oral contraceptive pill and had a pregnancy 2 years previously, which had been terminated at 8 weeks.

On examination, there was a mucoid vaginal discharge and green mucus emerging from the internal os. There was a small ectropion, which bled profusely after swabbing. On bimanual examination, the uterus was anteverted and mobile. There was cervical motion tenderness, bilateral adnexal tenderness and right hypochondrial tenderness.

The diagnosis of PID with presumptive perihepatitis was made and she was prescribed doxycycline 100 mg twice a

day for 3 weeks with metronidazole 400 mg twice a day for 5 days. A test for *Chlamydia trachomatis* was positive and at review after 1 week and 3 weeks her symptoms had resolved. Both her new and her previous boyfriends tested positive for *C. trachomatis* when screened in the GUM clinic.

The woman presented 1 year later with right-sided pelvic pain and amenorrhoea of 6 weeks. An ectopic pregnancy was confirmed.

## Comment

- Both *Chlamydia* and *Neisseria gonorrhoeae* can be carried for months or years before symptoms develop.
- Postcoital and intermenstrual bleeding are common symptoms of cervicitis and endometritis. Their presence should instigate a search for infection in young, sexually active women.

- As many as 20 per cent of women with PID have signs of perihepatitis on laparoscopy. Sometimes right hypochondrial pain overshadows the pelvic symptoms.
- An episode of PID threatens a woman's future fertility, causing both ectopic pregnancy and tubal infertility.

- It is important that re-infection after treatment is prevented by pursuing partner notification vigorously.

## Urinary tract infection

See Chapter 16.

## Additional reading

Barton S, Hay P (eds). *The handbook of genitourinary medicine.* London: Arnold, 1999.

Centers for Disease Control and Prevention. 1998 Guidelines for treatment of sexually transmitted diseases. *MMWR* 1998; **47**: 1–118. Also available at <http://www.cdc.gov/publications.htm>.

Holmes KK, Mardh PA, Sparks PF, Wiener PJ (eds). *Sexually transmitted diseases*, 2nd edn. New York: McGraw Hill, 1990.

Medical Society for the Study of Venereal Disease. <http://www.mssvd.org.uk>.

Pastorek-II JG (ed.). *Obstetric and gynecological infectious disease.* New York: Raven Press, 1994.

# Urogynaecology

## OVERVIEW

Urogynaecological conditions include urinary incontinence, voiding difficulties, prolapse (see also Chapter 17), frequency and urgency, urinary tract infection and urinary fistulae. Increasingly it is recognized that the pelvic floor is one structure and this has led to increased understanding of faecal incontinence and to improvements in its treatment.

## CLINICAL CONDITIONS

### Introduction

Urinary incontinence is defined as the involuntary loss of urine that is objectively demonstrable and is a social or hygienic problem. It is increasingly prevalent as the ageing population expands. It affects an individual's physical, psychological and social well-being and is associated with a significant reduction in quality of life. The prevalence increases with age, with approximately 5 per cent of women between 15 and 44 years of age being affected, rising to 10 per cent of those aged between 45 and 64 years, and approximately 20 per cent of those older than 65 years. It is even higher in women who are institutionalized and may affect up to 40 per cent of those in residential nursing homes.

Urinary incontinence is classified according to pathophysiological concepts rather than symptomatology, but the following definitions of symptoms are commonly used.

### S Common symptoms associated with incontinence

- Stress incontinence is a symptom and a sign and means loss of urine on physical effort. It is not a diagnosis.
- Urgency means a sudden desire to void.
- Urge incontinence is an involuntary loss of urine associated with a strong desire to void.
- Overflow incontinence occurs without any detrusor activity when the bladder is over-distended.
- Frequency is defined as the passing of urine seven or more times a day, or being awoken from sleep more than once a night to void.

## Urethral causes

### Urodynamic stress incontinence

Urodynamic stress incontinence (USI), previously called genuine stress incontinence, is noted during filling cystometry, and is defined as the involuntary leakage of urine during increased abdominal pressure in the absence of a detrusor contraction.

#### Symptoms

Stress incontinence is the usual symptom, but urgency, frequency and urge incontinence may be present. There may also be an awareness of prolapse. On clinical examination, stress incontinence may be demonstrated when the patient coughs. Vaginal examination should assess for prolapse and, in particular, the vaginal capacity and the woman's ability to elevate the bladder neck, as this may alter management. It is quite usual to find a cystourethrocele in women with stress incontinence.

Urodynamic studies will define the cause of incontinence and are particularly important when there has been a previous, unsuccessful continence operation or if the symptomatology is complex (these factors are covered later in this chapter).

### P Understanding the pathophysiology

The likely causes of USI are as follows.

- Abnormal descent of the bladder neck and proximal urethra, so there is failure of equal transmission of intra-abdominal pressure to the proximal urethra, leading to reversal of the normal pressure gradient between the bladder and urethra, with a resultant negative urethral closure pressure.
- An intra-urethral pressure which at rest is lower than the intravesical pressure; this may be due to urethral scarring as a result of surgery or radiotherapy. It also occurs in older women.
- Laxity of suburethral support normally provided by the vaginal wall, endopelvic fascia, arcus tendineus fascia and levator ani muscles acting as a single unit results in ineffective compression during stress and consequent incontinence (Fig. 16.1).

The aetiology of USI is thought to be related to a number of factors.

- Damage to the nerve supply of the pelvic floor and urethral sphincter caused by childbirth leads to progressive changes in these structures, resulting in altered function. In addition, mechanical trauma to the pelvic floor musculature and endopelvic fascia and ligaments occurs as a consequence of vaginal delivery. Prolonged second stage, large babies and instrumental deliveries cause the most damage.
- Menopause and associated tissue atrophy may also cause damage to the pelvic floor.
- A congenital cause may be inferred, as some nulliparous women suffer from incontinence. This may be due to altered connective tissue, particularly collagen.
- Chronic causes, such as obesity, chronic obstructive pulmonary disease, raise interabdominal pressure and constipation may also result in problems.

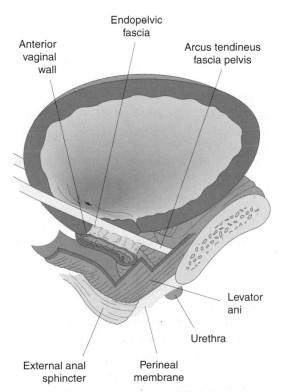

**Figure 16.1** Diagram showing the suburethral support mechanism.

### Detrusor over-activity

Detrusor over-activity, previously called detrusor instability, is a urodynamic observation characterized by involuntary detrusor contractions during the filling phase which may be spontaneous or provoked.

**P   Understanding the pathophysiology**

**P   Understanding the pathophysiology**

**Detrusor over-activity**
The pathophysiology of detrusor over-activity is poorly understood and the aetiological factors require substantiation. Poor toilet habit training and psychological factors have been implicated.

The largest group of women with this condition have an idiopathic variety. Neuropathy appears to be the most substantiated factor. Incontinence surgery, outflow obstruction and smoking are also associated with detrusor over-activity.

*Symptoms*

The presenting symptoms include urgency, urge incontinence, frequency, nocturia, stress incontinence, enuresis and, sometimes, voiding difficulties.

**Classification of incontinence**

**Urethral causes**
- Urethral sphincter incompetence (urodynamic stress incontinence)
- Detrusor over-activity or the unstable bladder – this is either neuropathic or non-neuropathic
- Retention with overflow
- Congenital causes
- Miscellaneous

**Extra-urethral causes**
- Congenital causes
- Fistula

*Examination*

Any masses that cause compression of the bladder must be excluded and prolapse must be examined for, as this may cause some of the symptoms. If there is vaginal atrophy, this may also cause some urgency and frequency.

Investigations are considered later in the chapter.

## Retention with overflow

Insidious failure of bladder emptying may lead to chronic retention and finally, when normal voiding is ineffective, to overflow incontinence. The causes may be:
- lower motor neurone or upper motor neurone lesions,
- urethral obstruction,
- pharmacological.

The patient may be aware of and present with increasing difficulty in bladder emptying or she may present only with frequency. Ultimately normal emptying stops and a stage of chronic retention with overflow develops.

*Symptoms*

Symptoms include poor stream, incomplete bladder emptying and straining to void, together with overflow stress incontinence. Often there will be recurrent urinary tract infection.

Cystometry is usually required to make the diagnosis, and bladder ultrasonography or intravenous urogram may be necessary to investigate the state of the upper urinary tract to exclude reflux.

## Congenital

Epispadias, which is due to faulty midline fusion of mesoderm, results in a widened bladder neck, shortened urethra, separation of the symphysis pubis and imperfect sphincteric control.

The patient complains of stress incontinence which may not be apparent when lying down but is noticeable when standing up. The physical appearance of epispadias is pathognomonic, and a plain X-ray of the pelvis will show symphysial separation.

It is unlikely that a conventional suprapubic operation to elevate the bladder neck will be sufficient. It may be wiser to proceed straight to urethral reconstruction or an artificial urinary sphincter.

## Miscellaneous

Acute urinary tract infection or faecal impaction in the elderly may lead to temporary urinary incontinence. A urethral diverticulum may lead to post-micturition dribble, as urine collects within the diverticulum and escapes as the patient stands up.

## Extra-urethral causes of incontinence

### Congenital

*Bladder exstrophy and ectopic ureter*
In bladder exstrophy there is failure of mesodermal migration with breakdown of ectoderm and endoderm, resulting in absence of the anterior abdominal wall and anterior bladder wall. Extensive reconstructive surgery is necessary in the neonatal period.

An ectopic ureter may be single or bilateral and presents with incontinence only if the ectopic opening is outside the bladder, when it may open within the vagina or onto the perineum. The cure is excision of the ectopic ureter and the upper pole of the kidney that it drains.

### Fistula

A urinary fistula is an abnormal opening between the urinary tract and the outside (Fig. 16.2). Urinary fistulae have obstetric and gynaecological causes. The former include obstructive labour with compression of the bladder between the presenting head and the bony wall of the pelvis. The gynaecological causes are associated with pelvic surgery or pelvic malignancy or radiotherapy.

Whatever the cause, the fistula must be accurately localized. It can be treated by primary closure or by surgery and can be delayed until tissue inflammation and oedema have resolved at about 4 weeks. The surgical techniques involve isolation and removal of the fistula tract, careful debridement, suture and closure of each layer separately and without tension and, if necessary, the interposition of omentum, which brings with it an additional blood supply.

## Frequency and urgency

Frequency and urgency are two common urinary symptoms that present singularly or combined. Approximately 15–20 per cent of women have frequency and urgency. Clinical examination and investigation can be directed towards discriminating between the common causes. These include masses that cause compression and prolapse. Investigations should rule out infection, stones and malignancy. A simple urinary diary may show signs of increased fluid intake or evidence of ingestion of too much caffeine.

## Voiding difficulties

Voiding difficulty and acute and chronic urinary retention represent a gradation of failure of bladder emptying. Of women attending a urodynamic clinic, 10–15 per cent may have voiding difficulties. The underlying mechanism is either failure of detrusor contraction or sphincteric relaxation, or urethral obstruction, and this may be due to causes such as an impacted retroverted gravid uterus.

### Symptoms

The main symptoms are poor stream, incomplete emptying and straining to void. As the residual of urine increases in amount, frequency occurs and urinary tract infection develops. Incontinence may follow, and chronic retention and overflow may develop.

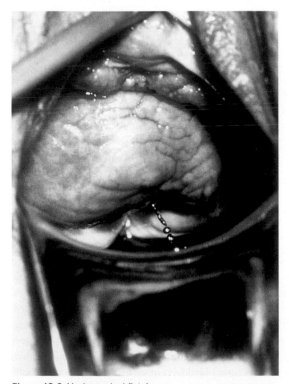

**Figure 16.2** Vesicovaginal fistula.

## Examination

A full bladder may be palpated and there may be the primary signs of the cause of voiding difficulty. Investigations include uroflowmetry, cystometry and a lumbar sacral spine X-ray. Part of the assessment involves taking an accurate drug history, as drugs such as anticholinergic agents may have been taken and the patient may be predisposed to retention.

### Urinary tract infection

Acute and chronic urinary infections are important and avoidable sources of ill-health among women. The short urethra, which is prone to entry of bacteria during intercourse, poor perineal hygiene and the occasional inefficient voiding ability of the patient and unnecessary catheterizations are all contributory factors.

A significant urinary infection is defined as the presence of a bacterial count >105 of the same organism/mL of freshly plated urine. On microscopy there are usually red blood cells and white blood cells. The common organisms are *Escherichia coli*, *Proteus mirabilis*, *Klebsiella aerogenes*, *Pseudomonas aeruginosa* and *Streptococcus faecalis*. These gain entry to the urinary tract by a direct extension from the gut, lymphatic spread via the bloodstream or transurethrally from the perineum. Symptoms include dysuria, frequency and occasionally haematuria. Loin pain and rigors and a temperature above 38 °C usually indicate that acute pyelonephritis has developed.

A culture and sensitivity of mid-stream specimen of urine is required. Intravenous urography or renal ultrasonography may be required in patients with recurrent infection to define anatomical or functional abnormalities.

With acute urinary infection, once a mid-stream urine specimen has been sent for culture and sensitivity, antimicrobial therapy can begin. If the patient is ill, the treatment should not be delayed and an antimicrobial drug regimen can be started immediately. The regimen can be changed later according to the results of the urine culture and sensitivity. Commonly used drugs include trimethoprim 200 mg twice daily or nitrofurantoin 100 mg four times daily or a cephalosporin.

Recurrent urinary tract infection for which an identifiable source has not been found may be managed by long-term low-dose antimicrobial therapy, such as trimethoprim. Recently, ciprofloxacin and norfloxacin have proved effective.

It is important to treat urinary tract infections effectively, especially in younger women. The development of acute pyelonephritis during pregnancy can be a cause of faecal morbidity.

### INVESTIGATIONS

An accurate and detailed history and examination provide a framework for the diagnosis, but there is often a discrepancy between the patient's symptoms and the urodynamic findings. The aim of urodynamic investigations is to provide accurate diagnosis of disorders of micturition and they involve investigation of the lower urinary tract and pelvic floor function.

Investigations range from simple procedures performed in the GP's surgery to sophisticated studies only available in tertiary referral centres. The clinician should pursue a streamlined yet meticulous evaluation, tailoring the investigations to the patient's clinical findings.

### Mid-stream urine specimen

Urinary infection can produce a variety of urinary symptoms, including incontinence. A nitrate stick test can suggest infection, but a diagnosis is made from a clean mid-stream specimen. The presence of a raised level of white blood cells alone suggests an infection and the test should be repeated. Invasive urodynamics can aggravate infection, and test results are invalid when performed in the presence of infection.

### Urinary diary

A urinary diary is a simple record of the patient's fluid intake and output (Fig. 16.3). Episodes of urgency and leakage and precipitating events are also recorded. There is no recommended period for diary keeping; a suggested practice is 1 week. These diaries are more accurate than patient recall and provide an assessment of functional bladder capacity. In addition to altering fluid intake, urinary diaries can be utilized to monitor

| Time | Day 1 Input | Day 1 Output | | Day 2 Input | Day 2 Output | | Day 3 Input | Day 3 Output |
|------|------|--------|---|------|--------|---|------|--------|
| 0700 hrs | 250 | 150 | | 200 | 160 | W | 250 | 170 |
| 0800 hrs | | 75 | W | | 50 | | | 75 |
| 0900 hrs | 200 | 140 | | 200 | 55 | | 150 | 60 |
| 1000 hrs | | 100 | | | 70 | | | |
| 1100 hrs | 150 | | | 150 | | W | 200 | 55 |
| 1200 hrs | | 60 | W | | 100 | | | 60 |
| 1300 hrs | 100 | 55 | | 100 | 50 | | | |
| 1400 hrs | | 75 | | | | | | |
| 1500 hrs | | | W | 100 | | | | |
| 1600 hrs | 100 | | | | | | | |
| 1700 hrs | | | | | | | | |
| 1800 hrs | | | | | | | | |

**Figure 16.3** Urinary diary. (W = wet episode.)

conservative treatment, e.g. bladder re-education, electrical stimulation and drug therapy.

## Pad test

Pad tests are used to verify and quantify urine loss. The International Continence Society pad test takes 1 hour. The patient wears a pre-weighed sanitary towel, drinks 500 mL of water and rests for 15 minutes. After a series of defined manoeuvres, the pad is re-weighed; a urine loss of more than 1 g is considered significant. If indicated, methylene blue solution can be instilled intravesically prior to the pad test to differentiate between urine and other loss, e.g. insensible loss or vaginal discharge. The popularity of 24-hour and 48-hour pad tests is increasing because they are believed to be more representative. The woman performs normal daily activities and the pad is re-weighed after the preferred period.

## Uroflowmetry

Uroflowmetry is the measurement of urine flow rate and is a simple, non-invasive procedure that can be performed in the outpatient department (Fig. 16.4). It provides an objective measurement of voiding function and the patient can void in privacy.

Although uroflowmetry is performed as part of a general urodynamic assessment, the main indications are complaints of hesitancy or difficulty voiding in patients with neuropathy or a past history of urinary retention. It is also indicated prior to bladder neck or radical pelvic cancer surgery to exclude voiding problems that may deteriorate afterwards.

The normal flow curve is bell shaped. A flow rate <15 mL/s on more than one occasion is considered abnormal in females. The voided volume should be >150 mL, as flow rates with smaller volumes are not reliable. A low peak flow rate and a

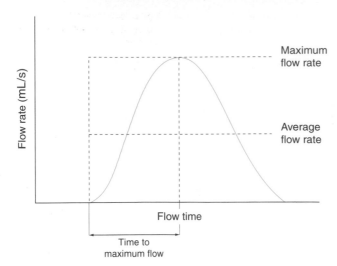

**Figure 16.4** Normal uroflowmetry.

prolonged voiding time suggest a voiding disorder. Straining can give abnormal flow patterns with interrupted flow. Uroflowmetry alone cannot diagnose the cause of impaired voiding; simultaneous measurement of voiding pressure allows a more detailed assessment.

## Cystometry

Cystometry involves the measurement of the pressure–volume relationship of the bladder. It is still considered the most fundamental investigation. It involves simultaneous abdominal pressure recording in addition to intravesical pressure monitoring during bladder filling and voiding. Electronic subtraction of abdominal from intravesical pressure enables determination of the detrusor pressure (Fig. 16.5).

Cystometry is indicated for the following.
- Previous unsuccessful continence surgery.
- Multiple symptoms, i.e. urge incontinence, stress incontinence and frequency.
- Voiding disorder.
- Neuropathic bladder.
- Prior to primary continence surgery: this is still debatable if stress incontinence is the only symptom.

Prior to cystometry, the patient voids on the flowmeter. A 12 French gauge catheter is inserted to fill the bladder and any residual urine is recorded. Intravesical pressure is measured using a 1 mm diameter fluid-filled catheter, inserted with the filling line, connected to an external pressure transducer.

A fluid-filled 2 mm diameter catheter covered with a rubber finger cot to prevent faecal blockage is inserted into the rectum to measure intra-abdominal pressure. Microtip transducers can be used but are more expensive and fragile. The bladder is filled (in sitting and standing positions) with a continuous infusion of normal saline at room temperature. The standard filling rate is between 10 and 100 mL/min and is provocative for detrusor instability. During filling, the patient is asked to indicate her first and maximal desire to void and these volumes are noted. The presence of symptoms of urgency and pain and systolic detrusor contractions are noted. Any precipitating factors such as coughing or running water are recorded. Pressure rises during filling or standing are also noted. At maximum capacity, the filling line is removed and the patient stands. She is asked to cough and any leakage is documented. The patient then transfers to the uroflowmeter and voids with pressure lines in place. Once urinary flow is established, she is asked to interrupt the flow if possible.

The following are parameters of normal bladder function.
- Residual urine of $<50$ mL.
- First desire to void between 150 and 200 mL.
- Capacity between 400 and 600 mL.
- Detrusor pressure rise of $<15$ cmH$_2$O during filling and standing.
- Absence of systolic detrusor contractions.
- No leakage on coughing.
- A voiding detrusor pressure rise of $<70$ cmH$_2$O with a peak flow rate of $>15$ mL/s for a volume $>150$ mL.

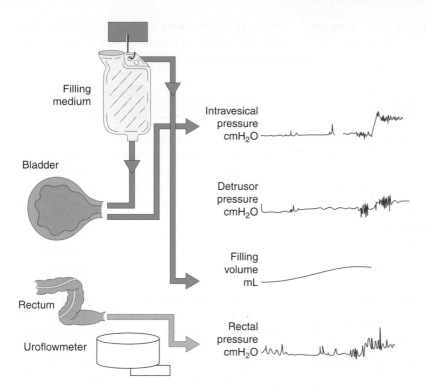

**Figure 16.5** Schematic representation of subtracted cystometry.

Filling medium

Bladder

Rectum

Uroflowmeter

Intravesical pressure cmH$_2$O

Detrusor pressure cmH$_2$O

Filling volume mL

Rectal pressure cmH$_2$O

Detrusor over-activity is diagnosed when spontaneous or provoked detrusor contractions occur which the patient cannot suppress. Systolic detrusor over-activity is shown by phasic contractions, whereas low compliance detrusor instability is diagnosed when the pressure rise during filling is >15 cmH$_2$O and does not settle when filling ceases. Urodynamic stress incontinence is diagnosed if leakage occurs as a result of coughing in the absence of a rise in detrusor pressure.

## Videocystourethrography

If a radio-opaque filling medium is used during cystometry, the lower urinary tract can be visualized by X-ray screening with an image intensifier. There are only a few situations in which videocystourethrography (VCU) provides more information than cystometry. During bladder filling, vesico-ureteric reflux can be seen. As the screening table is moving to the erect position, any detrusor contraction and leakage can be noted. In the erect position the patient is asked to cough; bladder neck and base descent and leakage of contrast can be evaluated. During voiding,

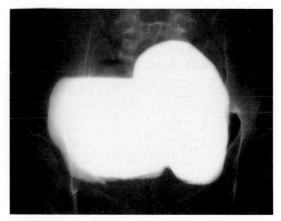

**Figure 16.6** Videocystourethrography showing bladder diverticulum.

vesico-ureteric reflux, trabeculation and bladder and urethral diverticulae can be noted (Fig. 16.6).

## Intravenous urography

This investigation provides little information about the lower urinary tract but is indicated in cases of haematuria, neuropathic bladder and suspected uretero-vaginal fistula.

## Ultrasound

Ultrasound is becoming more widely used in urogynaecology. Post-micturition urine residual estimation can be performed without the need for urethral catheterization and the associated risk of infection. This is useful in the investigation of patients with voiding difficulties, either idiopathic or following postoperative catheter removal. Urethral cysts and diverticula can also be examined using this technique.

## Magnetic resonance imaging

Magnetic resonance imaging (MRI) produces accurate anatomical pictures of the pelvic floor and lower urinary tract and has been used to demarcate compartmental prolapse. Although still mostly experimental, the use of endopelvic coils allows fine detail imaging, which may be useful in visualizing damage to the urethral sphincter mechanism.

## Cystourethroscopy

Cystourethroscopy establishes the presence of disease in the urethra or bladder. There are few indications in women with incontinence.
- Reduced bladder capacity.
- Short history (<2 years) of urgency and frequency.
- Suspected urethrovaginal or vesicovaginal fistula.
- Haematuria or abnormal cytology.
- Persistent urinary tract infection.

## Urethral pressure profilometry

To maintain continence, the urethral pressure must remain higher than the intravesical pressure, and various methods have been devised to measure urethral pressure. Urethral pressure profiles can be obtained using a catheter tip dual sensor microtransducer. Measurement of intraluminal pressure along the urethra at rest or under stress (e.g. coughing) appears to be of little clinical value because of a large overlap between controls and women with USI.

## Ambulatory monitoring

During ambulatory monitoring, fine microtip transducers are inserted into the bladder and rectum and data are recorded and stored in a portable device carried by the patient. The pressures are recorded for 4–6 hours with physiological bladder filling and emptying. The data are subsequently downloaded on to computer software and a chart recording is produced. It has become apparent that differences exist between values obtained for artificial and natural filling urodynamic systems in relation to pressure rise during filling and voiding. Ambulatory monitoring appears to be more sensitive than cystometry in the detection of detrusor over-activity.

## TREATMENT

Simple measures such as exclusion of urinary tract infection, restriction of fluid intake, modifying medication (e.g. diuretics) and treating chronic cough and constipation play an important role in the management of most types of urinary incontinence.

## Urodynamic stress incontinence

### Prevention

Shortening the second stage of delivery and reducing traumatic delivery may result in fewer women developing stress incontinence. The benefits of hormone replacement therapy have not been substantiated. The role of pelvic floor exercises either before or during pregnancy needs to be evaluated.

### Conservative management

Physiotherapy is the mainstay of the conservative treatment of stress incontinence. The rationale behind pelvic floor education is the reinforcement of cortical awareness of the levator ani muscle group, hypertrophy of existing muscle fibres and a general increase in muscle tone and strength.

With appropriate instruction and regular use, between 40 and 60 per cent of women can derive benefit from pelvic floor exercises to the point where they decline any further intervention.

Premenopausal women appear to respond better than their postmenopausal counterparts. Motivation and good compliance are the key factors associated with success. The use of biofeedback techniques, e.g. perineometry and weighted cones, can improve success rates. Maximal electrical stimulation is gaining popularity. A variety of devices have been used but have not been very successful.

## Surgery

For women seeking cure, the mainstay of treatment is surgery. The aims of surgery are:
- restoration of the proximal urethra and bladder neck to the zone of intra-abdominal pressure transmission,
- to increase urethral resistance,
- a combination of both.

The choice of operation depends on the clinical and urodynamic features of each patient, and the route of approach. The colposuspension operation (Fig. 16.7) is associated with the highest success rates in the hands of most surgeons. The success rate is over 95 per cent at 1 year, falling to 78 per cent at 15-year follow-up. However, for the elderly or frail patient with a scarred, narrowed vagina, a bladder neck bulking injection may be more appropriate because it is less invasive and is performed as an office or day-case procedure. Laparoscopic colposuspension may be performed, and in the best hands gives equivalent results to the open procedure but takes longer and does not appear to offer advantages in terms of postoperative recovery.

When the bladder neck is adequately elevated and aligned with the symphysis pubis, it is presumed that the incontinence is due to a defect in the sphincteric mechanism producing a low-resistance, poorly functioning, drainpipe urethra. The procedures to increase outflow resistance in these circumstances are the artificial urinary sphincter and peri-urethral injections, but suburethral slings are also used.

The artificial sphincter has been used since 1972. It is used where conventional surgery has failed and the patient is mentally alert and manually dexterous. It is a major procedure, performed only in tertiary referral centres because of the level of expertise required. Most of the procedures have been performed on patients with neuropathic bladders, but success rates for persistent female stress incontinence range from 66 to 85 per cent.

Peri-urethral bulking has attracted considerable interest because of the inherent simplicity of the

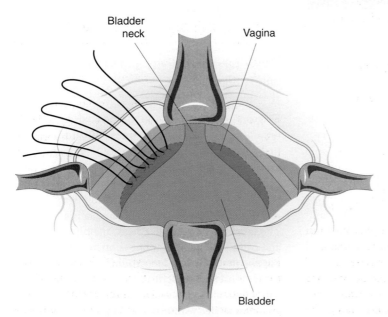

**Figure 16.7** Diagram showing colposuspension.

Bladder neck

Vagina

Bladder

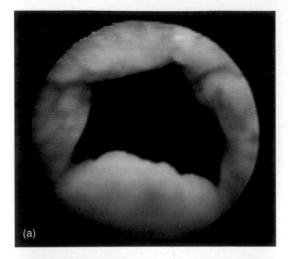

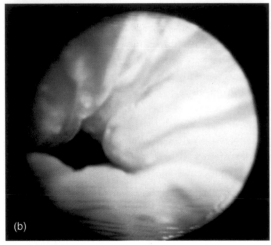

**Figure 16.8** The bladder neck (a) before and (b) after collagen injection.

Early success at 3-month follow-up ranges from 80 to 90 per cent, but there is a time-dependent decline to approximately 50 per cent at 3–4 years. Complications are uncommon and minor. Dysuria, urinary tract infection and retention requiring overnight catheterization are occasionally encountered. Newer bulking agents are also being utilized. When injectables fail, other bladder neck surgery can be performed without additional problems.

The move towards evidence-based medicine has shown colposuspension to be the most widely practised and most effective operation for stress incontinence. The anterior repair and end-stage bladder neck suspensions are not good operations in the medium or long-term for this condition. The most important point is that the primary operation provides the best chance of achieving success, as the success rate falls with subsequent attempts.

A new operation called a tension-free vaginal tape (TVT), which is based on the theory of suburethral support, has been developed. This involves insertion of a Prolene tape underneath the mid-urethra, through a very small vaginal incision with two tiny abdominal incisions. The novel aspect is that the tape is self-retaining and does not require fixation. Early and medium-term results are very encouraging and TVT is as effective as colposuspension at 2-year follow-up. There is a short operative time and the procedure can be performed under local anaesthetic and may be one of the major advances in surgery for stress incontinence of recent times.

## Detrusor over-activity and voiding difficulty

Detrusor over-activity can be treated by bladder retraining, biofeedback or hypnosis, all of which tend to increase the interval between voids and inhibit the symptoms of urgency. These methods are effective in between 60 and 70 per cent of individuals. Anticholinergic agents such as oxybutynin 2.5 mg twice daily or tolterodine 2 mg twice daily can be equally as effective. The latter has fewer side effects, mainly dry mouth and constipation. Imipramine is often used for enuresis and desmopressin (an antidiuretic hormone analogue) is useful for nocturia.

Neuropathic and non-neuropathic detrusor instability can be treated with anticholinergic drugs, and when

technique, its applicability in cases where other surgery has failed and its use in the frail patient. With increasing consumer demand, it is being used as a first-line surgical therapy for stress incontinence. Contigen collagen, subcutaneous fat, and microparticulate silicon (Macroplastique) have all been evaluated in the last decade. Subcutaneous fat, although cheap, has poor efficacy and therefore has lost popularity.

Contigen collagen is usually injected paraurethrally and Macroplastique transurethrally. Most surgeons inject collagen under local anaesthetic and Macroplastique under general anaesthetic. The principle is to inject the agents into the peri-urethral tissues at the level of the bladder neck, aiming for bladder neck coaptation (Fig. 16.8).

symptoms are resistant, intravesical therapy can be used.

At the end stage, bladder augmentation can be performed or even a ureterostomy. Bladder emptying can be achieved either by the use of clean intermittent self-catheterization or by an indwelling suprapubic or urethral catheter. Drug therapy to encourage and aid detrusor contraction or relax the urethral sphincter is relatively ineffective.

## New developments

There is increasing evidence that pre-pregnancy incontinence and pregnancy play a part in the aetiology of urinary stress incontinence, not just childbirth itself. There is a wide variety of suburethral tape operations now available and these are currently undergoing evaluation. The most novel of these uses the obturator fossae as an approach route to insert a tape.

There are several new pharmaceutical agents being evaluated for the treatment of urge incontinence, and a new drug for stress incontinence, duloxetine, will be launched soon.

### Key Points

- Urinary incontinence has a high prevalence, affecting approximately 20–30 per cent of the adult female population.
- The most common causes are USI and detrusor over-activity.
- The mainstays of treatment for USI are physiotherapy and surgery.
- The most appropriate treatment for detrusor over-activity includes bladder retraining and anticholinergic medication.
- Urinary tract infection must always be excluded, as it can cause most urinary symptoms.
- Women with voiding difficulty may present with similar symptoms to women with USI or detrusor over-activity.
- Subtracted cystometry is the most useful investigation for the management of the incontinent patient.
- Surgery for incontinence should be the patient's choice and must be tailored to clinical and urodynamic findings.

## CASE HISTORY

Mrs U is a 54-year-old married Caucasian weighing 95 kg. She is a non-smoker and works as a library administrator.

She presents with a long history of stress incontinence, since the birth of her first child, which has worsened recently. She also has urgency and urge incontinence, but these are not as severe as the stress incontinence. She has daytime frequency and nocturia but no history of voiding difficulty. She has had a previous total abdominal hysterectomy for menorrhagia.

Mrs U has four children; the first was a forceps delivery. The heaviest birth weight was 4 kg.

She is very fit and well but drinks a lot of coffee. She is sexually active.

Examination reveals a normal vaginal capacity and mobility, the bladder neck can be elevated and there is no sign of any major prolapse.

### Discussion

*What is the most likely diagnosis?*
This patient has mixed symptoms but probably has urodynamic stress incontinence. Urodynamics will help to elucidate the cause.

*What treatments can she be offered?*
Conservative measures would include weight loss and also reduction in caffeine intake. It would be beneficial to advise her about pelvic floor exercises first, before considering surgery. If surgery was to be considered, as the bladder neck can be elevated, the operation of choice might be a colposuspension or TVT. Anterior repair carries much lower success rates and therefore should not be considered.

## Additional reading

Stanton SL, Monga A (eds). *Clinical urogynaecology*. London: Harcourt Publishers, 2000.

# Uterovaginal prolapse

## OVERVIEW

Uterovaginal prolapse is extremely common, with an estimated 11 per cent of women undergoing at least one operation for this condition. Conservative management involves the use of pessaries, but surgery is the most appropriate option for the physically fit woman.

## Definition

A prolapse is a protrusion of an organ or structure beyond its normal confines (Fig. 17.1). Prolapses are classified according to their location and the organs contained within them.

### Classification

**Anterior vaginal wall prolapse**
- Urethrocele: urethral descent
- Cystocele: bladder descent
- Cystourethrocele: descent of bladder and urethra

**Posterior vaginal wall prolapse**
- Rectocele: rectal descent
- Enterocele: small bowel descent

**Apical vaginal prolapse**
- Uterovaginal: uterine descent with inversion of vaginal apex
- Vault: post-hysterectomy inversion of vaginal apex

## Prevalence

It is estimated that prolapse affects 12–30 per cent of multiparous and 2 per cent of nulliparous women. In the UK, approximately 30 000 prolapse operations are performed each year and in the USA the number is 400 000. A woman has an 11 per cent lifetime risk of having an operation for prolapse.

## Grading

Three degrees of prolapse are described and the lowest or most dependent portion of the prolapse is assessed whilst the patient is straining:
- 1st: descent within the vagina
- 2nd: descent to the introitus
- 3rd: descent outside the introitus.

In the case of uterovaginal prolapse, the most dependent portion of the prolapse is the cervix, and careful examination can differentiate uterovaginal

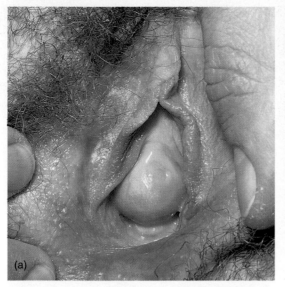 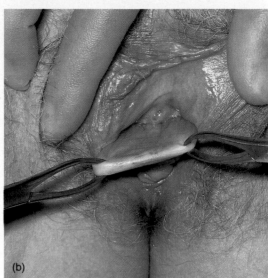

**Figure 17.1** (a) A cystourethocele. (b) A vaginal vault prolapse.

descent from a long cervix. Third-degree uterine prolapse is termed procidentia and is usually accompanied by cystourethrocele and rectocele.

## Aetiology

The connective tissue, levator ani and intact nerve supply are vital for the maintenance of position of the pelvic structures, and are influenced by pregnancy, childbirth and ageing. Whether congenital or acquired, connective tissue defects appear to be important in the aetiology of prolapse and urinary stress incontinence.

### Congenital

Two per cent of symptomatic prolapse occurs in nulliparous women, implying that there may be a congenital weakness of connective tissue. In addition genital prolapse is rare in Afro-Caribbean women, suggesting genetic differences exist.

### Childbirth and raised intra-abdominal pressure

The single major factor leading to the development of genital prolapse appears to be vaginal delivery.

Studies of the levator ani and fascia have shown evidence of nerve and mechanical damage in women with prolapse, compared to those without, occurring as a result of vaginal delivery.

Parity is associated with increasing prolapse. The World Health Organization (WHO) Population Report (1984) suggested that prolapse was up to seven times more common in women who had more than seven children compared to those who had one. Prolapse occurring during pregnancy is rare but is thought to be mediated by the effects of progesterone and relaxin. In addition, the increase in intra-abdominal pressure will put an added strain on the pelvic floor and a raised intra-abdominal pressure outside of pregnancy (e.g. chronic cough or constipation) is also a risk factor.

### Ageing

The process of ageing can result in loss of collagen and weakness of fascia and connective tissue. These effects are noted particularly during the post-menopause as a consequence of oestrogen deficiency.

### Postoperative

Poor attention to vaginal vault support at the time of hysterectomy leads to vault prolapse in approximately

**P** **Understanding the pathophysiology**

There are three components that are responsible for supporting the position of the uterus and vagina:
- ligaments and fascia, by suspension from the pelvic side walls,
- levator ani muscles, by constricting and thereby maintaining organ position,
- posterior angulation of the vagina, which is enhanced by rises in abdominal pressure causing closure of the 'flap valve'.

Damage to any of these mechanisms will contribute to prolapse.

Endopelvic fascia is derived from the paramesonephric ducts and is histologically distinct from the fascia investing the pelvic musculature, although attachments exist between the two. It is a continuous sheet that attaches laterally to the arcus tendineus fascia pelvis and levator ani muscles and extends from the symphysis pubis to the ischial spines. This network of tissue lies immediately beneath the peritoneum, surrounds the viscera and fills the space between the peritoneum above and the levators below; in parts it thickens to form ligaments, e.g. the uterosacral–cardinal complex. This complex is probably the most important component of the support. The segment of fascia that supports the bladder and lies between the bladder and vagina is known as pubocervical fascia, and that which prevents anterior rectal protrusion and lies between the rectum and posterior vagina is termed rectovaginal fascia.
(The levator muscles are described in Chapter 1.)

1 per cent of cases. Mechanical displacement as a result of gynaecological surgery such as colposuspension may lead to the development of a rectocele or enterocele.

## Clinical features

### History

Women usually present with non-specific symptoms. Specific symptoms may help to determine the type of prolapse. Aetiological factors should be enquired about.

Abdominal examination should be performed to exclude organomegaly or abdominopelvic mass.

**S** **Symptoms**

- **Non-specific**: lump, local discomfort, backache, bleeding/infection if ulcerated, dyspareunia or apareunia. Rarely, in extremely severe cystourethrocele, uterovaginal or vault prolapse, renal failure may occur as a result of ureteric kinking.
- **Specific**: cystourethrocele – urinary frequency and urgency, voiding difficulty, urinary tract infection, stress incontinence.
- **Rectocele**: incomplete bowel emptying, digitation, splinting.

## Vaginal examination

Prolapse may be obvious when examining the patient in the dorsal position if it protrudes beyond the introitus; ulceration and/or atrophy may be apparent.

Vaginal pelvic examination should be performed and pelvic mass excluded.

The anterior and posterior vaginal walls and cervical descent should be assessed with the patient straining in the left lateral position, using a Sims' speculum. Combined rectal and vaginal digital examination can be an aid to differentiate rectocele from enterocele (Fig. 17.2).

## Differential diagnosis

- Anterior wall prolapse: congenital or inclusion dermoid vaginal cyst, urethral diverticulum.
- Uterovaginal prolapse: large uterine polyp.

## Investigations

There are no essential investigations. If urinary symptoms are present, urine microscopy, cystometry and cystoscopy should be considered. The relationship between urinary symptoms and prolapse is complex. Some women with cystourethrocele have concurrent incontinence; as the prolapse increases in severity, urethral kinking may restore continence but lead to voiding difficulty (see Chapter 16). Should renal failure be suspected, serum urea and creatinine should be evaluated and renal ultrasound performed.

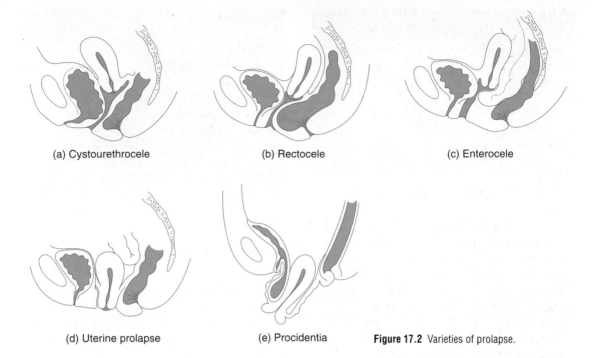

(a) Cystourethrocele     (b) Rectocele     (c) Enterocele

(d) Uterine prolapse     (e) Procidentia     **Figure 17.2** Varieties of prolapse.

## Treatment

The choice of treatment depends on the patient's wishes, level of fitness and desire to preserve coital function.

Prior to specific treatment, attempts should be made to correct obesity, chronic cough or constipation. If the prolapse is ulcerated, a 7-day course of topical oestrogen should be administered.

### Prevention

Shortening the second stage of delivery and reducing traumatic delivery may result in fewer women developing a prolapse. The benefits of episiotomy and hormone replacement therapy at the menopause have not been substantiated.

### Medical

Silicon-rubber-based ring pessaries are the most popular form of conservative therapy. They are inserted into the vagina in much the same way as a contraceptive diaphragm and need replacement at annual intervals (Fig. 17.3). Shelf pessaries are rarely used but may be useful in women who cannot retain a ring pessary (Fig. 17.4). The use of pessaries can be complicated by vaginal ulceration and infection. The vagina should therefore be carefully inspected at the time of replacement.

### Indications for pessary treatment

- Patient's wish
- As a therapeutic test
- Childbearing not complete
- Medically unfit
- During and after pregnancy (awaiting involution)
- While awaiting surgery

### Surgery

The aim of surgical repair is to restore anatomy and function. There are vaginal and abdominal operations designed to correct prolapse, and choice often depends on a woman's desire to preserve coital function (Fig. 17.5).

#### Cystourethrocele

Anterior repair (colporrhaphy) is the most commonly performed surgical procedure but should be avoided if there is concurrent stress incontinence.

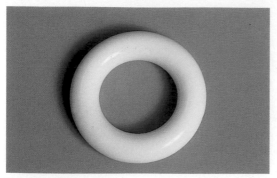

**Figure 17.3** Ring pessary.

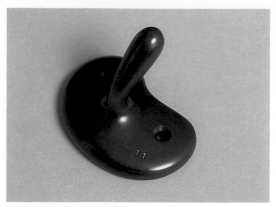

**Figure 17.4** Shelf pessary.

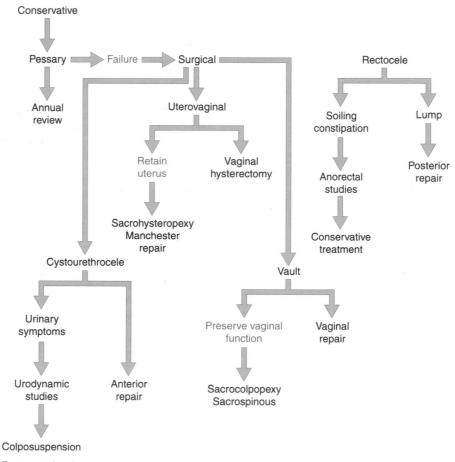

**Figure 17.5** Treatment of prolapse.

An anterior vaginal wall incision is made and the fascial defect allowing the bladder to herniate through is identified and closed. With the bladder position restored, any redundant vaginal epithelium is excised and the incision closed.

## Rectocele

Posterior repair (colporrhaphy) is the most commonly performed procedure. A posterior vaginal wall incision is made and the fascial defect allowing the rectum to herniate through is identified and closed.

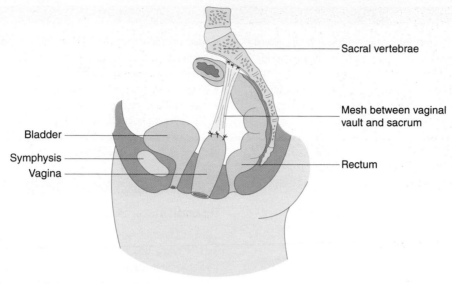

**Figure 17.6** Sacrocolpopexy.

Labels: Sacral vertebrae; Mesh between vaginal vault and sacrum; Bladder; Symphysis; Vagina; Rectum

With the rectal position restored, any redundant vaginal epithelium is excised and the incision closed.

### Enterocele

The surgical principles are similar to those of anterior and posterior repair but the peritoneal sac containing the small bowel should be excised. In addition, the pouch of Douglas is closed by approximating the peritoneum and/or the uterosacral ligaments.

### Uterovaginal prolapse

If the woman does not wish to conserve her uterus for fertility or other reasons, a vaginal hysterectomy with adequate support of the vault to the uterosacral ligaments is sufficient. If uterine conservation is required, the Manchester operation and sacrohysteropexy are alternatives.

The Manchester operation involves partial amputation of the cervix and approximation of the cardinal ligaments below the retained cervix remnant. (It is usually combined with anterior and posterior repair.) Sacrohysteropexy is an abdominal procedure and involves attachment of a synthetic mesh from the uterocervical junction to the anterior longitudinal ligament of the sacrum. The pouch of Douglas is closed.

### Vault prolapse

Sacrocolpopexy (Fig. 17.6) is similar to sacrohysteropexy but the inverted vaginal vault is attached to the sacrum using a mesh and the pouch of Douglas is closed. Sacrospinous ligament fixation is a vaginal procedure in which the vault is sutured to one or other sacrospinous ligament.

## New developments

Collagen metabolism in vaginal skin from premenopausal women with and without uterovaginal prolapse has been compared. There was a significant reduction in total collagen and an increase in immature cross-linking in women with prolapse compared to controls. Activity of matrix metalloproteinases (enzymes that break down collagen) was elevated. This suggests that the primary problem in genitourinary prolapse is increased collagen degradation causing a decrease in the mechanical strength of supporting fascia.

A variety of operations is described for the correction of prolapse; most of them use either fascial or muscle plication or attachment to ligaments to support the vagina in its presumed original position. The recognition of specific fascial defects at three different levels of vaginal support resulting in different combinations of incontinence and prolapse has prompted the development of surgical techniques aiming to repair these site-specific defects. These repairs can be performed under local anaesthesia.

To reduce the recurrence rates after surgery for prolapse, the use of reinforcement utilizing a variety of synthetic and organic meshes is being evaluated.

## Key Points

- A prolapse is a protrusion of an organ or structure beyond its normal confines; prolapses are extremely common in multiparous women.
- Damage to the major supports of the vagina, i.e. ligaments, fascia and levator ani muscles, leads to prolapse.
- Childbirth injury is the major aetiological factor.

- Most women with prolapse present with non-specific symptoms such as a lump and backache.
- Women with cystourethrocele often have urinary symptoms.
- Women with rectocele often have bowel symptoms.
- Diagnosis is made by clinical examination.
- Surgery is the mainstay of treatment.

## CASE HISTORY

Mrs PS is a 48-year-old married, sexually active Caucasian, weighing 89 kg. She is a non-smoker and works as a nursing assistant in a nursing home. She suffers from asthma and uses salbutamol and Becloforte inhalers.

She presents with an 8-month history of 'feeling a lump down below' and backache. The lump is bigger when she has been on her feet all day. She also complains of poor urinary stream and a feeling of incomplete emptying of her bladder. She admits to no urinary incontinence or bowel symptoms. She had a total abdominal hysterectomy 3 years previously for menorrhagia.

Mrs PS has two children, aged 22 and 24 years. Both were delivered vaginally; the heaviest at birth weighed 3.8 kg.

### Discussion

*What is the most likely diagnosis?*
Anterior vaginal wall prolapse is the most likely diagnosis in view of her urinary symptoms. However, vault prolapse and rectocele can also cause obstructive urinary symptoms.

*What risk factors does she have for the development of prolapse?*
- Vaginal delivery of a large infant can cause damage to pelvic nerves, endopelvic fascia and levator ani, which can result in prolapse.
- She is overweight and this will increase the effect of abdominal pressure on the pelvic floor.
- She has a chronic cough and her job involves heavy lifting. Both these factors increase abdominal pressure.

## Additional reading

Jackson SR, Avery NC, Tariton JF, Eckford SD, Abrams P, Bailey A. Changes in metabolism of collagen in genitourinary prolapse. *Lancet* 1995; **347**: 1658–61.

Mallett VT, Bump RC. The epidemiology of female pelvic floor dysfunction. *Curr Opin Obstet Gynaecol* 1994; **6**: 308–12.

# Menopause

## OVERVIEW

The term menopause is often misapplied and it is therefore worthwhile to define its origin and precise meaning. A derivation of the ancient Greek words *menos* (month) and *pausos* (ending), the term means the end of the monthly or menstrual cycle, the central external marker of human female fertility. A natural menopause, therefore, is deemed to have occurred after 6 months of secondary amenorrhoea in a woman aged 45 years or over. The central event leading to the menopause is the obligatory mid-life ovarian failure, which results from exhaustion of available oocytes.

## Introduction

The menopause takes place at a modal age of 51 years in developed countries – and therein lies the central demographic problem, for life expectancy in the UK is now at a modal age of 81 years for women. Thus, a woman at menopause today can expect to live for some 30 years, or 40 per cent of her life, in a state of relatively profound oestrogen deficiency (Fig. 18.1).

The considerable concentration of births in the late 1940s and early 1950s – popularly known as the baby boom – has resulted in some 40 per cent of the female population of the UK now being perimenopausal or postmenopausal. Hence, any symptomatic or metabolic disturbance consequent on menopause that requires medical investigation will impose a significant effect upon the public health and a significant call upon the public purse in the form of National Health Service (NHS) resources.

The menopause, as defined above, is simply one event in the whole range of anatomical, physiological and psychological events that contribute to the climacteric, a term also worthy of definition. Derived from the Greek *klimakter* (rung of a ladder), the climacteric

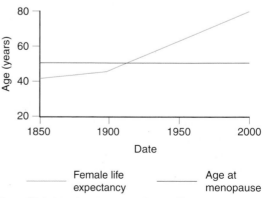

**Figure 18.1** Age of menopause and mean life expectancy in women in the UK since 1850.

was so termed to describe a major movement on life's ladder. It is the global expression for what the general public succinctly calls 'the change'. This is the transition from fertility to infertility, and occupies that decade, from 45–55 years, when a woman passes from her reproductive into her post-reproductive years. It is attended by a wide variety of symptoms, signs and metabolic adjustments, the ultimate cause of which is a major reduction in the level of circulating oestrogen.

## Pathophysiology

### Premature ovarian failure

Secondary amenorrhoea – due to a failure of the ovaries to generate sufficient oestrogen – may occur at any age and, if below the age of 45 years, is described as premature. Such patients exhibit low plasma oestradiol (E2) (usually <150 pmol/L), high levels of follicle-stimulating hormone (FSH) and luteinizing hormone (LH) and a symptom pattern suggestive of oestrogen deficiency. The term resistant ovary syndrome describes a group of such women in whom the biological appearances of the ovary are normal, with abundant primordial follicles. In premature ovarian failure (POF), by contrast, the appearances are those of a postmenopausal ovary. POF may be associated with other autoimmune endocrinopathies and in about half of patients other autoantibodies are present. However, the precise site of action of an antibody attack on the hypothalamo–pituitary–ovarian axis is unknown.

### Surgical menopause

Obviously, if for any reason both ovaries need to be surgically removed, an obligatory menopause is immediate. Following hysterectomy in premenopausal patients, even if both ovaries are conserved, a POF may supervene. Studies have indicated that the median age of menopause in such cases is 47–48 years, in contrast to the expected age of 51 years. No prediction can be given at the time of operation as to which patients may or may not be affected. Such a menopause is, of course, occult due to the postoperative amenorrhoea and therefore must be diagnosed on symptomatic and endocrine grounds.

A considerable debate still continues as to whether in women over the age of 45 oophorectomy should accompany hysterectomy. The principal argument for oophorectomy is the absolute prevention of subsequent ovarian cancer, and the principal argument for conservation is the retention of the steroid output from developing follicles until natural menopause, and from the ovarian stroma thereafter.

**P  Understanding the pathophysiology**

The human ovary basically consists of an outer cortex containing follicles at various stages of development, and a central medulla, which is heavily vascularized. Both cortex and medulla contain stroma of mesenchymal origin, which, in addition to their supportive function, are actively involved in steroid synthesis, principally of androgens. Stromal cells are recruited to form the thecal cells, which surround the follicles.

The primordial follicles number some 1.5 million at birth, the number having sharply declined from a peak of 7 million midway through gestation (Fig. 18.2). The vast majority of these primordial follicles become atretic (non-functional) and, in the reproductive lifetime of a healthy woman, only some 400 of the 400 000 follicles present at puberty will progress to ovulation. It is important to realize that it is the cells of the developing follicle that produce the bulk of the E2 circulating in the plasma of a premenopausal woman, the median level of which is usually between 400 and 500 pmol/L. Synthesis is principally from androstenedione and testosterone to E2 in the granulosa cells, which form the internal lining of

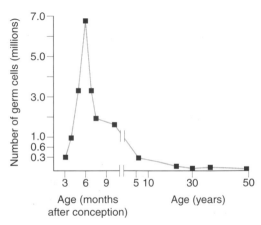

**Figure 18.2** Total number of oocytes in the human ovary at different ages.

the follicle. The androgen to oestrogen conversion is catalysed by the aromatase enzyme cascade and is promoted by FSH. Theca cells also produce E2 from androgens whose elaboration from cholesterol is stimulated by LH.

The first sign of approaching menopause is a decline in fertility, in which a downturn is apparent after the commencement of the fourth decade in most studies. The first endocrine change is a fall in inhibin production by the ovary. This glycoprotein inhibits the production of FSH by the anterior pituitary and hence, with this loss of restraint, the plasma FSH concentration begins to rise above the premenopausal upper limit of $<5\,IU/L$. The rise in LH values above the premenopausal limit of $12\,IU/L$ is of later onset. Plasma values of both gonadotrophins remain elevated into old age. It is important to state that a significant amount of the postmenopausal androgen production is stimulated, in the ovarian stroma, by FSH and LH, whereas the principal site of oestrogen production – by androstenedione conversion to oestrone – is in adipose tissue.

The cessation of cyclic bleeding takes many forms. The menstrual cycle may stop abruptly or may cease after a prolonged stage of oligomenorrhoea. Even after a substantial period of amenorrhoea, a further cycle may occur which, if more than 6 months from the last, will be correctly classed as postmenopausal bleeding and will therefore require investigation.

## Other causes of menopause

Suppression of ovarian steroid output is physiologial during lactation, when the recurrent surges of prolactin, released by suckling, inhibit the gonadotrophin drive to the ovaries and, possibly, intra-ovarian steroidogenesis. Therapeutically, the use of gonadotrophin-releasing hormone agonists (GnRH analogues) in the treatment of endometriosis or in the preoperative containment of leiomyomata (fibroids) results in virtually complete suppression of ovarian steroid output. Such treatment, if given continuously for more than 6 months, may result in major metabolic consequences such as significant loss of skeletal tissue.

The management of malignant disease in young women may provoke menopause in two ways. In premenopausal women with breast cancer radiation, menopause may still be used to suppress oestrogen output, although this management may be superseded by pure oestrogen antagonists, such as aromatase inhibitors, in future. The use of chemotherapeutic agents in conditions such as breast cancer or lymphoma may suppress and indeed arrest ovarian cyclic activity. Patients entering the management of such conditions should have the implications for their fertility and ovarian hormonal output fully discussed.

## Symptoms of menopause

It is important to realize that the symptoms of oestrogen deficiency, loosely termed menopausal symptoms, may begin long before the actual cessation of menstruation, which, as noted above, defines the menopause itself. These symptoms are often triggered by a relative fall in circulating E2 and hence may afflict the patient before the absolute level of circulating E2 reaches the levels of the fully developed post-menopause at $<100\,pmol/L$. The physical symptoms of menopause include the classical vasomotor symptoms of hot flushing and night sweats. These are common and occur in at least 70 per cent of peri-menopausal women. Their frequency varies widely from a few to several dozen per day, and the duration may be from a few weeks to many years. Hot flushes are not contemporaneous with LH pulses and are essentially a vascular response to a central disturbance of the thermoregulatory centre in the hypothalamus. There is a downshift of the set-point of this centre such that there is a frequent central misapprehension that body temperature is too high. This in turn leads to activation of the physiological mechanisms such as cutaneous flushing and perspiration, which result in heat loss by radiation and by the loss of the latent heat of vaporization. If the episode occurs at night, the patient, in addition to the vasomotor discomfort, may experience repeated awakening from sleep with consequent loss of sleep quantity and quality. In turn, this chronic incursion into the deep sleep/rapid eye movement (REM) sleep/deep sleep rhythm may promote certain pyschological symptoms, such as irritability and short-term memory impairment, of which menopausal women frequently complain.

## S Symptoms

**Physical**
- Tiredness
- Hot flushes
- Night sweats
- Insomnia
- Vaginal dryness
- Urinary frequency

**Psychological**
- Mood swings
- Anxiety
- Loss of short-term memory
- Lack of concentration
- Loss of self-confidence
- Depression

Vaginal dryness is a vitally important symptom of menopause, not least because it is frequently missed. Some patients find it difficult to give a sexual history and thus a gentle, courteous but full enquiry should be made regarding the presence of dryness and associated dyspareunia. The latter can lead to significant disharmony between partners in a relationship. The vaginal skin is dependent on oestrogen for the depth and lubrication of its squamous epithelium and, with loss of plasma oestrogen, the skin becomes thin and poorly moisturized.

The physical symptoms of menopause are partnered by a set of psychological symptoms that can be equally distressing and disabling. The degree to which these symptoms are due to a lack of oestrogen per se or to chronic sleep deprivation is not clear. In addition, the perimenopausal years are often marked by life events such as divorce, departure of children, death of partner or parents and other stressful occurrences that may contribute to the overall psychological picture. Intrinsic personality type may also exert an influence, with the symptoms being more marked among those with a tendency to anxiety and low self-esteem. There does not, however, appear to be a true increase in formal psychiatric disorders at this time.

Overall, it should be stressed that the severity, duration and nature of menopausal symptoms are highly variable. Symptoms may be absent, they may be fleeting and mild, or they may be severe and continue for years. The duty of the clinician is to assess the global effect of the symptom complex presented and to decide whether or not an exogenous replacement of the lost oestrogen is likely to result in a significant reduction in the symptom load.

## Urinary symptoms

Menopausal women often complain of frequency, dysuria and urgency, symptoms which suggest urinary tract infection (UTI) but which are not associated with a positive urine culture. The presence of oestrogen receptors in the trigone and proximal urethra may explain certain symptoms, which should only be assigned to menopause if other causes have been excluded. Similarly, stress incontinence is also a common symptom at this time and, in the absence of interovaginal prolapse, may be attributed to oestrogen deficiency. However, direct experimental evidence of a true relationship is absent.

## Skeletal system

The skeleton consists of 203 bones but of only two types of bone. Some 80 per cent of the skeleton is compact bone, which is found, for example, in the shafts of the long bones. It is relatively insensitive to oestrogen. The remaining 20 per cent of bone is, in contrast, highly oestrogen sensitive and is named after its trabecular structure. It is found at such sites as the vertebrae, the distal radius, the femoral neck and the calcaneus. The relationship between oestrogens and trabecular bone is complex and intimate.

In summary, oestrogen acts as a physiological restraint on bone turnover and to hold the balance between bone resorption and bone formation. Over a 4-month period, each of the half million or so bone turnover sites in the skeleton moves through the unvarying sequence of bone removal and then bone replacement (Fig. 18.3). It is obvious that these processes should be balanced or be coupled to preserve bone mass.

However, with the loss of circulating oestrogen after menopause, a decoupling takes place that is characterized by a greater bone resorption than formation against the background of a general increase in the activation of new bone turnover sites on bone surfaces. Trabecular bone, with its high surface area, is thus particularly at risk. Trabecular bone is shock-absorbing

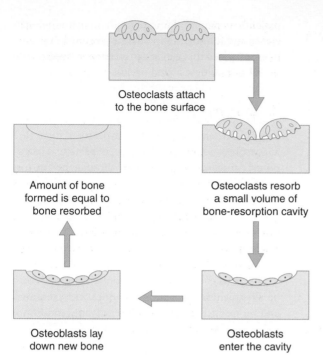

Osteoclasts attach
to the bone surface

Amount of bone
formed is equal to
bone resorbed

Osteoclasts resorb
a small volume of
bone-resorption cavity

Osteoblasts lay
down new bone

Osteoblasts
enter the cavity

**Figure 18.3** The bone remodelling cycle shown clockwise from top. Some 0.5 million sites are operational simultaneously and each cycle takes approximately 5 months to complete.

bone. Its central function is to absorb, dissipate and dispense incident kinetic energy. This it accomplishes by means of the vast network of interconnecting trabeculae or struts that comprise its internal architecture. Hence, when this network is degraded by the progressive loss of trabecular number, thickness and interconnection (Fig. 18.4), the bone becomes more liable to fracture after minimal or moderate trauma. The net result is that after menopause there is a progressive rise in the incidence of fracture of the trabecular sites. Traumatic fracture affects the distal radius and femoral neck, whereas non-traumatic fracture affects the vertebrae (Fig. 18.5).

## Cardiovascular system

The function of the heart and great vessels is now known to be affected by the presence and by the relative absence of E2. It has been known for many years that the incidence of such clinical events as myocardial infarction is much lower in premenopausal women than in men of the same age, but a precise elucidation of the protective role of oestrogen has been slow to emerge. The decline in plasma oestrogen is attended by changes in the lipid profile that are conducive to atherogenesis.

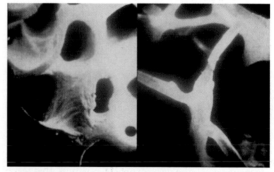

**Figure 18.4** Normal bone is shown on the left. Osteoporotic bone is shown on the right. Note the reduction in trabecular number, breadth and connectivity.

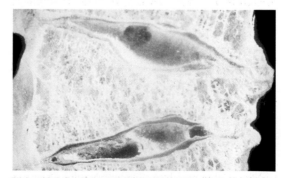

**Figure 18.5** Sagittal section of human osteoporotic thoracic vertebrae. Note the wedging effect due to collapse of the trabecular structure anteriorly.

- Total cholesterol: ↑
- High-density lipoprotein (HDL) cholesterol: ↓
- Low-density lipoprotein (LDL) cholesterol: ↑
- Triglycerides: ↔

In addition to the lipid effects, oestrogen is now known to exert direct effects on the vessel wall. Oestradiol is known to stimulate the enzyme nitrogen synthase, whose product, nitric oxide, is both a vasodilator and an oxidant for lipoprotein accumulating in the subintima. Loss of oestrogen can thus result in a promotion of both atherogenesis and vasoconstriction.

Initially, observational results from cohort and case-control studies indicated a major reduction in cardiovascular system disease among treated women. However, recently published data from more rigorous randomized controlled trials have shown no benefit and found an early excess of events such as myocardial infarction and stroke. Hormone replacement therapy (HRT) is not indicated for the treatment or prevention of cardiovascular system disease.

## Hormone replacement therapy

Strong and opposing views on HRT are held by professional and lay groups, extending from the view that the menopause is natural and physiological, and thus requires no intervention, to the view that it is a true hormonal deficiency state and thus should be treated with replacement therapy for life. Between these views is the compromise position that each patient should be examined and counselled on the individual nature of her problems, with HRT being offered when the presence of symptoms or effects of oestrogen deficiency are such as to interfere with her personal, marital or occupational welfare. What is vital is that the woman herself has the final say in whether or not she will initiate and continue with such therapy.

### Consultation

A full history is taken, with concentration on those symptoms that are, or are likely to be, due to oestrogen deficiency – as listed above. Not only the presence of these symptoms but also their impact upon the patient's personal, domestic and occupational efficiency and fulfilment should be ascertained. It should be emphasized that gentle and courteous enquiry into sexual difficulties, including loss of libido and dyspareunia, should be made. In view of the longer-term effects of oestrogen deficiency, the family history should include any history of cardiovascular disease, particularly angina pectoris, myocardial infarction and stroke, and of skeletal disease, in particular osteoporosis manifested in relatives through height loss and low-trauma fracture to wrist, hip and other sites. The presence of Alzheimer's disease or other neurogenerative disease in the family is of relevance. The history of any gastrointestinal or liver disease that might interfere with the normal pharmacodynamics of oestrogen therapy must also be sought.

The gynaecological history should include a record of all previous medical and surgical interventions, and in particular the presence of any conditions influenced by ambient plasma oestrogen, such as leiomyomata or endometriosis. A history of benign or malignant breast disease must be sought. Histological reports on any breast biopsy material should be scrutinized to determine whether or not cellular atypia was present, as this may affect future management. The patient's mammographic record should be ascertained and she should be encouraged to accept all triennial recalls from age 50 to 64 in the National Breast Screening Campaign. Any heavy, or persistently irregular, bleeding should be further investigated by pelvic ultrasonic examination, proceeding, if required, to hysteroscopy and endometrial biopsy.

### Examination

Any patient who is being considered for HRT must have a physical examination by a qualified practitioner. This is principally to identify the presence of potentially oestrogen-sensitive tumours in breast or pelvis. Thus, the patient should have a breast examination not as a routine, but if it is indicated from the foregoing history. She should also be advised, if necessary, on the techniques of breast awareness and self-examination. A pelvic examination should be performed – again, not routinely, but when clinically indicated – and a record made of any abnormality, particularly uterine enlargement, the presence of fibroids and any signs suggestive of past or present endometriosis. Adnexal palpation to seek any ovarian turnover completes the examination. The blood pressure should be checked in the semi-recumbent position.

## Modes of treatment

Oestrogen and the progestogens may be delivered by many routes. Most common in the UK is the oral route, where the oestrogen is absorbed from the stomach and duodenum and is therefore passed up the portal system and through the liver en route to its other target sites. Oestradiol is largely converted in the liver parenchyma into oestrone, which is then released via the hepatic veins. This results in an E2:oestrone ratio of 1:2, which is the reverse of the normal premenopausal position. Oral oestrogen can be taken at any time of the day. It is cheap and convenient and is usually well tolerated.

The oral route does, however, result in the activation by oestrogen of certain hepatic enzymes, resulting in the synthesis and release of such proteins as thyroid-binding globulin, resin substrate and sex hormone-binding globulin. Patients taking thyroxine, for example, should have their dosage reviewed after starting oral HRT in case adjustment is required. No pronounced effects upon hepatic production of the proteins of the coagulation cascade have been observed. Nevertheless, some effect on this system is likely, since there has been a recently confirmed increase in the risk of venous thromboembolism (VTE), from approximately 1.5 to approximately 3.5 per 10 000 per year. Formerly, oral oestrogen was given for 3 weeks out of 4, as in the combined oral contraceptive pill, but the modern practice is to give oestrogen daily, thus mimicking the premenopausal daily release of hormone by the ovary. The oral oestrogens in common use are:

- oestradiol valerate 1 mg or 2 mg
- conjugated equine oestrogen 0.625 mg or 1.25 mg
- oestrone 1.25 mg.

### Transdermal oestrogen

The advent of transdermal oestrogen, first by reservoir and now by matrix patches, is a further attempt to mimic the physiology of the premenopause. The oestrogen, which, being lipid soluble, may transit across the epidermis, passes directly into the systemic circulation, thus avoiding the hepatic first pass which is an obligatory feature with the oral route. This maintains the E2:oestrone ratio of 2:1 and is thus highly physiological. The reservoir patch in which the oestrogen is linked to an alcohol carrier may cause skin irritation and is being superseded by the matrix patch, in which the E2 is incorporated into an adhesive matrix lined by a backing membrane. Skin reactions are few and absorption is steady, with therapeutic plasma levels of E2 being achieved within 4 hours. Patches are available in varying strengths, usually delivering 28, 50, 75 or 100 μg of E2 per day, and can be tailored to the individual patient's needs. Seven-day patches are now also available.

Transdermal HRT is of particular use in the older patient with, for example, osteoporosis in whom a very gradual build-up of oestrogen is required in order to avoid adverse start-up effects. Thus, the patient can be given a 25 μg patch for 3 months before advancing, if required, to the 50 μg therapeutic level. In general terms, the 50 μg patch has been found to have effects equivalent to 0.625 mg of conjugated equine oestrogen and 2 mg of oral E2.

A variant of the transdermal patch is the percutaneous gel. In this mode of HRT delivery, E2 is spread onto a convenient surface such as an upper arm, the metered dose from the container being some 2.5 g. Absorption produces therapeutic plasma levels within 4 days of commencement and the treatment is well tolerated.

### Subcutaneous implantation

This mode of delivery is restricted in the UK to patients who have undergone hysterectomy with or without oophorectomy. The procedure involves the positioning of a pellet of E2 in the subcutaneous tissue, usually of the lower abdomen, under sterile conditions and local anaesthetic. Implants are available at 25, 50 and 100 mg strengths and are usually reviewed at intervals of 6 months. They are very well tolerated and, of course, they obviate the need for daily or weekly action by the patient. Reports of tachyphylaxis have appeared in which patients are described as requesting re-implantation at progressively shorter intervals. In practice, however, this is rare, but nevertheless re-implantation should be preceded by an annual check on plasma E2, which should not be allowed to rise above 1000 pmol/L.

This mode of treatment successfully treats menopausal symptoms and also protects against bone loss. Indeed, there is now evidence that long-term E2 implantation may be associated with a significant gain in bone mass at hip and spine.

**Table 18.1** Progestogens used in conjunction with oestrogen (minimum treatment 12 days/month)

| Progestogen | Daily dose (mg) |
|---|---|
| **C-21 group** | |
| Micronized progesterone | 200 |
| Medroxyprogesterone acetate | 10 |
| Dydrogesterone | 10 |
| **C-19-*nor* group** | |
| Norethisterone | 1 |
| Norgesterel | 0.15 |

## Progestogens

In the premenopausal state, progesterone from the corpus luteum transforms the oestrogen-primed endometrium, which then sheds when progesterone production fails. In the 1970s, early attempts to give oestrogen alone resulted in a significant degree of endometrial hyperplasia and neoplasia, and it was realized that, again, the physiology of the premenopause would have to be mimicked. To this end, studies showed that the administration of a progestogen for 12 days per month resulted in the secretory transformation of the endometrium and in satisfactory shedding (Table 18.1).

Unfortunately, the use of progestogens, particularly those of the 19-*nor* group which are derived from testosterone, may cause adverse effects which may be of sufficient severity for the patient to give up treatment. These adverse effects include bloating, mastalgia and a premenstrual syndrome (PMS)-like syndrome involving irritability and mood swings. When one considers that these are the very symptoms for which HRT is often prescribed in the first place, the necessary use of progestogen in women with a uterus is seen to be a major potential problem.

In one method of avoiding cyclic progestational effects, the progestogen is given daily combined with the oestrogen in oral or transdermal therapy. This continuous combined approach has the effect of suppressing oestrogen receptor production in the endometrium, thus preventing proliferation and rendering the patient free of the cyclic bleeding which many find unacceptable. Some 80 per cent of 50-year-old women in the UK retain their uterus and should receive continuous or cyclic progestogen if being treated with HRT. Progestogen is not necessary in hysterectomized patients.

The progestogens commonly used for 12 days per month include a C-21 group derived from native progesterone and a C-19-*nor* group derived from testosterone.

## Tibolone

This is a synthetic steroid that exhibits oestrogenic, progestogenic and androgenic activity. Given in a dose of 2.5 mg per day to women at least 1 year after menopause, it results in suppression of symptoms and the prevention of bone loss. Mild androgenic side effects may occur, but in general the preparation is well tolerated and the amenorrhoea that is present in 80 per cent of patients by 6 months is usually warmly welcomed. Some patients report a significant increase in libido with tibolone.

# Contraindications to HRT

## Contraindications to HRT

**Absolute**
- Present or suspected pregnancy
- Suspicion of breast cancer
- Suspicion of endometrial cancer
- Acute active liver disease
- Uncontrolled hypertension
- Confirmed VTE

**Relative**
- Presence of uterine fibromyomata
- Past history of benign breast disease
- Unconfirmed VTE
- Chronic stable liver disease
- Migraine

The presence of any of the conditions listed in the box in a patient being considered for HRT should result in a specialist referral so that further investigations can refine the balance between indication and contraindication. For example, the presence of benign breast fibrocytic disease but without atypia may allow treatment to proceed. Similarly, the presence of a normal thrombophilic screen in a patient with a history of unconfirmed deep venous thrombosis (DVT) may allow oestrogen to be given.

## Management of the patient receiving HRT

The first essential in management is the preparation of the patient for those symptoms that mark the re-introduction of oestrogen and progestogen into the circulation. The longer the elapsed time since menopause, the more likely these symptoms are to arise. Forewarned is forearmed and, equipped with the knowledge that the start-up symptoms are likely to be temporary and to remit by 3 months, the patient is more likely to persevere over the first 12 critical weeks.

The similarity with certain symptoms of early pregnancy is striking and useful. Parous women will remember these symptoms and the fact that they tend to remit at about 12–14 weeks' gestation. If a patient is not so forewarned, the occurrence of, say, breast tenderness will distress and alarm her and she will be minded to stop treatment.

---

**S Symptoms**

The start-up symptoms of HRT include:
- breast tenderness
- nipple sensitivity
- appetite rise
- weight gain
- calf cramps.

---

Thus the time for the first critical review is at 3 months. At this stage, enquiry should be made about the resolution of menopausal symptoms and of start-up effects. At 3 months, the incidence of vasomotor symptoms reaches baseline and hence a critical review prior to this time may falsely indicate that treatment is failing. If no untoward effects are encountered, the patient may be reviewed 6 months later and thereafter annually.

### Annual review
There is no general agreement as to the constitution of an annual review.

### Breast
The patient's participation in the national campaign should be verified. If the patient is breast aware, performing self-examination regularly, and in the mammographic programme, a full clinical breast examination is probably not necessary. If, however, there is any doubt about her breast awareness, and if she complains of breast pain or swelling, an examination should be performed. Recent results from cohort studies, such as the Million Women study in the UK, indicate that long-term use of oestrogen alone and of oestrogen plus progestogen is associated with a small but measurable increase in the risk of breast cancer.

### Blood pressure
This should be checked at least annually.

### Pelvic examination
If the patient is amenorrhoeic on a continuous combined oestrogen/progestogen or tibolone treatment or if she is bleeding on time and with normal flow on a cyclic regimen, routine pelvic examination is unlikely to disclose an abnormality. However, unscheduled bleeding, especially if it is heavy, prolonged or recurrent, should always trigger a specialist consultation with a view to hysteroscopy and biopsy if indicated. Further information may be obtained from ultrasonic evaluation of the pelvis either abdominally or, preferably, transvaginally, when leiomyomata or endometrial polyps may be identified.

## Central nervous system

The favourable impact of HRT upon the psychological symptoms of oestrogen deficiency has prompted enquiry into its possible role in the prevention and treatment of Alzheimer's disease and other related neurodegenerative disorders. The physiological basis for such studies rests upon the known ability of oestrogen to enhance cerebral blood flow, its action as a monoamine oxidase inhibitor, and the presence of oestrogen receptors in key areas of the central nervous system, such as the hippocampus, which is the point of interface between short-term and long-term memory.

To date, cognitive function has been shown to improve in symptomatic but not in asymptomatic perimenopausal women. A recent meta-analysis of ten observational studies addressing the incidence of dementia concluded that the prior use of oestrogen was associated with a decrease in incidence of about one-third. These observations held firm after adjustment for potentially confounding variables such as ethnic group, education and APO-E genotype, which confers added risk.

The true relationship between HRT exposure and subsequent Alzheimer's disease and related dementia now urgently requires testing by an interventional study, such as a randomized placebo-controlled trial. Treatment of established Alzheimer's disease with oestrogen has been reported in several studies. No evidence of benefit has emerged and hence the use of HRT in the established condition is not indicated. At present, HRT products are not licensed for the prevention of neurodegenerative disease.

## Local oestrogens

The treatment of symptoms originating in the lower genital tract and in the bladder and urethra may be approached through the use of locally applied oestrogen. In the form of a cream, pessary or vaginal tablet, oestrogen may be inserted into the upper vagina, where it will disperse and engage the local receptors. This route of delivery is suitable for those women whose symptoms are of genitourinary origin and in whom systemic delivery of oestrogen is unacceptable or hazardous. For example, in patients with a past history of breast cancer, it may be beneficial to relieve local symptoms without elevating the plasma E2.

## Other sites of action

The oestrogen receptor is now known to be of extremely wide distribution and it is likely that its presence in a specific tissue implies, but does not mandate, a role for the hormone in the optimal function of the tissue concerned.

The clinical importance of postmenopausal oestrogen deficiency and the usefulness of HRT have yet to be established in the majority of these tissues, but several promising clinical leads are now to hand. It has repeatedly been reported that the incidence of colonic cancer in HRT-treated women is lower than would have been expected in a control population.

### New developments

#### Selective oestrogen receptor modulators (SERMs)

Clinical trial data have now begun to appear concerning the SERMs. These agents are special or, in other words, specific. They do not engage the oestrogen receptor in all tissues but do so selectively, with the central object of retaining the protective oestrogenic actions on the skeleton while avoiding the two key adverse effects of conventional HRT that are disincentives to its acceptance – namely, vaginal bleeding and fear of breast cancer.

The first SERM, raloxifene, is now licensed in the USA and the European Union for the prevention and treatment of bone loss. In summary, raloxifene is a benzothiophene and is related to tamoxifen. It engages the oestrogen receptor and locks into the ligand-binding cavity at its

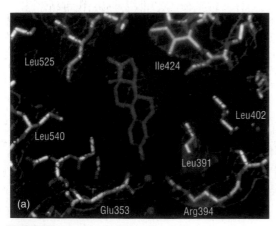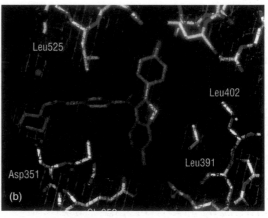

**Figure 18.6** Electron crystallographic image of the ligand-binding domain of the oestrogen receptor with (a) oestradiol and (b) raloxifene occupying the central cavity.

core (Fig. 18.6). However, in doing so, the side chain of raloxifene disables one of the activation function domains of the receptor (the AF-2 domain) necessary for oestrogen action at certain tissues, such as breast and uterus. The other activation function domain (AF-1) is unaffected, and at sites such as the skeleton where its action is required, raloxifene behaves like an oestrogen. A significant reduction in the risk of breast cancer has now been found in osteoporotic women receiving raloxifene in clinical trials.

Raloxifene does not reduce, and indeed may exacerbate, the vasomotor symptoms of menopause and its use will initially be restricted to patients at risk of developing osteoporosis, such as those with premature menopause, steroid therapy and positive family history.

## 🔑 Key Points

- The modal age of menopause is 51 years in the UK.
- The central change is a tenfold reduction in plasma E2.
- Oestrogen's activities range far beyond the reproductive system.
- Premenopausal amenorrhoea of >6 months should be investigated.
- Physical and/or psychological symptoms should be treated if causing distress to the patient.
- Bone loss after menopause may be arrested by exogenous oestrogen.
- Progestogen is required for endometrial protection.
- SERMs avoid withdrawal bleeding and breast cancer risk.
- A careful breast and pelvic examination should precede HRT treatment.
- Withdrawal bleeding and fear of breast cancer impede acceptance and continuance with HRT.

## CASE HISTORY

Mrs CJ is a 54-year-old Caucasian who works as a staff nurse. She presents with a history of early menopause at the age of 44 years, accompanied by vasomotor symptoms, which have now ceased. Vaginal dryness and dyspareunia persist. She is overweight but not obese (with a body mass index [BMI] of 29) and smokes occasionally. A breast biopsy 3 years ago led to local resection of a fibromyoma with atypia. Her mother died following a femoral neck fracture at the age of 83 and had previously lost height. Her father died of a myocardial infarction. She lives with a partner and is sexually active.

### Discussion

The patient presents several risk factors for osteoporosis, including premature menopause, positive family history and cigarette smoking. A bone mineral density scan to include hip and spine is indicated.

### Treatment

The absence of vasomotor or psychological symptoms of oestrogen deficiency together with the prior breast histology mitigate against the use of systemic oestrogen. However, for relief of the lower genital tract dryness, locally applied E2 by tablet or cream may be used.

If the densitometry scan confirms osteopenia (bone density was 1–2.5 standard deviations below the mean for young adults), treatment with a SERM may be considered. Alternatively, bone loss may be prevented by means of a weekly bisphosphonate such as alendronate or risedronate. Dietary intake of calcium should be established and if <1000 g/day, should be supplemented. A weight-bearing physical exercise programme of 20 minutes three times per week should be encouraged.

## Additional reading

Carr BR. Disorders of the ovary. In: Wilson JD, Foster DW (eds), *Williams' textbook of endocrinology*. Philadelphia: WB Saunders, 1992, 733–98.

Panney J. Management of the menopause. In: Grossman A (ed.), *Clinical endocrinology*. Oxford: Blackwell, 1998, 769–86.

Rees M, Purdie DW (eds). *The British Menopause Society handbook*. (Available from BMS Offices, Marlow, Bucks SL7 2NB.)

# Psychological aspects of gynaecology

## OVERVIEW

A woman is likely to experience a variety of changes to her body throughout her life: puberty, the menstrual cycle, pregnancy and the menopause are all states defined by physical change. The ability to adapt to these and other life events is important and if there are difficulties, the woman's sense of well-being may be adversely affected, which, in turn, may have an effect on her ability to function in other areas of her life. Understanding the psychosocial aspects of gynaecology is therefore important and will help to ensure that a holistic approach is adopted, integrating physical, psychological and cultural dimensions.

## Introduction

### Puberty

With puberty there are enormous physical changes and the young woman must come to terms with her changing body shape, menstruation and awareness of her own femininity and sexuality. Through the phase of adolescence that follows, the main tasks are separation from the family, formation of identity and coming to terms with sexuality and its attendant demands for decisions about sexual orientation, behaviour and relationships. Risk-taking behaviour is a natural part of this growing-up process. Not all adolescents complete identity formation in a healthy and safe way. Some remain dependent and insecure, while others make identity decisions too early, either to comply or to rebel against decisions imposed on them by significant adults in their lives.

### Transition to parenthood

With parenthood comes responsibility and loss of freedom. Depression and sexual difficulties are common following childbirth. A woman's withdrawal from her partner, both emotionally and sexually, may be an expression of her perceived inadequacy in the face of extra responsibility.

### Menopause

At the time of the menopause, stress may come from several sources. Loss of oestrogen may cause physical discomfort or symbolize the loss of youth and potential.

The woman's relationship with her partner may need to adjust to health problems or retirement. Elderly parents become dependent or die, and the sense of personal mortality grows. Children leave home and a new purpose in life needs to be found.

## Menstrual problems

Emotional problems can affect the menstrual cycle. Most women experience this at some time, such as missing a period when anxious about exams. The emotional disturbance can be more protracted and can lead to amenorrhoea, e.g. in anorexia nervosa.

Menorrhagia and psychosomatic factors may interact in one of the following ways.

- Heavy periods and consequent anaemia may lead to considerable distress and lethargy.
- Anxious or depressed women may be less tolerant of their periods and therefore report menorrhagia or dysmenorrhoea more frequently as an acceptable symptom to obtain medical help.
- Chronically anxious or depressed women may unconsciously use the complaint of menorrhagia to avoid sexual intimacy or pregnancy.

Psychosocial factors from the history should alert the gynaecologist to the possibility of an emotional disturbance underlying the presentation of menorrhagia and other gynaecological problems. These are:

- multiple social problems,
- relationship problems,
- recent life stress, e.g. divorce, bereavement,
- dysfunctional family background,
- history of self-abuse, e.g. alcohol, drugs, self-harm, eating disorders,
- symptoms suggestive of chronic anxiety or depression.

If several of these factors are present in the history, together with normal findings on examination and investigation, it is important to refer the woman to a counsellor or psychologist and not to resort to surgery in the first instance. Some women will not accept that there could be a psychological component to their problem and, as part of this denial, will insist that surgery is the answer. It is easy for the gynaecologist to collude and perform a hysterectomy only to find that the underlying depression gets worse. The woman may then be dissatisfied after surgery and may look for other surgical solutions to remove her unacceptable psychic pain.

Referral for psychological help can be very threatening for women who have a heavy investment in denial. They may feel they are being accused of malingering and that people think their problem is 'all in the mind'. It is important that the gynaecologist does not give the impression that he or she thinks the woman is malingering, but instead is able to accept and believe the woman's story and empathize with the importance and reality of her symptoms. At the same time a non-judgemental link between psychological distress and physical illness can be made, which may help her to doubt her previously held belief in a purely physical cause for her problem and accept a more holistic therapeutic approach.

## Premenstrual syndrome

Research has shown that women who keep diaries about premenstrual symptoms and who are aware of the purpose of the diary over-report psychological symptoms compared to women who are ignorant of the purpose of the diary. Under these conditions a correlation between the premenstrual phase and negative mood has not been made so readily. The only symptoms consistently linked to the premenstrual phase are pain and water retention and not the psychological ones.

Psychological symptoms are more likely to present in women with pre-existing psychological or social problems. Evidence suggests that in a society where women are expected to be emotionally out of control premenstrually, negative emotions expressed premenstrually will be attributed to being governed by female hormones. The danger in attributing negative feelings to internal uncontrollable forces is that women may avoid solving situational and relationship problems.

Gynaecologists should be wary of colluding in this avoidance. It is too easy to prescribe hormones or other drug therapies without attending to the woman's background or current environment.

Transactional analysis (TA), originated by the American psychiatrist Eric Berne in the 1960s, is a model for understanding human personalities, relationships and communication. Using TA concepts, Stephen Karpman devised a model for looking at

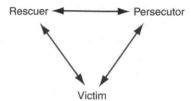

**Figure 19.1** The drama triangle.

dysfunctional relationships. He proposed that people who play games might be in one of three roles: persecutor, rescuer or victim. A persecutor is someone who discounts other people by putting them down. A rescuer is someone who discounts other people by helping them because he or she assumes they are incapable of helping themselves. Victims discount themselves and will agree with the put-down or the concept that, as a victim, they are helpless. These three roles together form the drama triangle (Fig. 19.1).

Women with premenstrual mood disturbance tend to adopt the role of rescuer during the first half of their cycle when they feel full of energy. They experience lower energy levels as they approach their next period and change to feeling put upon by others (victim role). They become resentful of doing everything for their friends and family and turn into the irritable persecutor. A psychological approach to working with women with premenstrual syndrome (PMS) can therefore help the sufferer to gain insights into these shifts and to learn assertiveness skills and relaxation techniques. These will reduce the tendency to rescue others in the first half of the cycle and be aggressive in the second.

## Menopause

Attitudes to the menopause range from relief to acute dread. It is reasonable to assume that no one wishes to get older and lose their physical and mental abilities. Since the menopause is often seen as the beginning of these changes, it is likely that the woman who affects indifference will be denying her anxiety. If the denial worked, it would be a satisfactory way of dealing with the anxiety, but it often fails and anxiety emerges in other ways, such as physical symptoms or as excessive emotional reactions to ordinary situations.

For many women, the menopause coincides with a variety of stressful life events that can affect how they perceive and cope with the physical changes:
- empty nest syndrome
- retirement
- divorce
- bereavement
- elderly parents
- teenage children
- moving home.

Hormone replacement therapy (HRT) can be used for the short-term alleviation of unpleasant symptoms. Some women also see it as a means of retaining youth or of denying the stress of coexisting life events. Inability to adjust to the reality of ageing can lead to depression, especially when long-term HRT is withdrawn as new evidence about its safety changes its pattern of use.

## Subfertility

Subfertility is very stressful, with cycles of continual hope and disappointment (loss). Life centres around having a baby. Nothing else seems important, and partners blame each other and become frustrated and guilty.

The more advanced technology becomes, the more difficult it is to accept subfertility, and it is partly the gynaecologist's role to help a patient judge when to withdraw from what may become an obsession. By the very nature of her problems, the subfertile woman becomes increasingly divorced from any normal doubts about having a child. The more it seems she may be denied her natural right as a woman, the more desperate she becomes in her efforts to obtain it. Paradoxically, it is the woman who always wanted children who is best able to accept disappointment and to adopt, or to seek fulfilment by working with children. The woman who originally did not want children may become desperate, depressed and unable to face life without a child. There are many unconscious reasons why some women do not want a child:
- their mother's life was drudgery; therefore, motherhood is to be avoided,
- hatred of younger siblings displacing them, leading to a fear that they hate babies,
- a successful career is valued more highly than motherhood,

- avoidance of having a child of a gender that is hated or feared,
- desire to have been born a boy: motherhood is the ultimate proof they are 'only a woman'.

The question of adoption can give insight into these problems, and much can be learned from the woman's response to the idea of adoption. The woman who knows she has much to offer as a parent and realistically wants a baby will consider adoption. Those who will not consider adoption may unconsciously want a baby to prove some point about themselves, or may be ambivalent towards motherhood.

## Fertility choice and control

The responsibility of controlling conception and choosing when to conceive ideally rests with the couple, although frequently women take it on as their sole responsibility.

Women need a sense of positive self-worth and the ability to make decisions in order to exercise this responsibility. It is not uncommon for personal issues relating to low self-esteem and impulse control to present as contraceptive problems or unwanted pregnancy. It is important to be aware of the possibility of such problems in women who present with multiple symptoms that prevent them settling with one contraceptive method. When method failure has been excluded, an unwanted pregnancy is likely to be the end result of some inner conflict over an unconscious need:

- to love or be loved,
- to right the wrongs of their own childhood experiences,
- to establish control by rebelling,
- to be successful at something.

## Chronic pelvic pain without pathology

Chronic pelvic pain is a common symptom presenting in the gynaecology outpatient clinic.

Following laparoscopy, about two-thirds of women will be found to have no pathology, but even the presence of pathology does not mean that the cause of the pain has been found. It may be a somatic expression of psychic pain, the unconscious pay-off being avoidance of conflict relating to issues such as sex, intimacy or pregnancy.

Self-monitoring and a heightened awareness of pain are particularly apparent in women who have a past history of pelvic pathology or who have a family history of pelvic disease. This increased awareness leads to distress and the discomfort is relabelled pain, which heightens the distress and sets up a vicious circle. Family members can reinforce the distress.

## Sexual problems

Sexual intimacy is a fundamental aspect of humanity, which is of much deeper significance than the reproductive element. Sexual problems in women can be primary, secondary, situational or total and may occur in any of the phases of the sexual response cycle. Sexual dysfunctions are difficult to classify and several dysfunctions may overlap. Common precipitating and predisposing factors for sexual problems are summarized in Table 19.1.

Sexual expression is complex. There is interaction between:

- the instinctive reproductive drive
- emotional responses
- thought processes
- physical actions
- physiological changes.

**Table 19.1**  Common precipitating and predisposing factors underlying causes for sexual problems

| Precipitating factors | Predisposing factors |
|---|---|
| Parenthood | Physical, emotional |
| Illness | or sexual abuse in |
| Random failure | childhood |
| Life stresses | Restrictive upbringing |
| e.g. bereavement, | Lack of information |
| redundancy, relationship | Uncertain sexual |
| problems | identity |
| Performance pressure | Poor self-esteem |
| Traumatic sexual | Poor body image |
| experience | Communication |
| Psychiatric illness | problems |

The possibility of conflict surrounding sexual expression may be due to:

- lack of information
- belief in sexual myths
- poor communication skills
- expectations from past generations leading to guilt
- expectations from current generation leading to performance pressure.

Difficulty in any of these areas can interfere with the final integration of responses necessary for the sexual fulfilment of two people. Failure in any aspect of the sexual response is likely to feed a fear of failure on future occasions, thus perpetuating a vicious circle.

## Female sexual behaviour

The 1990 and 2000 Sexual Attitudes and Lifestyles Surveys have extended understanding of female sexual behaviour in Great Britain.

- Women are experiencing first intercourse at a younger age.
- Vaginal intercourse is the most common activity.
- Non-penetrative sex, including fellatio and cunnilingus, contribute to the sexual experiences of the majority of the female population.
- Anal sex is a minority but increasingly reported activity.
- Younger women tend to have more partners than older women.
- Serial monogamy remains the main pattern.
- Homosexual activity is reported by a minority of women: 4.5 per cent sexual attraction, 3.5 per cent sexual contact, and 1.5 per cent genital contact. Other studies indicate that:
- 85 per cent of women have masturbated,
- most women find it easier to reach orgasm through clitoral stimulation rather than coitus.

## The sexual response cycle

Sex drive underlies the sexual response cycle, which consists of five phases:

1. drive
2. desire
3. arousal
4. orgasm
5. resolution.

On average, women take longer than men to reach the peak of arousal. Recent research has indicated that some women do not experience desire before arousal but that the two phases are experienced together. This may be more evident after the menopause. Before the menopause, women have a biological drive to initiate sex as well as a motivational drive to initiate sex to please themselves or please their partner. With the menopause, the biological drive ceases and the motivation to initiate or participate in sex may not be sufficient on its own. Other effects of ageing are that the time to reach the peak of arousal increases further and intensity of orgasm may decline.

---

### P Understanding the pathophysiology of sexual problems

**Physiological/organic or iatrogenic factors**

- Physiological, e.g. childbirth, menopause and ageing.
- Disease directly affecting the sexual response, e.g. diabetic autonomic neuropathy.
- Alteration of genital anatomy, e.g. post-surgery or post-radiotherapy for gynaecological cancers.
- Mobility for sexual activity affected, e.g. spinal cord injury, cerebrovascular accident.
- Musculoskeletal pain limiting sexual activity, e.g. rheumatoid arthritis.
- Genital pain limiting sexual activity, e.g. vestibulitis, episiotomy scar.
- General ill-health leading to fatigue, e.g. anaemia, renal failure.
- Secondary to medication side effects, e.g. antidepressants, antihypertensives.

It is important to remember that although organic or iatrogenic factors can affect sexual function, a psychological component usually coexists. Loss of previous sexual function can lead to a grief reaction and loss of confidence because of a poor self/body image.

**Psychosocial factors**

Lack of, or incorrect, information about sex.
Many adults still lack knowledge about sexual anatomy, physiology and behaviour. They may have received inadequate information due to a restrictive upbringing, incorrect information from peers or a false impression of sexual behaviour from the media.

## Sexual myths and taboos

Our value systems, beliefs and attitudes develop within our family and from social, cultural and religious experiences. Myths and taboos about sexual behaviour evolve within different cultural frameworks and perpetuate guilt and shame about sexual activity.

Examples of sexual myths include:

- performance is everything,
- the man is responsible for the woman's orgasm,
- the woman is responsible for the man's erection,
- good sex is spontaneous sex,
- only loose women initiate sexual activity,
- sex equals intercourse,
- mind reading: when in love, one doesn't need to tell one's partner what is wanted because they already know.

## Communication problems

Talking about sex can be embarrassing. The man may think he can mind-read the woman's sexual needs, and the woman may fear upsetting her partner by telling him he has got it wrong and that his sexual technique is not pleasurable. This failure of honest communication can also occur the other way round, with the man finding it hard to ask for what he wants from the woman. Also fear, anger, resentment or guilt can build up in a relationship because of general communication problems, and these can be acted out as sexual avoidance.

## Predisposing, precipitating and perpetuating factors

Past experiences, life events and behaviour patterns for dealing with problems can all contribute to the onset and maintenance of sexual problems.

## Differing and unrealistic expectations

Problems can arise when partners have a different need for sexual expression, particularly if they have different levels of sex drive. Problems can also arise due to unrealistic expectations, which lead to performance pressure and fear of failure.

Examples of unrealistic expectations include:

- no change in sexual interest when ill, tired or bereaved,
- always to achieve orgasm during intercourse,
- mutual orgasm on every occasion,
- to return to the same interest in sex after childbirth,
- performance to remain unchanged by age.

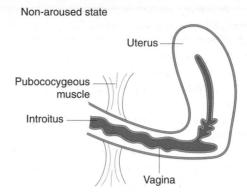

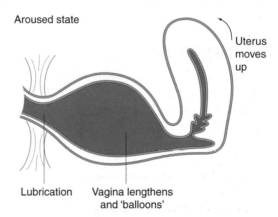

**Figure 19.2** Physiological changes occurring in the female genitalia during the sexual response cycle.

The physiological changes occurring in the female genitalia during the sexual response cycle are summarized in Figure 19.2 and Table 19.2.

## Classification of sexual disorders

The *Diagnostic and Statistical Manual of Mental Disorders IV* of the American Psychiatric Association (DSM IV) classification is as follows.

- Sexual desire disorders
  - hypoactive sexual desire
  - sexual aversion disorder
  - excessive sexual desire
- Arousal disorder
- Orgasmic disorder
- Sexual pain disorder
  - dyspareunia
  - vaginismus

**Table 19.2** Physiological changes occurring in the female genitalia during the sexual response cycle

|  | Excitement | Plateau | Orgasm | Resolution |
|---|---|---|---|---|
| Labia | – | Vasocongestion red $\gg$ burgundy | – | 10–15 s |
| Clitoris | Vasocongestion | Retracts flat under hood | – | 5–10 s |
| Vagina | Lubrication Vasocongestion Ballooning of inner two-thirds | The same plus orgasmic platform of outer third | Contracts 0.8 s $\times$ 3–15 | 10–15 s |
| Uterus | Engorged Rises from pelvic floor | Completes ascent | Cervix opens and contracts | 20–30 min |

## Prevalence

The prevalence of female sexual problems is unknown. Various scientific and unscientific studies involving general or clinic populations have attempted to quantify the frequency of sexual problems and it appears that about 60 per cent of women will have a sexual problem at some time.

The most commonly presenting problems are:
- decreased frequency due to either low desire or avoidance,
- problems with penetration,
- problems with orgasm.

## Assessment

### Taking a sexual history
The first concern of the doctor in history taking must be accurately to identify the area of difficulty, i.e. emotional or physical, since it is easy for trouble in one area to be mistaken for trouble in the other. Experience shows that when symptoms seem to be physical there is a risk that the more elusive and difficult emotional cause may be ignored. Taking a sexual history therefore requires sensitivity, careful attention to detail and good communication skills.

Whenever there is a sexual problem, the patient is likely to be embarrassed when talking about it. It is

### Sexual history

**Childhood and adolescent experiences**
- Family background and relationships
- Cultural and religious background
- Family attitudes to sexuality, intimacy and expression of emotion
- Traumatic sexual or other life experiences
- Sex education
- Experience of puberty
- Sexual opportunities, masturbation, non-coital and coital experiences

**Adult experiences**
- Past relationships
- Traumatic life events

**Current experiences**
- History of the presenting problem
- Details of the current sexual dysfunction
- Present sexual practices and preferences, including masturbation
- Present relationship(s)
- Sexual orientation
- Use of fantasy, erotic material or sex aids

**Medical history**
- Past medical and surgical history
- Past gynaecological and obstetric history
- Drug history, both social and therapeutic
- Contraception/infertility

therefore important that health professionals develop an open, non-judgemental style that encourages talking about such sensitive matters as sexual orientation, masturbation, fantasies and affairs. It is important to be confident about the use of language and sexually explicit words and to check a patient's understanding of these words. The patient's verbal and body language can be a window into his or her belief systems, fears and shame.

### Examination

It is important always to offer women a chaperone and to document this. When examining a woman with a sexual problem, it is important to progress at a pace she can cope with. This is particularly important for women who have been sexually abused, as they need to feel in control of the situation. The way in which a woman responds to the genital examination can give insight into how she feels about her sexuality. This insight can be used diagnostically and therapeutically.

### Investigations

Investigations (Table 19.3) should be performed selectively depending on the possible underlying causes of a sexual problem (see 'Understanding the pathophysiology').

## Sexual therapy/psychosexual counselling

All health professionals should be trained to offer first-line education, advice and guidance, especially if they work in a specialty that deals specifically with aspects of sexuality, such as gynaecology.

Outcome research in the field of sex therapy is notoriously difficult. Many couples and individuals present with more than one dysfunction and with mixed organic and psychogenic factors. The variables involved are complex and confuse outcome results. Further confusion has arisen because of failure to define dysfunctions by internationally agreed classifications. Finally, a successful outcome defined by the patient may not be a resolution of the dysfunction. Sometimes individuals or couples find ways of adapting to the dysfunction and therefore satisfaction with the outcome may be more relevant than 'success'.

## Management of sexual problems due to physiological or pathological change

Most National Health Service (NHS) clinics that work with sexual problems offer general management such as:
- education, advice and guidance – including recommendation of self help-books,

**Table 19.3** Investigations to consider for a sexual problem

| Sexual problem | Disorder/condition | Investigation |
| --- | --- | --- |
| Loss of desire | Anaemia | FBC |
| | Renal disease | U&Es |
| | Liver disease | LFTs |
| | Hyperprolactinaemia | Prolactin |
| | Hypothyroidism | TFTs |
| | Hypogonadism | Testosterone |
| | | Oestradiol |
| | Menopause | FSH |
| Superficial dyspareunia | Genital infections | STI screen |
| | Dermatological problem | Skin biopsy |
| Deep dyspareunia | Urinary tract infection | MSU/IVU |
| | Pelvic inflammatory disease | STI screen, ultrasound/laparoscopy |

FBC, full blood count; U&Es, urea and electrolytes; LFTs, liver function tests; TFTs, thyroid function tests; STI, sexually transmitted disease; MSU, mid-stream urine; IVU, intravenous pyelogram.

- physical treatments as appropriate,
- brief counselling/therapy – this may be with individuals or couples.

If long-term counselling or psychotherapy is required, patients will need referral to a counsellor or psychotherapist who can undertake this work either within the NHS or privately.

In the following sections, sexual problems are considered with specific management options that are additional to the general management outlined above.

### Post-childbirth

Many women experience reduced interest in sex in the first 6 months after childbirth and do not return to previous sexual activity until 1 year later (if at all). Exhaustion and sleep deprivation play a part, as may the raised prolactin and low oestrogen levels in women who are breastfeeding. Following vaginal delivery, physical changes to the labia minora and introitus may affect the woman's ability to grip the penis and achieve the same sensations during penetration as before. This reduces the indirect stimulation to the clitoral head from the tugging effect on the clitoral hood produced by the thrusting penis, thus the woman's ability to achieve orgasm with penetration may be reduced. Other adverse factors after childbirth can be painful scars or temporary incontinence of urine, flatus or even faeces. Fear of pain or embarrassment may lead to sexual avoidance.

Specific management will include the following.
- The female superior position and the simultaneous manual stimulation of the clitoris may overcome a difficulty with achieving coital orgasm.
- Added lubrication and the female superior position may help overcome fear of pain (see 'Dyspareunia' below).
- Pelvic floor muscle tone can be improved with pelvic floor exercises.

### Post-menopause

The loss of oestrogen and testosterone has been linked psychologically with loss of sexual interest. Physical factors such as night sweats and atrophic changes to the urogenital tissues can lead to sexual avoidance because of exhaustion or fear of pain. Women may present problems with arousal or orgasm because with ageing it takes longer to become aroused and orgasm becomes less intense. Some women have described either hypersensitivity or hyposensitivity to touch with the menopause that leads to sexual avoidance.

Stress incontinence can also present at this time and this also leads to sexual avoidance.
Specific management will include:
- short-term HRT for night sweats, atrophic urogenital changes and touch impairment,
- topical vaginal oestrogen for atrophic urogenital changes,
- testosterone implant, gel or tibolone for loss of interest,
- strengthening pelvic floor muscles for stress incontinence,
- surgery for persistent stress incontinence.

### Organic/iatrogenic factors

Organic disease can lead to sexual problems because of physical and psychological factors (see 'Understanding the pathophysiology', above).

Specific management comprises:
- treatment of the specific pathological condition,
- information about the disease and/or treatment effect on the sexual response,
- practical advice to adapt sexual activity to the limitations of the disease process,
- couple therapy can be helpful to open up communication about the sexual relationship that may otherwise be avoided for fear of hurting or being hurt.

## Management of specific sexual problems

### Desire phase
Lack or loss of desire
The problem may have always existed or may develop after a period of normal sexual interest. It is possible for low desire to exist in isolation, but commonly it is secondary to some other sexual problem, so that repeated unsatisfactory experiences lead to a loss of desire. Deep-seated personal problems, sexual orientation dilemmas or relationship difficulties often present in this way. Chronic physical illness frequently leads to low desire because of fatigue, loss of self-esteem, altered body image or as a side effect of medication.

Specific management will involve the following.
- Exclude physical factors or, if they exist, recognize their significance to the maintenance of the sexual problem and manage appropriately.
- Self-pleasuring or sensate focus exercises to improve understanding and communication of sexual needs (see p. 230).

- Management of hypoprolactinaemia.
- Testosterone implants, gel or tibolone for postmenopausal women (especially if the menopause occurs prematurely through a natural or iatrogenic loss of ovarian function).
- Antidepressants if clinically depressed. (Caution: antidepressants can also affect the sexual response, e.g. selective serotonin reuptake inhibitors [SSRIs] may reduce desire or delay the orgasmic response.)

### Sexual aversions and phobias

Problems may stem from receiving negative messages about sex so that sex is feared as it leads to feelings of guilt or shame. They can also be the result of some traumatic sexual experience. Sexual aversion may be confused with low desire because both present with reduced frequency of sexual activity. There is a difference between sexual interest being present but the activity avoided and no interest and therefore no activity. Sexual aversion and phobias can be total, in which case all sexual activity is avoided, or situational, when specific sexual activities trigger the aversion or phobic response, e.g. masturbation, penetration, breast stimulation or oral sex. The sense of impending loss of control with mounting arousal can also trigger a panic response.

Specific management includes the following.

- Individual therapy is usually required to help to discover the predisposing or precipitating factors.
- Abuse resolution therapy when there is a history of past sexual abuse.
- Gradual desensitization to sexual activities that lead to the aversive response.
- SSRIs can reduce the physical phobic response.

### Excessive sexual desire

This sexual problem is also referred to as sexual addiction. Sexual behaviour in this condition is self-destructive and compulsive and, like other addictions, can lead to loss of family, money, job and even life. Most sexual addicts come from dysfunctional families and were abused as children, sexually, physically or emotionally. Many exhibit other addictions such as alcohol, drugs or gambling. Sexual addicts are powerless to control their compulsion to be sexual despite the negative consequences.

Specific management covers the following.

- Long-term individual therapy.
- Group therapy: most groups function along lines similar to those of Alcoholics Anonymous, with a 12-step recovery programme.

## Arousal phase

### Failure of genital response

The physiological arousal response in the female is invisible, unlike the male erection. Most men and women know that vaginal lubrication indicates arousal but have no knowledge of the pelvic congestion and ballooning of the inner two-thirds of the vagina that occur with high arousal (see Fig. 19.2). Sometimes problems arise because the woman allows her partner to penetrate her too soon because she is too shy to communicate her need for longer foreplay. Arousal problems can present as painful sex, which can trigger avoidance. Lack of lubrication leads to superficial dyspareunia and lack of vaginal ballooning can lead to deep dyspareunia.

Arousal requires:

- positive 'turn-ons' and not negative 'turn-offs',
- enhancement by that what you see, hear, smell, taste and touch,
- a time and place that will enhance sexual feelings,
- positive tactile stimuli to genital and other sensual areas,
- switching off distracting thoughts.
Specific management includes the following.
- Self-pleasuring exercises (see p. 229).
- Sensate focus (see p. 230).
- Exploring the use of fantasy, erotic material or vibrators.
- Topical oestrogen if oestrogen deficiency is a factor in failure of lubrication.
- Lubricants, e.g. KY jelly, Astroglide, Sylk or Replens.

## Orgasmic phase

### Orgasmic dysfunction

There is controversy about whether all women are potentially orgasmic or whether some women are unable to reach an orgasm. Studies suggest that 5–10 per cent of women never experience an orgasm. The female orgasm is not essential for fertility, and anorgasmia is linked with late-onset menarche and chronic constipation, which suggests possible physiological explanations. Psychologically, anorgasmia is related either to inadequate stimulation or to difficulty in losing control. It is often situational, so that orgasm may occur with masturbation but not with a partner. Half of the women who are orgasmic find it easier to achieve orgasm with manual stimulation rather than during coitus.

Specific management includes the following.

- The same solutions as for arousal problems.
- Nipple stimulation during sexual arousal may help enhance the orgasmic response due to oxytocin release.

### Sexual pain disorders

#### Vaginismus

Vaginismus is caused by an involuntary spasm of the pubococcygeus muscle. The muscle tightens in anticipation of pain and if penetration is forced through the tight muscle, pain is experienced, re-enforcing the problem. The involuntary tightening of the vaginal muscle can be likened to closing the eyelids tight to protect the eye from anticipated pain, i.e. vaginismus is like 'vaginal blinking'. Women with vaginismus frequently enjoy full non-penetrative sex to orgasm.

#### Aetiology of vaginismus

- Growing up with negative experiences or with relationships leading to fear of intimacy or loss of control (avoidance of psychological pain).
- Growing up with cultural, religious or romanticized messages about relationships leading to a belief that sex is dirty or shameful.
- Women of small stature who believe that their vagina is too small.
- Fear of pain, either primary or secondary after childbirth.
- Traumatic past sexual experiences.
  Specific management involves the following.
- Gradual desensitization can help, as it does in other phobic situations.
- The vagina can 'learn' to accept items of progressively increasing size, e.g. cotton buds, tampon covers, one finger, two fingers etc. (plenty of lubrication helps). Alternatively, there are specifically designed vaginal trainers in different sizes, e.g. Amielle trainers (Fig. 19.3).
- Desensitization using visualization techniques.
- Transition to penile penetration – best achieved in gradual steps with the woman maintaining control. She is likely to feel most relaxed in the female superior or side-to-side position.
- SSRIs may be useful to overcome a phobic response if this is blocking progress.

#### Dyspareunia

Dyspareunia can be either superficial or deep. There can be an organic component and therefore a full

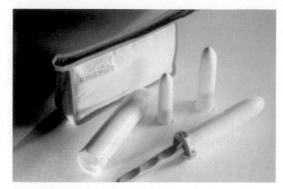

**Figure 19.3** Amielle trainers.

medical history, examination and appropriate investigations are necessary. It can be particularly difficult when minimal or no abnormality is found on examination (see 'Chronic pelvic pain without pathology', p. 221). Superficial dyspareunia can be part of the vulval pain syndromes of vulval vestibulitis (VV) and dysaesthetic vulvodynia (DV). VV is typically characterized by pain when pressure is applied to the vestibule, so that penetrative sex, fitting tampons or wearing tight clothing can trigger the pain. The cause of VV is frequently unknown, and treatments vary from the use of local anaesthetic jelly to topical steroids or low-dose tricyclic antidepressants for neuropathic pain. DV is typically a problem of older women and is characterized by constant vulval burning and soreness. It is due to neuropathic pain and is likely to respond partially or completely to drugs that alter pain fibre impulses, such as amitriptyline or gabapentin. For both VV and DV, sexual problems are common, as they can trigger sexual avoidance and/or vaginismus and spiral downwards into relationship problems when the avoidance is interpreted as rejection.

Emotional (non-organic) pain related to penetrative sex can also be expressed as genuine physical pain. Non-organic dyspareunia can be divided into type I (intrapersonal) and type II (interpersonal). In type I, the presentation involves guilt, misinformation, previous traumatic experiences or previous physical factors such as episiotomy. Type I responds well to permission giving and desensitisation, as outlined in the section on vaginismus.

In type II dyspareunia, relationship problems exist and dyspareunia is an expression of unconscious fear or anger in the relationship providing an excuse to avoid sex. Type II requires individual or couple therapy.

Specific physical management options for dyspareunia are as follows.

- Vaginal trainers.
- Adaptation of sexual positions to minimize pain.
- Adequate lubrication is essential and the use of artificial lubricant is beneficial.
- Treatment for candidiasis or other genital infections.
- Treatment of other pelvic organ problems when these are the cause of deep dyspareunia, e.g. irritable bowel syndrome, chronic pelvic infection, chronic cystitis.
- Low-dose amitriptyline may be beneficial in vulvodynia or vestibulitis.
- Topical steroids may help if dermatological problems exist.
- Topical oestrogens may improve atrophic changes.
- Local anaesthetic gel applied to the painful area.
- For many couples, the task is to find strategies that help them to maximize sexual enjoyment while managing the dyspareunia and grieving (then accepting) the loss of sexual freedom they previously enjoyed.

## Specific sex therapy concepts and strategies

### The sexual response staircase

The sexual response staircase can be used educationally, diagnostically and therapeutically. Information about the human sexual response is given as an analogy to going up stairs (Fig. 19.4).

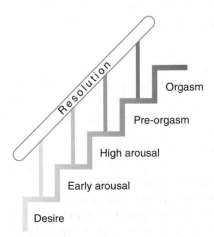

**Figure 19.4** The sexual response staircase.

- Ground level: non-sexual.
- Step 1: desire without any physical change.
- Step 2: arousal begins. The woman begins to lubricate; for the man the penis begins to get firm, but not firm enough for penetration.
- Step 3: arousal progresses. For the woman there is more lubrication and vaginal ballooning; for the man there is a firm erection that could achieve penetration.
- Step 4: orgasm is recognized as being imminent.
- Step 5: orgasm itself.
- Sliding down the banisters is the process of resolution and is accompanied by all the thoughts and feelings from that particular sexual encounter. It is possible to choose to climb on to the banister from any step on the staircase.

It is normal for both men and women to spend time going up and down the steps and not go directly to step 5 in one dash up the stairs. Men and women often progress up the stairs at different rates. Physiologically a man on step 3 can penetrate a woman who can still be on step 1 or even on the ground level. The reverse is impossible. A common problem occurs when the man is ahead of his partner and reaches step 5 to slide down the banisters, leaving her to feel frustrated still on step 1 or 2.

The important concept for both partners to understand is that each is responsible for his or her own progression up the staircase. The woman is responsible for her orgasm and the man for his. Communication is therefore essential. There is no need to aim for synchronicity. What is important is that each individual feels comfortable with his or her own progress, and if they do not wish to reach orgasm on that occasion, this is also acceptable. For sex to be seen as a positive experience, the thoughts and feelings that predominate when returning down the banisters need to be those of fulfilment and contentment, not anger, resentment or a sense of failure.

### Self-discovery and self-pleasuring

Information about the physiology of the sexual response cycle is given. With this knowledge, a woman can embark on learning about her own body and sexual needs through a process of self-discovery and self-pleasuring. She can experiment at home in private through a series of exercises that will give her insights into her sexual likes and dislikes. The information gained can then be communicated to her partner.

## Sensate focus

This is an extension of the self-discovery programme into couple work. It is a strategy for overcoming sexual problems by addressing all the possible blocks (turn-offs) to arousal. 'Homework' assignments are set for the couple and can be tailor-made to meet specific needs.

### Step 1

Sexual intercourse is banned, thus removing performance pressure. The couple sets aside two or three 1-hour sessions during the week to be together. Difficulty in finding the time may highlight other issues such as privacy or a busy schedule, indicating that time for intimacy has a low priority or is being avoided. Setting the scene is important. Attention is paid to ensuring privacy, and selecting an environment will enhance the experience. The couple takes turns to touch and be touched in all areas of the body excluding the breasts and genitals. Focusing on the sensation of touch and being touched helps overcome distracting thoughts. Each individual focuses on getting pleasure from the experience for himself or herself, but not at the expense of the partner. In this way each person takes responsibility for his or her own enjoyment but also cares about the other person's enjoyment. If talking is difficult, feedback can be given by the receiver moving the hands of the giver to achieve the desired effect.

### Step 2

Once the couple is comfortable with step 1, they can move on to introduce genital touching. Arousal is still not the goal, and it is important for the couple to discuss what they will do, should the exercise lead to arousal in one or other of the partners. The ban on sexual penetration is continued, so that the couple experiences the pleasure of arousal for its own sake and trust is maintained.

### Step 3

The final step is to remove the ban on intercourse and bring back the concept of pleasure leading to arousal. When there has been a problem with penetration, a further sequence of gradual steps may be required before full penetrative sex can be achieved.

## New developments

There is a need for research into problems of desire and drive in women – testosterone gel may help women with low drive/desire.

Dihydroepiandrostenedione (DHEA) may have a role in helping postmenopausal loss of libido in oestrogenized women. 5-Phosphodiesterase inhibitors such as sildenafil citrate (Viagra) are not licensed for use in women, but evidence suggests they may help arousal phase dysfunction and, secondarily, improve the ability to achieve orgasm or improve libido if loss of libido is secondary to arousal or orgasmic difficulties. The benefit appears to be best for premenopausal women. Advances in understanding and managing neuropathic pain may help women with vulval pain syndrome.

### Key Points

- Treat the whole person and consider psychological causes and consequences of gynaecological and sexual problems.
- Good communication skills: talk openly, be non-judgemental and avoid jargon. Observe non-verbal messages. Listen carefully and avoid assumptions.
- Know your professional limitations and resources for referral.

## CASE HISTORY

Mrs AV, a 33-year-old teacher, presents with superficial dyspareunia leading to loss of interest in sex since the difficult assisted delivery of her first child 2 years previously. She has been married for 4 years to a busy lawyer. Sex prior to the pregnancy was satisfactory. Six months after the birth of her son, she returned to work as a part-time supply teacher. Her husband's legal practice seems to have got busier and he spends long hours at work. Their relationship is under stress and separation is possible if the sexual problem is not resolved.

### Discussion

*What is the most likely diagnosis?*
Is it dyspareunia leading to sexual avoidance, or sexual avoidance leading to dyspareunia? There may have been organic factors such as initial high prolactin and low

oestrogen levels if she was breastfeeding, or a painful episiotomy scar. Alternatively it could be psychosocial, with her symptoms secondary to fear of a further pregnancy and delivery, coming to terms with her new role as a mother, or a relationship problem if she resents the time her husband spends at work or is suspicious he is having an affair.

*Management options*

Include brief individual or couple therapy to give information and improve general and sexual communication. Attention should also be paid to exclude organic factors and, if found, to manage them appropriately.

## Additional reading

Cooper E, Guillebaud J. *Sexuality and disability.* Oxford: Radcliffe Medical Press, 1999.

Leiblum S, Daniluk J. *Women's sexuality across the lifespan: challenging myths, creating meanings.* New York: Guilford Press, 1998.

Skrine R. *Blocks and freedoms in sexual life.* Oxford: Radcliffe Medical Press, 1997.

Skrine R, Montford H (eds). *Psychosexual medicine. An introduction.* London: Arnold, 2001.

Wellings K, Field J, Johnson M, Wadsworth J. *Sexual behaviour in Britain – the National Survey of Sexual Attitudes and Lifestyles.* London: Penguin, 1994. (This book, published in 1994, details the findings of the 1990 survey; the findings of the 2000 survey are currently in press.)

# Common gynaecological procedures

## Hysteroscopy

Hysteroscopy involves passing a small-diameter telescope, either flexible or rigid, through the cervix to directly inspect the uterine cavity. Excellent images can be obtained. A flexible hysteroscope may be used in the outpatient setting, with carbon dioxide as a filling medium. Rigid instruments employ circulating fluids and therefore can be used to visualize the uterine cavity even if the woman is bleeding.

### Indications

Any abnormal bleeding from the uterus can be investigated by hysteroscopy, including:
- postmenopausal bleeding,
- irregular menstruation, intermenstrual bleeding and postcoital bleeding,
- persistent menorrhagia,
- persistent discharge,
- suspected uterine malformations,
- suspected Asherman's syndrome.

### Complications

- Perforation of the uterus.
- Cervical damage – if cervical dilatation is necessary.

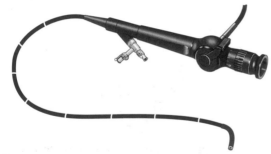

**Figure 1** Flexible fibreoptic hysteroscope.

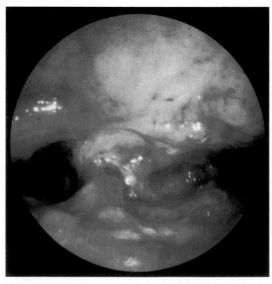

**Figure 2** Hysteroscopic view of endometrial cavity.

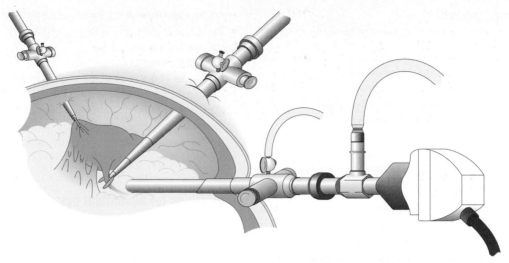

**Figure 3** Schematic diagram showing laparoscope.

- If there is infection present, hysteroscopy can cause ascent.

  An operating hysteroscope can also be used to resect endometrial pathology such as fibroids and polyps.

## Laparoscopy

Laparoscopy allows visualization of the peritoneal cavity. This involves insertion of a needle called a Veress needle into a suitable puncture point in the umbilicus. This allows insufflation of the peritoneal cavity with carbon dioxide so that a larger instrument can be inserted. The majority of instruments used for diagnostic laparoscopy are 5 mm in diameter, and 10 mm instruments are used for operative laparoscopy. More recently, a 2 mm laparoscope has become available.

## Indications

- Suspected ectopic pregnancy.
- Undiagnosed pelvic pain.
- Tubal patency testing.
- Sterilization.

  Operative laparoscopy can be used to perform ovarian cystectomy or oophorectomy and to treat endometriosis with cautery or laser. Reversal of sterilization is also possible using laparoscopy.

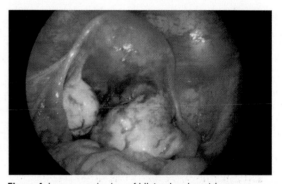

**Figure 4** Laparoscopic view of bilateral endometriomas.

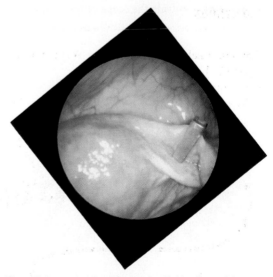

**Figure 5** Laparoscopic view showing Fishie clip on right Fallopian tube.

## Complications

Complications are uncommon, but include damage to any of the intra-abdominal structures, such as bowel and major blood vessels. The bladder is always emptied prior to the procedure to avoid bladder injury. Incisional hernia has been reported.

## Abdominal and vaginal hysterectomy

Vaginal hysterectomy is associated with a much quicker recovery than abdominal hysterectomy and is preferred for that reason. However, vaginal hysterectomy is not indicated when there is malignancy, as the ovaries often need to be removed and lymph nodes examined and sampled. If the uterus is larger than that of a 12-week pregnancy and has outgrown the pelvis, an abdominal hysterectomy is usually preferred and is thought to be safer. The main reason vaginal hysterectomy is associated with faster recovery is the lack of abdominal incision.

Most abdominal hysterectomies are performed through a Pfannenstiel incision, which is a low (bikini line) suprapubic transverse incision. Patients recover more quickly from this incision than from than a midline incision and the cosmetic result is more acceptable. For larger masses and malignancies, a midline incision is utilized.

Although a complete description of abdominal hysterectomy is outside the scope of this chapter, the procedure involves taking three pedicles:

- the infundibulopelvic ligament, which contains the ovarian vessels,
- the uterine artery,
- the angles of the vault of the vagina, which contain vessels ascending from the vagina; the ligaments to support the uterus can be taken with this pedicle or separately.

In the vaginal hysterectomy, the same steps are taken but in the reverse order.

## Indications for abdominal hysterectomy

- Uterine, ovarian, cervical and Fallopian tube carcinoma.
- Pelvic pain from chronic endometriosis or chronic pelvic inflammatory disease where the pelvis is frozen and vaginal hysterectomy is impossible.
- Symptomatic fibroid uterus greater than 12-week size.

## Indications for vaginal hysterectomy

- Menstrual disorders with a uterus less than 12 weeks in size.
- Microinvasive cervical carcinoma.
- Uterovaginal prolapse.

## Complications

Specific complications of hysterectomy include:
- haemorrhage
- ureteric injury
- bladder and bowel injury.

## Cystoscopy

Cystoscopy involves passing a small-diameter telescope, either flexible or rigid, through the urethra into the bladder. Excellent images of both these structures can be obtained. A cystoscope with an operative channel can be used to biopsy any abnormality, perform bladder neck injection, retrieve stones and resect bladder tumours.

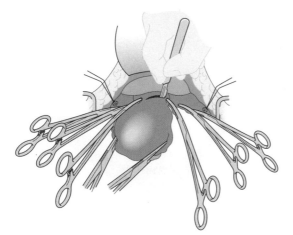

**Figure 6** Total abdominal hysterectomy with clamps on.

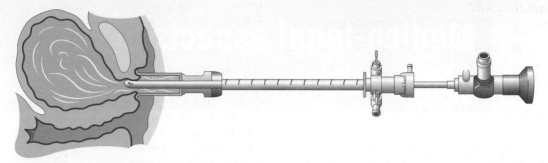

**Figure 7** Diagram showing the cystoscopic procedure.

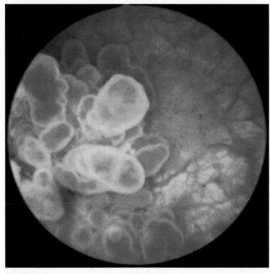

**Figure 8** Cystoscopic view of bladder papilloma.

## Indications

- Haematuria.
- Recurrent urinary tract infection.
- Sterile pyuria.
- Short history of irritative symptoms.
- Suspected bladder abnormality (e.g. diverticulum, stones, fistula).
- Assessment of bladder neck.

## Complications

- Urinary tract infection.
- Rarely, bladder perforation.

# Medico-legal aspects of gynaecology

## Litigation

Litigation has become a major feature of medical practice over the last two decades. Not only has the frequency of claims escalated, but also the basis for these claims has changed. Complications that were once viewed as acceptable hazards of common surgical procedures are now commonly the source of litigation. In other words, the Bolam Principle that has provided the guidelines for judgements about negligence in the past is no longer being applied. The fact that actions taken by a doctor may be considered to be reasonable by a significant number of medical colleagues is no longer always a defence, and in reality a complication is increasingly taken as evidence that there has been substandard practice. It is therefore important, both as a basis for good practice and to avoid litigation, to minimize the risk of complications.

Case records are medico-legal documents and whilst they are of great importance in the general care of the patient, they also provide the basis for the defence of a case in medico-legal claims. Case records should be kept for a minimum of 7 years in gynaecology and 25 years in obstetrics. It is essential to remember that case records may be scrutinized in a court case line by line, so they should contain nothing that is not accurate, factual and contemporaneous.

All entries in case notes must be dated and signed in a legible fashion. Too often it is impossible to decipher the signature after a case note entry and, as medical staff in the training grades commonly move on to other jobs, it can be subsequently very difficult to trace the personnel in an individual case. The same principle applies to entries that are made into computer records, although it may be easier to trace the authors through their access codes.

If it is necessary to alter or modify an entry in the case notes, it is important to countersign and date any modifications so that the alteration is seen to be a deliberate act. Important reports, such as histopathology reports, should be signed and dated at the time of receipt and when they are placed in the records to demonstrate that the report has been noted and the appropriate action taken.

## Consent

The following is the legal definition of consent as laid down by the Medical Defence Union.

*The competent adult patient has a fundamental right to give, or withhold, consent to examination, investigation or treatment. This right is founded on the moral principle of respect for autonomy.*

*An autonomous person has the right to decide what may or may not be done to him (or her). Any treatment or investigation or, indeed, even deliberate touching, carried out without consent may amount to battery. This could result in an action for damages, or even criminal proceedings, and in a finding of serious professional misconduct by the healthcare professional's registration body.*

Consent must be informed or it becomes invalid. In obtaining consent, it is important that the patient understands the nature of any procedure that is to be performed and the attendant risks of that procedure.

In most instances, consent is obtained in writing, but consent may be implied by the patient's actions or by oral consent. Material risks must be made clear to the patient and the consent form must be signed before premedication is given. However, there is no longer any certainty about what constitutes a 'material risk'.

The consent form should be signed by the patient and, ideally, by the surgeon who will perform the procedure. It must, however, be emphasized that consent forms are only of value if it is evident that the consent is informed.

## Consent for minors

The legal age for consent for medical and surgical treatment is 16 years or above. Under the age of 16 years, the situation is more complex. When an underage child consents to treatment, the doctor may proceed with that treatment. If the child refuses treatment, that refusal can be over-ridden by someone with parental authority.

# Index

Compiled by Indexing Specialists (UK) Ltd (www.indexing.co.uk)
*Italic* page numbers refer to figures, tables and appendices.